FRIENDSHIPS IN CHILDHOOD
AND ADOLESCENCE

The Guilford Series on Social and Emotional Development

Claire B. Kopp and Steven R. Asher, Editors

Friendships in Childhood & Adolescence

CATHERINE L. BAGWELL
MICHELLE E. SCHMIDT

THE GUILFORD PRESS
New York   London

© 2011 The Guilford Press
A Division of Guilford Publications, Inc.
72 Spring Street, New York, NY 10012
www.guilford.com

Printed in the United States of America

This book is printed on acid-free paper.

Last digit is print number: 9 8 7 6 5 4 3 2 1

Library of Congress Cataloging-in-Publication Data

Bagwell, Catherine.
  Friendships in childhood and adolescence / Catherine L. Bagwell, Michelle E. Schmidt.
    p. cm. — (The Guilford series on social and emotional development)
  Includes bibliographical references and index.
  ISBN 978-1-60918-646-3 (hbk.)
  1. Friendship in children.   2. Friendship in adolescence.   I. Schmidt, Michelle E.
II. Title.
  BF723.F68B34 2011
  302.3′4083—dc22
                                                              2011012647

For Noah, William, and Ada—
wishing you all the joys of good friends

About the Authors

Catherine L. Bagwell, PhD, is Associate Professor in the Department of Psychology at the University of Richmond in Virginia. Her primary research interests are peer relationships in childhood and adolescence and the developmental significance of friendship. She is investigating the importance of having friends, friendship quality, and the characteristics of friends. Dr. Bagwell's interest in the peer relations of children with disruptive behavior disorders led to her second area of research, on attention-deficit/hyperactivity disorder and the social and emotional correlates and outcomes that are associated with this disorder.

Michelle E. Schmidt, PhD, is Associate Professor and Chair of the Department of Psychology at Moravian College in Bethlehem, Pennsylvania. She also serves as Director of Academic Leadership Programs. Her primary research interests include friendship, peer relationships, and peer victimization. Along with Dr. Bagwell, she is investigating the importance of having friends, friendship quality, and the characteristics of friends. Dr. Schmidt is also involved in two large studies of peer victimization—one in a group of high-risk public schools and the other in an independent school—studying children and adolescents from prekindergarten through the high school years.

Preface

Think of a book you enjoyed as a child or an adolescent. Chances are good that one of the main themes in the book you chose is friendship. Indeed, friendship is often considered a sine qua non of childhood. Classic children's books like A. A. Milne's *Winnie the Pooh* series and E. B. White's *Charlotte's Web*, novels like Mark Twain's *Adventures of Tom Sawyer*, and modern tales like J. K. Rowling's *Harry Potter* series describe in vivid detail the adventures, mishaps, and highs and lows of friendships in childhood and adolescence.

What makes these relationships special? Why are they important to the protagonists—Winnie, Tigger, and Christopher Robin; Wilbur the pig and Charlotte the spider; Tom and Huck; Harry, Ron, and Hermione? How do experiences in these friendships affect the protagonists' current and future development? How are these specific friendships similar to and different from relationships with other peers? How does the broader context in which these relationships flourish—the Hundred Acre Wood, the Zuckermans' barn, mid-19th-century small-town Missouri, modern-day England and the magical world of Hogwarts school—help determine their nature and meaning?

The study of friendship is as old as ancient Greek philosophy and as new as recent studies of microsocial processes in friends' interactions. Writers and scholars have been interested in this topic for centuries, yet empirical investigation of children's relationships with friends is relatively recent. There are a few empirical studies of friendship from the first half of the 20th century (e.g., Challman, 1932). However, an

explosion of research on peer relations began in the late 1970s and early
1980s. Much of this research focused on the causes and consequences of
acceptance or rejection by the peer group (for reviews, see Asher & Coie,
1990; Newcomb, Bukowski, & Pattee, 1993). At the same time, however, scholars recognized that the close, affective, mutual ties children
form with a friend—distinguished from peer relations more generally—
also have important implications for their well-being and development.
We know that children spend a great deal of time with their friends, and
adolescents spend even more; that children show greater positive affect
with friends than with other children; that youth with friends are more
socially competent than youth without friends; that friends get into fights
and arguments with one another; that children and adolescents turn to
their friends in times of stress; that friendships vary in their characteristic
features; and that even aggressive and generally disliked youth often have
a close friend. The overarching question of almost all of the research on
friendship is, What is the developmental significance of friendship? In
other words, how does friendship contribute to social, emotional, and
cognitive development, and how is the context of friendship significant
for adjustment and well-being? This is the primary question that our
book addresses, as we seek to provide a comprehensive account of friendship's significance for children and adolescents.

The book consists of nine chapters, divided into four parts, which
explore different aspects of the study of friendship in childhood and adolescence. Part I sets the stage for understanding the significance of friendship from nomothetic and idiographic perspectives. Chapter 1 demonstrates how friendship is a unique aspect of children's peer relations, how
it is conceptualized across several disciplines, and how it is considered
as a developmental context from both a nomothetic and an idiographic
perspective. Chapter 2 is specifically focused on the multiple strategies
for assessing friendships and presents a model of what to assess when
studying friendships.

The two chapters in Part II present the normative experience of
friendship, and each examines a particular developmental period—from
the beginnings of friendship during childhood in Chapter 3 and from
early through late adolescence in Chapter 4. In these chapters, the guiding theme is whether and how children's and adolescents' friendships are
developmentally significant and unique. We discuss both how friendships
change as children age and what developmental processes might contribute to those changes.

Part III focuses on individual differences in the experience of friendship, the relationships themselves, and the resulting effects on outcomes.
Chapter 5 highlights associations among individual behaviors and characteristics and relationship processes. Chapter 6 considers how and why

friendships differ in their quality and the effects of friendship quality on adjustment and well-being.

The final three chapters comprise Part IV and are written to be forward-looking. Chapter 7 examines how the broader cultural context affects friendship and describes cross-cultural similarities and differences in this relationship. Chapter 8 builds from earlier discussions and considers interventions to help children who have trouble forming and maintaining positive friendships. In it, we review current intervention efforts and provide ideas for future directions for intervention work with children and adolescents. Chapter 9 provides a conclusion to the book that offers a conceptual framework for understanding friendship and its significance for children and adolescents.

Together, we believe that the information in this book has the potential to serve a number of purposes. First, it provides researchers on children's peer relations and related areas with a comprehensive summary of the friendship literature with a focus on the significance of friendships in childhood and adolescence. Second, this book may serve as a resource for clinicians and others (even teachers or parents) who work with children on a daily basis and could benefit from a better understanding of the meaning and significance of children's friendships as well as ideas about the potential for intervention with children who experience difficulties in friendships. In the end, we hope the content of the book will encourage additional basic research on friendships using diverse methods and from multiple perspectives (e.g., psychology, sociology, anthropology) and will inspire applied research aimed at helping children successfully navigate the peer world.

Acknowledgments

We are grateful to many people without whom this book could not have been written. We thank colleagues, students, and administrators at the University of Richmond and Moravian College for their support of us and this project in many ways. Richmond and Moravian provided us with sabbatical leaves, summer research funding (including a University of Richmond Summer Research Fellowship and Moravian College SOAR grants), and wonderful colleagues who offer excellent models of seamlessly combining teaching and scholarship. Thanks, too, to our many talented undergraduate students at Richmond and Moravian, who gave us research assistance and insight and humorous anecdotes about their own experiences with friends and peers. We extend special thanks to Emily Jenchura, who worked with us on Chapter 7, and then went on to study friendships cross-culturally on a Fulbright Fellowship in Trinidad and Tobago.

We are both fortunate to have had excellent teachers and mentors throughout our careers. The work of many of them is cited in the book, but their formative influence goes well beyond specific references to their work. For their dedication to asking and answering important questions about children's social world with peers, their commitment to their students, and their singular influence on our own development, we thank John Coie and Steve Asher at Duke University, Susanne Denham and Elizabeth DeMulder at George Mason University, and Bill Bukowski at Concordia University. We are especially grateful to Andy Newcomb at the University of Richmond, who introduced us both to the wonder of studying children's friendships—Catherine as an undergraduate and Michelle as a postdoc at Richmond—and who, most importantly, introduced us to one another.

We are honored that this book is part of The Guilford Series on Social and Emotional Development alongside important works by authors we admire for their intelligence, excellent writing, and significant contributions to developmental psychology. Claire Kopp served as our editor, and we are grateful to her for her ideas and suggestions throughout the writing process. We also thank Rochelle Serwator and Kristal Hawkins at The Guilford Press for their help and guidance and Marion Underwood for introducing us to Guilford. Thanks as well to the anonymous reviewers for their insightful comments.

During the time we were working on this book, peer relations researchers lost one of our most valued colleagues, Duane Buhrmester, far too early. We are indebted to him for the richness of his contributions to our understanding of children's friendships and their significance.

Most of all, we thank our families for their unending support while we wrote this book and always. Our parents, Fred and Ann Bagwell and Irene Stroffolino Estelle, and our siblings, Todd Bagwell and Lisa Bader, have always encouraged us in our education and careers. Catherine offers special thanks to her husband, Doug Hicks, who provided the emotional and instrumental support and the friendship that allowed her to focus on this book, even as he pursued his own successful career and their family experienced the chaos and joy that comes with young children.

Over the course of writing this book, we have grown as parents and researchers as our sons have progressed from preschool to elementary school and Catherine's daughter from infancy to preschool. Watching their social worlds blossom has given us new perspectives on many of the topics we discuss in the book, and we are grateful to them for the opportunities they have given us to see children's friendships through their eyes. Thank you to Noah and Ada Hicks and William Schmidt for the happiness they provide us every day.

Contents

PART III. INDIVIDUAL DIFFERENCES IN THE EXPERIENCE OF FRIENDSHIP

PART IV. IMPLICATIONS AND LOOKING FORWARD

FRIENDSHIPS IN CHILDHOOD
AND ADOLESCENCE

PART I

THE NATURE
OF FRIENDSHIP

Chapter 1

What Is Friendship?

Consider a variety of friendships as reflected in these vignettes.

> Leah (age 2) and Olivia (almost 3) attend the same home-based day care with a few other children. The girls spend nearly every weekday together and have been doing so for the past 18 months. They love to play with one another in the pretend kitchen, and they both like to draw pictures. They sit next to each other at lunch, take naps on cots side by side, and are concerned if the other is crying or upset. One of Leah's very first words was "Livy," the name she uses for Olivia.

> Mark and Jeremy are in the same second-grade class. Mark is active and impulsive, and he is often aggressive toward his classmates—pushing to be first on the slide, grabbing toys away from others, hitting when he does not get his way. Most of the other children in his class avoid playing with him and even actively exclude him when they can. Jeremy is a bit of a loner who often plays by himself. He also acts aggressively toward his peers when he is frustrated or upset by them. Whenever the second graders need to pick partners for an activity, Mark and Jeremy choose each other. On the playground, they play together more often than either of them plays with any other child.

> Johnny and Dave are friends who live in the same neighborhood and are in the sixth grade. They both wait at the same bus stop for the school bus to pick them up each morning. Some of the

older boys at the bus stop like to pick on Dave and make fun of him. Johnny, who is a strong and athletic boy, sticks up for his friend and frequently tells the other boys to leave Dave alone. The older boys usually listen to Johnny, and Dave and Johnny work on their homework together or trade baseball cards or make up games to play as they wait for the bus.

Amy is in high school and her parents are going through a messy divorce. She spends a lot of time at her friend Mary's house, having dinner with Mary's family and staying for sleepovers on many weekend nights. Amy often talks with Mary about her concerns about her parents and what will happen to her and her younger brothers when her parents' divorce is finalized. There is no one else with whom she shares her worries. Mary is a good listener and tries to comfort her friend when she is feeling down about her family.

When they were in the fifth grade, James and Thomas nominated each other as best friends on a sociometric assessment. Twelve years later, they were asked to describe what their relationship had been like in fifth grade. Thomas said, "We've spent nearly all our waking hours together in the past 23 years." James said, "He lived near me. We would ride our bikes. We were together *constantly.*" On rating scales, they both described their relationship as highly enjoyable, supportive, intimate, and satisfying. On the same sociometric assessment, Katie nominated Jennifer as her best friend, but 12 years later, Katie couldn't remember who her best friend had been in the fifth grade. When asked specifically about Jennifer, Katie said, "Oh, yeah, Jennifer. She was just someone to talk to. I had nothing better to do so we would sometimes talk ... she was someone to call to do things when I didn't want to go by myself."

At first blush, these stories describe very different relationships, yet we refer to them all as friends. What do they have in common? What is it that sets these relationships apart from other relationships the children may have? What do the children bring to the friendships based on previous life experiences and personal characteristics? What are the concurrent and long-term implications of these friendships for the children involved in them? On the one hand, each of these children has a friend. On the other hand, the most salient features of the relationship differ from child to child and from friendship to friendship, and the quality of the relationship likely differs as well. The children bring to the relationship their own characteristics and relationship histories. These characteristics and histories will determine the nature and dynamics of the friendship and will contribute to the future pathways of the individuals in the friendships. Thus, recognizing the significance of friendship requires linking past, present, and future to understand what determines whether children have a friend and what that friend (and that relationship) are like, how the relationship affects the child's current adjustment and well-being, and whether there are long-term implications of the child's experience in that relationship.

The first tasks in specifying the developmental significance of friendship are to define the relationship clearly and to differentiate it from other important relationships with peers. This introductory chapter considers both of these issues. We define friendship from the perspectives of psychology, sociology, and anthropology and briefly describe key theories of friendship. Then we distinguish friendship from popularity and from social networks. Finally, we discuss four assumptions that guide the remainder of the book.

DEFINITIONS OF FRIENDSHIP

Friendships in childhood and adolescence have been studied most extensively by developmental psychologists, but sociologists, anthropologists, and other scholars have also investigated friendships. Unfortunately, research from these various disciplines has most often proceeded in parallel with only rare intersection. In order to integrate the research from these disciplines, it is first necessary to understand the ways in which the definition of friendship and the assumptions about this relationship differ from one discipline to another. Here, we will review how psychologists, sociologists, and anthropologists define and study friendship and also present some strengths and weaknesses of each approach.

Psychological Perspectives on Friendship

When developmental psychologists talk about friendship, they are most often referring to a specific kind of relationship with distinct properties. Their definition of friendship centers on friendship as a dyadic relationship. Friendships are often described as "horizontal" relationships because of the sense of equality that is at their core. Thus, they are unlike other close dyadic relationships, such as parent–child and sibling relationships, that are "vertical" in nature because the partners differ in age and developmental stage. Friendship is based on mutual affection or reciprocity of liking. When asked to describe a friend, most people, regardless of age, emphasize mutuality or reciprocity—including the expectations that friends support one another and that giving and taking are at the foundation of the relationship (Bigelow, 1977; Hartup & Stevens, 1997; Weiss & Lowenthal, 1975).

Hartup and Stevens (1997) distinguish between the deep structure and the surface structure of friendship. The deep structure, or essence of friendship, is reciprocity. This deep structure exists relatively unchanged across the lifespan. In contrast, the surface structure, or the actual exchanges and interactions that occur between friends, changes with age according to the developmental tasks associated with that period. Thus, while play and sharing are the social exchanges that define friendship among young children, social exchanges among adolescent friends center on intimacy (Hartup & Stevens, 1997). Hartup and Stevens are careful to identify reciprocity as the deep structure within friendships in Western cultures. As we discuss in more detail in Chapter 7, there are cultural differences in the meaning of friendship and the characteristics associated with friendship. For example, in Western cultures, a defining feature of friendship is that it is voluntary, unlike kinship relations, yet in other societies, strict social constraints may dictate who is able to be friends or whether and how relationships can be terminated (Krappmann, 1996). Nevertheless, psychological research on friendship is dominated by studies of children and adolescents in the United States, Canada, and Western European countries.

In the method section of most developmental psychology journal articles, considerable effort is given to a careful and thorough explanation of the specific definition of "friend" used in that study. Commonly, this involves asking children to name their best friends and then identifying friends as those pairs of children who reciprocally nominate one another. As we discuss in Chapter 2, reciprocal friendship nominations are the gold standard in developmental psychology research. This means, then, that psychological research usually focuses on specific identified friendship pairs. Comparisons of friends versus nonfriends may then be made by asking a child questions about a reciprocally nominated friend (vs. a classmate not named as a friend) or by observing pairs of friends together and comparing the features of their interactions to those of two classmates who do not nominate one another as friends. Friendship quality (discussed more thoroughly in Chapter 6) is often assessed as well, by giving a child a questionnaire that asks specific questions about the named best friend and asking the friend questions about the target child.

In studying friendship, developmental psychologists typically focus on the outcomes of friendship. This research identifies differences between children with and without friends, examines the effects of high- versus low-quality relationships, and considers how participation in friendship contributes to adjustment and functioning currently (e.g., cross-sectional studies) or in the near future (e.g., short-term longitudinal studies). There are, of course, notable exceptions to this focus on outcomes as more psychologists are now studying friendship processes, but the majority of the existing psychological work is outcome oriented.

As with any approach, there are strengths and weaknesses of the psychological approach to defining and studying friendship. The greatest strength is that when developmental psychologists identify friendships, they are likely capturing "real" friendships, due to the requirement of reciprocity and mutuality. These friendships can then be examined to determine, for example, what brings children together as friends, how they influence each other over the course of their friendship, the quality of the friendship, and the outcomes of the friendship (topics that are covered in Chapters 3, 4, 5, and 6). Methodologies that prioritize reciprocated friendships, however, may inadvertently miss important relationships (see Chapter 2 for a discussion of methodologies for identifying and studying friendships). Namely, children may change their choice of a best friend from month to month, week to week, or even day to day. Limited nominations may cause researchers to miss some mutual friendships, and typically only friendships with same-age schoolmates are identified. Another concern is that there is some inconsistency in how psychologists use the word *friend* and how others use the term. For example, teachers and parents may refer to all children's classmates as "friends." Despite potential shortcomings, the way psychologists define friendship allows for investigation of a particular relationship that is declared by two people as important and significant.

Sociological Perspectives on Friendship

Sociological research often focuses on the construction of friendship culture. This research examines the active role that children play in their own socialization. Drawing on symbolic interactionism (e.g., Mead, 1934), sociological research considers how social interactions with peers involve interpretation of self and others and how children produce and reproduce with peers and friends routines that they adopt and adapt from adult culture. This interpretive approach (Corsaro, 1985, 1992, 1994, 2003) assumes that children develop social competence and knowledge about social institutions, social structure, and the contexts in which they live through interactions in the peer culture (Crosnoe, 2000).

Sociological studies of friendship also examine how friendships fit within the larger social structure and how factors such as gender, race, and socioeconomic status organize friendships. For example, Thorne (1993) and Eder (1995) provide in-depth ethnographic studies of gender and peer culture. Allan (1989) argues that a sociological analysis of friendship should include an examination of the significance of friendship—not only on the support that friends provide individuals and the significance of these relationships for individual development as psychologists study—but more specifically on "the way in which friendships are incorporated into social organization, their social utility and their significance for social identity" (p. 10).

Sociological definitions of friendship are usually broad and inclusive. "Friends" are often assumed to be the peers with whom a child frequently interacts, and friends often include small groups of peers as opposed to dyads only (Adler & Adler, 1998; Corsaro, 1985; Rizzo, 1989). Sociological studies often do not define friendship explicitly and may leave it up to the children themselves to label other children as "friends" with no check on reciprocity. This emphasis fits with sociologists' focus on how children themselves define their relationships rather than on outsiders' views. Alternatively, in ethnographic studies, researchers themselves label some children as friends, and thus the term *friend* reflects the researchers' personal expectations of a friend that is likely based on frequency of interaction, participation in common activities, and observing the children who refer to one another as friends.

One key contribution of the sociological approach to studying friendship is in identifying friendships according to how the children themselves define friendship. Additionally, attention to how friendships fit into the larger social organization contributes to a greater understanding of the "social whole." Of course, leaving the definition of friendship up to the children studied or to the researcher's perspective means that different studies are not necessarily examining the same relationship. Another issue of concern may be the lack of attention to the dyad and various levels of friendships (friends vs. best friends, for example), but overall, there is great potential for understanding the place of friendship within children's social lives with the sociological perspective.

Anthropological Perspectives on Friendship

Anthropological study of friendship in childhood and adolescence is more scarce than either psychological or sociological investigation of these relationships. This stems from two factors: anthropologists have only rarely studied friendship (Bell & Coleman, 1999; cf. Allan, 1989), and studying children has generally remained at the margins of research in mainstream anthropology (Hirschfeld, 2002; Reed-Danahay, 1999). Nevertheless, recent interest in children's lives—called "childhood studies" or the "anthropology of childhoods" (Bluebond-Langner & Korbin, 2007; LeVine, 2007)—and recognition of children as active agents have encouraged anthropologists to attend to children's unique perspective on their social worlds (Bluebond-Langner & Korbin, 2007; James, 2007).

In studying friendship, anthropologists eschew a search for a universal definition of friendship and focus on how it emerges in particular social and cultural contexts (Bell & Coleman, 1999). Some anthropologists consider friendship an idiom of interaction (Smart, 1999) or an idiom of affinity and togetherness (Rezende, 1999). By referring to friendship in these terms, the authors allow for different understandings of friendship across cultures without imposing a set of specific criteria with which to define the relationship (cf. Carrier, 1999).

For example, the notion that friendships are voluntary relationships is taken as a given in psychological research, yet anthropologists have identified societies in which relationships with ties like friendship are understood through kinship terms. In still other societies, friendship is formalized and institutionalized through ceremonies and rituals that rigidly define appropriate behavior between friends (e.g., Allan, 1989; Banton, 1966). Consistent with the broader interests and emphases of the discipline, anthropological study of friendship has focused on how the social and economic structures and cultural practices of different societies allow for (or hinder) friendships and on how relationships such as friendships are organized and function to sustain the institutions and practices of different societies (Allan, 1989; Gaskins, 2006). These questions logically pull for a comparative perspective examining how friendships differ between societies and cultures.

Perhaps indisputably, the greatest strength of the work of anthropologists is the attention paid to culture. Too often we examine children in Western cultures and assume we understand the construct of friendship. There is much more to understand, however, and anthropologists provide us with fascinating and informative perspectives on cultures and societies around the globe. We should also note that the work of anthropologists is extraordinarily involved. Researchers must gain permission and enter societies that are not their own; they must become a part of the group they are studying in order to understand the nature of friendship in that group; and they must spend a great deal of time and energy studying these societies, without a "blueprint" methodology.

Summary

The importance of friendship is acknowledged across a number of disciplines, and each emphasizes different aspects of the relationship consistent with the overarching concerns, questions, and levels of analysis of the particular field of study. Although the discussions in this book draw most heavily on research within psychology, an integration of the findings and methods of study across disciplinary boundaries provides a richer, more complex and complete understanding of the importance of friendship in children's lives.

THEORETICAL PERSPECTIVES ON FRIENDSHIP

There is no single unified theory of friendship from psychology, sociology, or anthropology that describes its development, its features, and its significance; that yields clear testable hypotheses; and that provides a framework for organizing research. Nevertheless, the study of peer relations, and of friendship in particular, has made use of relevant theories in other areas of developmental, social, and personality psychology to guide research and explain discoveries about friendship.

Sullivan's Interpersonal Theory

The most often cited theoretical conceptualization of friendship is Harry Stack Sullivan's (1953) interpersonal theory. We describe it in detail here because of its importance in guiding empirical research, especially in the last several decades. Sullivan's theory is developmental in nature and is aimed at explaining how personality develops within interpersonal relationships. Central to his theory is the assumption that specific tensions or interpersonal needs arise at each period in development. Individuals are motivated to seek certain types of interpersonal situations to satisfy these social needs. Particular interpersonal relationships are best suited for the satisfaction of each need, and thus, these relationships are essential at the various stages or "developmental epochs."

Sullivan (1953) asserts that peer relations are central to adaptive development beginning in the juvenile period with the need for compeers. Sullivan describes the juvenile era as the "actual time for becoming social" (p. 227), and its beginning roughly corresponds to when children enter school. Interactions with peers provide children the opportunity to develop the social skills and competencies of competition, cooperation, and compromise. The need for acceptance and the desire to avoid the peer rejection that Sullivan labels ostracism also emerge at this time. Sullivan describes the formation of ingroups and outgroups as children compare themselves to one another, determine what characteristics, behaviors, abilities, and attitudes make valued companions, and then exclude those peers who do not meet these expectations.

Sullivan (1953) places singular importance on friendship. The beginning of preadolescence is "spectacularly marked" by the need for interpersonal intimacy that is satisfied through close friendship. Mutuality is the key to this relationship as a friend "becomes of practically equal importance in all fields of value" (p. 245). Sullivan eloquently describes friendship this way:

> All of you who have children are sure that your children love you; when you say that, you are expressing a pleasant illusion. But if you

will look very closely at one of your children when he finally finds a chum—somewhere between eight-and-a-half and ten—you will discover something very different in the relationship—namely, that your child begins to develop a real sensitivity to what matters to another person. And this is not in the sense of "what should I do to get what I want," but instead "what should I do to contribute to the happiness or to support the prestige and feeling of worth-whileness of my chum." (p. 245)

The friendships Sullivan describes are based on closeness and self-disclosure, reciprocity, similarity, and collaboration that requires sensitivity to the other person. This relationship thus represents a notable shift from peer relationships in the juvenile era when preferred playmates do not achieve this level of collaboration and intimacy.

In Sullivan's (1953) view, a primary outcome of preadolescent friendship is validation of self-worth. Through self-disclosure, children learn that their friends have similar interests, concerns, and values, and are reassured that they are important and worthy. Consensual validation of self-worth also occurs simply because children recognize (for the first time, Sullivan argues) that they are valued by another person. If children do not form a chumship, loneliness is an expected result.

As a psychiatrist, Sullivan (1953) was especially interested in friendship, not only for what it provides children currently and for the future, but also for the therapeutic potential of chumships for resolving problems from earlier periods. Isolated juveniles may avoid further isolation and loneliness by experiencing the consensual validation and collaboration of a chumship. Immature, irresponsible juveniles may "grow up" (p. 254) when the need for intimacy is satisfied with a friendship. Ostracized or rejected children may form a friendship with one another, and may "do each other a great deal of good" (p. 252) and improve their status in the group. Malevolent children may experience the closeness, caring, and tenderness of friendship, "whereupon the malevolent transformation is sometimes reversed, literally cured" (p. 253). Sullivan acknowledges that friendship does not always have these "curative" effects. He also does not provide specific hypotheses about the processes through which the therapeutic effects occur, though he suggests that consensual validation is of central importance.

Expansions of Sullivan's Theory and Other Viewpoints on Friendship

More recently, other theorists have built on Sullivan's ideas in related conceptualizations of friendship. In their neo-Sullivanian model, Duane Buhrmester and Wyndol Furman (1986) build on Sullivan's ideas by suggesting that social competence develops as children interact with others in a variety of relationships. They further outline the specific competencies that result from the key relationship at each developmental epoch, noting similarities and differences in the contributions of friendships and peer acceptance. The highly collaborative nature of chumships is expected to foster perspective-taking skills, empathy, and altruism.

James Youniss (1980) integrated Sullivan's ideas with Jean Piaget's theory of cognitive development, which also places great significance on social interactions. Youniss's Sullivan–Piaget thesis is that "relations with adults and peers serve equally important but distinct functions in children's social development" (p. 1). A central tenet of the thesis is that both Sullivan and Piaget view social maturity as stemming from interpersonal understanding and not from individual behavior. There is a special place in development, then, for peer relationships and particularly friendships according to this thesis. Reciprocity and cooperation are the cornerstones of children's peer relationships that explain their unique contributions to development.

Of all current researchers and theorists, Willard Hartup's name is most closely connected with the study of friendship. Hartup was active in the general resurgence in the interest in peer relations in the 1970s and 1980s. However, while others focused on peer interactions and peer acceptance and rejection, Hartup quickly moved to emphasizing the significance of the dyadic tie of friendship. His ideas about friendship are influenced by behaviorism, social exchange theories, cognitive theories, attachment theory, and interpersonal theory. Hartup's theory of friendship emphasizes its significance as a developmental context across the lifespan (e.g., Hartup & Stevens, 1997). In addition, Hartup's conceptualization of friendship emphasizes its multidimensional nature, including the three "faces" of friendship—having friends, friendship quality, and the identity of friends (Hartup, 1995, 1996a). This focus on multiple dimensions of friendship has been incredibly influential in guiding empirical research in the last two decades.

Other Theories Relevant to Friendship Research

The vast majority of empirical studies on friendship include an almost obligatory reference to Sullivan's theory, yet given that there is no unified theory of friendship, researchers must look to a variety of theories from diverse domains as the basis for many of their hypotheses and studies. Some of these come from the modifications and expansions of Sullivan's ideas, described above. Others come from theories that are not specific to friendship, yet they have in common attention to reciprocity, mutuality, and equality that are hallmarks of friendship. Several of these are described here.

Attachment Theory

Attachment theory as first proposed by John Bowlby in the 1930s (Bowlby, 1969, 1973, 1980, 1988) suggests that infants develop attachments with their primary caregivers who respond to their signals and behaviors. From these early experiences, mental representations of the self, others, and relationships, called *internal working models,* develop and guide future interactions and relationships. Attachment theory and its importance as a model for understanding friendships are discussed more thoroughly in Chapter 5.

Wyndol Furman and his colleagues (e.g., Furman & Buhrmester, 2009; Furman & Wehner, 1994) have proposed a behavioral systems conceptualization of close relationships that draws on attachment theory and neo-Sullivanian perspectives. This model proposes four behavioral systems—attachment, caregiving, affiliative, and sexual/reproductive. The first three systems emerge in the parent–child relationship but then develop further in other relationships, including friendships and romantic relationships. The affiliative system is of particular importance in friendships and involves play, cooperation, collaboration, and reciprocity. Individuals are expected to rely on different relationships to satisfy the goals of the different behavioral systems, and the particular relationship an individual turns to at any given time is expected to be determined by a variety of factors, including age and development and culture (Furman & Buhrmester, 2009).

Ecological Systems Theory

Ecological systems theory was proposed by Urie Bronfenbrenner in the 1970s (Bronfenbrenner, 1979, 2005) and was developed further over the next several decades. It is not a specific theory of friendship but is a model of studying human development. In brief, Bronfenbrenner suggests that development proceeds as a system of interactions and accommodations over the life course between a person and the changing settings and context in which the person lives. The model is often depicted as a series of concentric circles representing the complex system of relationships within multiple levels of the child's environment. The microsystem includes the child and reciprocal interactions in the child's immediate environment (e.g., parent–child relationships, friendships). The mesosytem involves interactions and connections between microsystems (e.g., ways in which out-of-school friends might influence children's relationships with others in school). The exosystem consists of settings that influence children's development but do not include them directly, and the macrosystem includes cultural values and customs. We consider the macrosystem in Chapter 7 regarding cultural influences on children's friendships. Finally, the chronosystem reflects the fact that the environment is ever changing. The focus on friendship as a context for development and the idea that children influence and are influenced by their environment are ways in which ecological systems theory guides friendship research.

Learning Theories and Theories of Interpersonal Attraction

Learning theories and various social psychological theories of interpersonal attraction and relationship development (see Kelley et al., 1983; Perlman & Fehr, 1986, for reviews) have been applied (though rarely) to friendships in childhood and adolescence. Findings of the importance of similarity, propinquity, reinforcement, and positive affect in friendship selection and maintenance fit with assumptions of these theories. For example, reinforcement theorists focus on the rewards received from others (e.g., Clore & Byrne, 1974; Lott & Lott, 1960, 1974). Exchange and equity theorists focus not only on the rewards received but also on what we invest in a particular relationship and how the rewards and costs of a particular friendship compare to others (e.g., Kelley & Thibaut, 1978; Rusbult, 1980; Thibaut & Kelley, 1959). These theories have been used extensively to describe adult relationships, including friendships, and they may hold promise as models to be applied to friendships in childhood and adolescence. For example, Hand and Furman (2009) considered exchange theory as a framework for evaluating adolescents' perceptions of costs and rewards in same-sex and opposite-sex friendships.

Summary

Although Sullivan's theory is the most often-cited theory in research on children's and adolescents' friendships, there are numerous others that focus specifically on friendship and still others that are more general theories but are relevant for friendship. Our current understanding of friendship, however, suggests that friendships may vary by age, gender, cultural group, and many other variables. It is not surprising, then, that no single model of friendship will likely "work" in all cases. Thus, it seems futile to search for one guiding theory that might explain all of the variables of interest related to friendships. Developing relevant "mini theories" of friendship, incorporating models and theories from other research areas, and more thoroughly and systematically investigating the theories we do have will serve to enrich the empirical research literature on friendship in the coming decades.

FRIENDSHIPS COMPARED TO OTHER PEER RELATIONS

One task in identifying what is special about friendships is to show how they are different from other types of peer relations. Current conceptualizations of the peer world emphasize that peer relations occur at different levels of social complexity—at the level of interactions, dyads, and groups (Hinde, 1979, 1997; Rubin, Bukowski, & Parker, 2006). It is important for us to present these distinctions early in the book so that it is clear what is meant by the term *friend* versus the term *peer*, especially because these terms are often used interchangeably outside of the research realm. When we use the term *friend*, we are referring to a particular type of peer relationship that is dyadic in nature and can be distinguished from other aspects of peer interactions and peer groups, namely peer acceptance and rejection and peer networks. These forms of peer relations do not necessarily involve specific relationships between two children.

Friendship and Peer Status

Peer Status

As the vignettes at the beginning of this chapter illustrate, children have different types of relationships with both their friends and their peers. There are some children in every classroom who are not liked and others who are popular and liked by many. A child's status in the peer group—called social status, peer status, or sociometric status—is a measure of how liked (accepted) or disliked (rejected) the child is. This status is a summary of how other children in a particular group, usually classmates or grade mates, feel about a child in terms of liking. Thus, it is a unilateral construct (unlike friendship) and only represents feelings of others toward the child. Although we often speak of "rejected children" or "popular children," peer rejection versus acceptance is not a characteristic that resides in the child and only makes sense in the context of the peer group (see Asher & Coie, 1990; Bierman, 2004; Newcomb et al., 1993; Rubin et al., 2006).

With respect to peer status, children who are well liked are more cooperative and socially competent than rejected children. They communicate well with others, regulate their emotions effectively, and show social sensitivity and a keen awareness of others. Children who are rejected by peers show low rates of these positive, prosocial behaviors and high rates of aggressive and disruptive behavior as well as impulsive and immature behavior (Bierman, 2004; Newcomb et al., 1993). Countless studies have shown that being rejected by the peer group is a risk factor for a host of adjustment problems both concurrently and in the future including loneliness, victimization, mental health problems, and antisocial behavior and delinquency (Bierman, 2004). Peer status is the dimension of peer relations that has received the most attention in the developmental literature.

In addition to continuous measures of acceptance versus rejection, social status is also indexed by placing children into five sociometric status groups based on their pattern of being liked and disliked (Coie, Dodge, & Coppotelli, 1982; Newcomb & Bukowski, 1983). The "rejected" group includes children who are highly disliked and not liked. Children in the "popular" group are highly liked and not disliked. The "neglected" group is comprised of children who are neither liked nor disliked by many peers, and the "controversial" group includes children who are both liked and disliked by many peers. Children who do not fall into one of these four extreme groups are considered to have "average" sociometric status. The rejected group has received the most attention because of the serious implications for poor adjustment associated with being disliked (Bierman, 2004; Rubin et al., 2006).

Distinctions between Peer Status and Friendship

Friendship differs from peer status because it defines a particular relationship between two individuals (see Bukowski & Hoza, 1989, for a review of differences between peer status and friendship). Although it also involves liking, the key difference is that the liking involved in friendships is *reciprocal*. Peer status and friendship are correlated, but their differences are clearly seen in the fact that not all popular children have friends, and many rejected children do. The numbers vary from study to study depending in part on how researchers measure the overlap between friendship and social status. In one sample, slightly less than half of low-accepted children had at least one mutual friend, but over 90% of high-accepted children had at least one friend (Parker & Asher, 1993). Using specific sociometric status categories, the distinctions between social status and friendship may be even more striking with nearly 40% of rejected children having at least one mutual friendship and at least 30% of popular children being friendless in one sample (Gest, Graham-Bermann, & Hartup, 2001).

Similarities across Peer Status and Friendship

Links between peer status and friendship are evident in several ways. Some of the social skills and competencies that help children make friends are also those that enhance their social acceptance. Thus, it is not surprising that peer acceptance predicts the number of reciprocal friends a child has (Erdley, Nangle, Newman, & Carpenter, 2001; Ladd, Kochenderfer, & Coleman, 1997; Parker & Asher, 1993). Better accepted, more popular children have more opportunities to form mutual friendships. In addition, popularity may temporally precede friendship. In several analyses, Bukowski and colleagues showed that popularity mediated the link between children's characteristics (e.g., aggression, competence) and participation in a mutual friendship (Newcomb, Bukowski, & Bagwell, 1999). Specifically, children's characteristics determined their popularity, and popularity determined the likelihood that the children had a mutual friend. In addition, children who were popular at one time were more likely to have a friend 6 months later, but having a friend did not predict later popularity (Bukowski, Pizzamiglio, Newcomb, & Hoza, 1996).

Friendship, Peer Status, and Adjustment

In terms of their association with adjustment, additional findings suggest that popularity, but not friendship, is directly related to children's feelings of belongingness. In contrast, friendship, but not popularity, is directly related to children's feelings of loneliness in early adolescence (Bukowski, Hoza, & Boivin, 1993). Popularity is associated with loneliness through its association with friendship—children who are more popular are more likely to have a friend and thus feel less lonely. Thus, popularity and friendship are conceptually and empirically linked to one another, yet they are also associated with different aspects of adjustment. This difference is evident even over the long term: Rejection in preadolescence (but not friendship) predicted school adjustment and aspiration level in early adulthood, yet having a friend in preadolescence (but not peer rejection) was associated with lower levels of depressive symptoms and higher self-worth in early adulthood (Bagwell, Newcomb, & Bukowski, 1998).

Moreover, the quality of children's friendships differs for popular and unpopular children. Children's own reports of the quality of their friendships do not yield straightforward conclusions about links between friendship and peer status. Parker and Asher (1993) found that low-accepted children had friendships with less validation and caring, more conflict and betrayal, less help and guidance, less intimate exchange, and less conflict resolution—in short, lower-quality friendships—than average-accepted and/or high-accepted children. In contrast, other evidence indicates that self-reports of friendship quality by rejected girls and their friends do not differ from those of average and popular girls with their friends (Lansford et al., 2006). There are very few observational studies of friendship quality. Nevertheless, two studies show compromised friendship quality for children who are not well accepted in the larger peer group. Rejected girls' interactions with their friends showed poorer conflict resolution and more immaturity as compared to higher-status girls with their friends (Lansford et al., 2006). In a study of both boys and girls, dyads of two low-accepted friends also showed less positive, coordinated, and sensitive interactions than two high-accepted friends (Phillipsen, 1999).

Summary

A complete picture of a child's experience in the world of peers requires understanding both the child's place in the larger peer group (i.e., peer status) and the child's relationships with specific peers (i.e., friendship). As we argue in this book, a child's participation in and experience of friendships throughout childhood and adolescence is significant. But so is the child's level of acceptance and rejection by others. Therefore, it is valuable to look within particular friendships to appreciate the significance, meaning, and implications of that relationship, but we should do so without ignoring an understanding of the child's place in the peer group as a whole.

Friendships and Larger Peer Groups

Peer Networks

Children typically have multiple friends, and they often spend time with multiple peers in cohesive peer networks, also called peer cliques. The peers in a network are tied by bonds of affection and association. They "hang around" together. Research on peer networks draws both from sociometric research, because it assumes that children are embedded in a peer context with a particular structure, and from friendship research, because it assumes that there are particular peers who are most important to a child and influence the child (Kindermann, 1993). Children may belong to more than one network, and networks may be overlapping. Often these groups are formed around activities the children enjoy or participate in together. Peer networks are usually identified by asking children with whom they hang around (Bagwell, Coie, Terry, & Lochman, 2000) or by asking children to identify naturally occurring peer groups in their class or grade with "Who hangs out together?" (Cairns,

Cairns, Neckerman, Gest, & Gariepy, 1988; Cairns, Xie, & Leung, 1998; Gest, Farmer, Cairns, & Xie, 2003; Kindermann, 1996). With this latter approach, children are expected to be able to report on the social networks in their class because these are children who are observed to spend time together frequently. Reports from multiple children are combined to identify peer networks according to how often children are named as hanging around other peers. With both approaches—self-report and peer informant—network membership is based on a consensus of peers about who belongs together in a clique.

Friendship and Peer Networks

Dyadic friendships are often embedded within peer networks, but a child does not necessarily have a reciprocal friendship with every other child in his or her peer network. Although there is some overlap between groups based on friendship versus affiliation (hanging around together), the groups are not identical (Rodkin & Ahn, 2009). Rodkin and Ahn (2009) found that networks based on dyads of friends are smaller and less stable than groups based on affiliative ties, and agreement in the placement of individual children using the two methods was modest. In one cohort of sixth-grade students, just over 40% of children nominated as one of three best friends were members of the child's peer network. Likewise, just over 40% of children in a child's peer network were nominated as a friend (Kindermann, 1996). In another sample of sixth- through twelfth-grade adolescents, over 90% of the best friends named by students were members of the same peer network, and from 50 to 70% of the friends named by adolescents in a list of 10 friends were in their peer network (Urberg, Değirmencioğlu, Tolson, & Halliday-Scher, 1995). In some cases, youth may not like all members of their network even though they frequently associate with them. In addition, not all members of a network hang around with others in their group with equal frequency, and this reflects a child's centrality in the peer network (Cairns et al., 1988). Some children are more peripheral members of their clique, and there are dominance hierarchies that suggest differences in the degree to which certain peers influence the activities and attitudes of other network members (Adler & Adler, 1995; Strayer, 1989).

Peer networks are an important dimension of peer relations because of the powerful socialization that occurs within the clique, yet they are distinct from friendships in both their form and function. Not only do networks provide a structure or social arrangement within the larger social world of childhood, but they are critical for the transmission of cultural knowledge (Adler & Adler, 1995, 1998; Harris, 1995). As such, participation within a particular network provides access to a set of behaviors and attitudes that are valued by at least a portion of fellow clique members. Indeed, network members are similar in both positive and negative qualities such as aggression and bullying; academic motivation, engagement, and achievement; leadership; popularity; and sports participation (Adler & Adler, 1998; Bagwell et al., 2000; Cairns et al., 1988; Cairns & Cairns, 1994; Duffy & Nesdale, 2009; Espelage, Holt, & Henkel, 2003; Kindermann, 1993, 2007; Salmivalli, Huttunen, & Lagerspetz, 1997; Sijtsema et al., 2010).

Crowds

In adolescence, crowds become more salient dimensions of the social world. Crowds are large reputation-based groups that are not based on affiliation and may include many peer networks (Brown, 1990; Brown & Lohr, 1987). Crowd members may interact with one another, but it is not necessarily the case that all adolescents in the same crowd know one another. Rather, they are linked only by being given the same label identifying stereotypic behaviors and attributes. Although particular crowds and the names for those groups differ from school to school, typical crowds include "brains" or "nerds," "jocks" or "athletes," "preps," "druggies" or "toughs," and "populars." Adolescents' crowd affiliation may be an important component of their sense of identity, yet among older adolescents, crowd affiliation is perceived as a hindrance to self-expression and the development of personal identities (Brown, 1990).

Friendship and Crowds

Youth view crowds as important for providing support and facilitating friendships (Brown, Eicher, & Petrie, 1986; Urberg, Değirmencioğlu, Tolson, & Halliday-Scher, 2000). In one sample of middle and high school students, 55–85% of their friendships were from their own or similar crowds (Urberg et al., 2000). The importance of affiliation with a crowd decreases across adolescence as older adolescents place more emphasis on their peer networks and are frustrated with the demands for conformity associated with crowd affiliation (Brown et al., 1986).

Summary

Friendships often exist within a larger peer network, and it is important not to lose sight of the context for the friendship that the larger network provides. To be sure, friendships are only one dimension of children's social world that also involves participation in peer interactions and social groups. Nevertheless, we contend that friendship is a unique relationship that holds importance for children's lives and makes independent contributions to their development and well-being.

FRAMEWORK FOR THE BOOK

The primary goal of the book is to use research from the past three decades to understand the developmental significance of friendship. In pursuing this goal, our perspective is guided by four primary assumptions that we describe more thoroughly below.

1. Friends are important.
2. Children's development influences friendships, and friendships influence children's development.
3. Friendships are a developmental context.
4. Friendships are best considered from both a normative and an idiographic perspective.

Friends Are Important

First and foremost is the assumption that friends matter, and they matter a lot. At least in most Western cultures, this statement is a truism. By describing friendships as important, we mean specifically that they have implications for children's development and adjustment. In other words, they are *developmentally significant.* Friends also matter simply because they are significant to children and adolescents. When children are asked to name others who are important to them, friends (along with parents) are named without hesitation (Blyth, Hill, & Thiel, 1982; Kiesner, Kerr, & Stattin, 2004). That alone may be reason to devote considerable effort to understanding friendships.

This assumption also recognizes that friends are important socialization agents who provide influences on development beyond those conveyed by parents, siblings, teachers, and other peers. To be sure, these influences are often similar or overlapping. An academically inclined child may receive support and encouragement to do well in school from parents. He or she may also have a best friend who is actively engaged in school, and with whom he or she enjoys working on homework. Prosocial, cooperative, easy-going children are likely to be well liked among their classmates and to have a close friend. They are also not likely to be lonely or depressed. Given the correlations among various socializing agents and socialization experiences and contexts, we place special emphasis on identifying ways in which friendships are unique in their contributions to development.

Furthermore, it is clear that there are multiple ways in which friendships affect development. Friendship may have a direct association with a particular outcome. Such would be the case if children without friends are more lonely or depressed than children with friends, controlling for as many potential confounding variables as possible (e.g., peer status, individual personality or adjustment variables, friendship network involvement, family experiences). Friendship may also affect development by serving as a moderator variable. One hypothesis is that having a good friendship buffers children against the negative effects of other peer experiences. For example, children with a friend may be less likely to suffer from depression and anxiety associated with rejection or victimization experiences (e.g., Hodges, Boivin, Vitaro, & Bukowski, 1999). In other words, having a good friend may serve a protective role.

Friendship and Development

Second, we assume that friendships are important *across* childhood and adolescence. Interactions with peers and potential friends begin as early as infancy and toddlerhood for many children (Dunn, 2004; Howes, 1983). By the preschool period, many children identify a particular "best" friend. Certainly, friendships change as children age. They become more complex, more strongly embedded in a broader social context, and more intimate. Yet, there are aspects of friendship, such as companionship and enjoying spending time together, that are at the core of friendships from very early childhood through adulthood.

A developmental perspective on friendship suggests that the effects of friendship are not the same at every age. Although their developmental significance may vary with age, friendships are nonetheless valued relationships across childhood and adolescence. Likewise, a developmental perspective requires considering ways in which children's social, emotional, and cognitive development affects friendships. For example, as children gain the ability to take another's perspective, their ability to resolve conflicts with friends may improve. In statistical terms, we can consider how friendships are both independent and dependent variables. As independent variables, friendships affect development. Indeed, this is the emphasis of most of the book. However, friendships are simultaneously dependent variables because developmental processes and other social experiences affect friendship.

Friendship as a Developmental Context

Third, we assume that friendships provide a context for social, emotional, and cognitive development. At the most basic level, friendship provides a setting or environment in which development occurs by virtue of the time children spend with friends and the activities they do together. Friendships provide different developmental contexts than other social relationships because they are voluntary and because they are horizontal in nature (i.e., friends are relatively equal in their degree of social power). Understanding friendships as developmental contexts requires specifying how friendships affect socialization—both what aspects of development are affected and what processes account for those effects (Hartup & Laursen, 1991, 1999).

To date, we know much more about the "what" of friendships. We know about their important features and how they differ from other relationships with peers. We know what children think about and expect from their friends. And we have some good ideas about what aspects of children's development and adjustment are most likely influenced by their relationships with friends. We know much less about the "how" and "why" of friendships. Why is it that children without friends are "worse off" than children with friends? How is it that friends contribute to one another's development of emotion regulation skills? These questions speak to the processes that occur within friends' ongoing interactions and how those processes determine the significance of friendship. Our assumption is that we need to move toward analyses of processes to better understand friendships as a developmental context.

Nomothetic and Idiographic Perspectives

Fourth, the framework we present for understanding friendship incorporates a nomothetic (or normative) approach and an idiographic (or individual differences) perspective. Specifically, it is possible to identify many aspects of friendship that seem to hold true for most children and adolescents. These include age-related changes in the features, functions, and meaning of friendship; ways in which friendships are embedded within larger social systems, such as peer groups, schools, and cultural context; and pathways through which friendships affect current and later functioning. At the same time, however, the experience of friendship and the context that a particular friendship provides may differ substantially across children. These individual differences are a function of the characteristics each child brings to the relationship, the interactions between the children, and features of the relationship itself, such as friendship quality. Most individual empirical studies of friendship proceed primarily from one of these approaches. As we study the normative development of friendships and the individual differences in friendships, we must take care to consider those who have negative interactions with friends and those who are friendless. Friendless children and those who choose the "wrong" friends, for example, may potentially benefit from efforts that seek to help children make friends or make the "right" friends. In sum, our fourth assumption presumes that the nomothetic and idiographic perspectives are complementary. They can and should be integrated for a richer understanding of friendship and its significance.

The remaining chapters of this book aim to shed light on the friendship experiences of children and adolescents. We consider research, for example, that will help us better understand the children and adolescents represented in the vignettes at the beginning of this chapter: why Leah and Olivia may have befriended one another during toddlerhood (see Chapter 3 for a discussion of the developmental significance of friendship in childhood); how Mark and Jeremy's friendship compares to their relationship with the larger peer group (see Chapter 5 for a discussion of the dark side of friendship and aggression, and Chapter 8 for a discussion of friendship interventions); how Johnny and Dave's friendship may serve a protective function for Dave in the face of his harassing peers (see Chapter 5 for a discussion of the protective role of friendship in the face of victimization); how positive friendship quality contributes to the wellbeing of two adolescent friends like Amy and Mary (see Chapter 6 for a discussion of the importance of high-quality friendships); and whether childhood and adolescent friendships like those of James and Thomas or Jennifer and Katie shape psychosocial functioning in later life (see Chapter 4 for a discussion of friendships in adolescence).

Friendship is complex and multifaceted—there is no "one size fits all" for how friendships are formed, maintained, or terminated—but several decades of research have helped us understand the significant contributions of friendship to child and adolescent development. Of course, there are several related and important topics that are beyond the scope of this book. Because of our focus on dyadic friendships, the book only peripherally covers the growing literature on social networks. Likewise, although we focus on the contributions of friendships to child and adolescent development, a complete analysis of processes of peer influence is not included. Much of this work focuses on larger peer groups and the peer network as a whole.

Chapter 2

Studying Friendship

We must view friendships as dynamic; as reactive and evocative; as predictor, outcome, and process; as links between individual lives and the larger world; as components of development and socialization throughout life.

—ROBERT CROSNOE (2000, p. 388)

At face value, identifying a child's friends seems like a fairly simple task—can't we just ask them? As this chapter describes, however, measuring or assessing friendships effectively is a complex task. In part, this is due to the fact that there are multiple dimensions of friendships to assess, and each is usually examined with a different strategy. There are two questions to consider when thinking about ways to study children's friendship experience—*what* to assess and *how* to assess it. Figure 2.1 shows a model to guide the first of these questions. The model highlights the multidimensional nature of friendships and specifies six domains for assessing the friendship experience of children and adolescents—the *what* to assess. These domains include the presence of friendship, the quality of the relationship, the characteristics of that friend, the characteristics of the child, the context of the friendship, and the child's interactions with that friend. Not all studies are likely to include assessments of all six domains. In addition, the six domains are not independent, and much can be learned by examining the intersections between domains. Each domain is described in further detail below with a discussion of methods for assessing each one—the *how* to assess it question. In addition, we include summaries of research findings that illustrate the complexity of assessing various components of friendship.

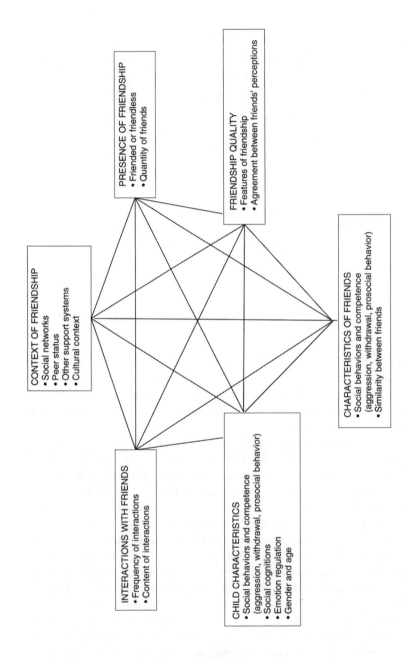

FIGURE 2.1. Model for assessment of children's friendship experience.

ASSESSING THE PRESENCE OF FRIENDSHIP

At the most basic level, assessing children's friendship experiences involves determining whether a particular child has a friend. Given the focus on friendship as a reciprocal, dyadic relationship, this process typically involves at least two steps—asking a child who his or her friends are and then determining whether the nominated friends also view the child as a friend. One of the most straightforward and commonly used methods is to ask children to nominate some number of classmates who are their friends, typically by selecting names from a class or grade-level roster. Each child's nominations are compared to the other children's nominations, and reciprocal nominations are evidence for a mutual friendship between those two children.

A variation to this procedure involves combining friendship nominations with a rating scale of how much children like peers in their classroom. Early studies by Berndt and colleagues assessing children's perceptions of specific relationships exemplify this approach (e.g., Berndt, 1981a, 1981b; Berndt & Perry, 1986; Berndt, Hawkins, & Hoyle, 1986). Children were asked to name five best friends in their grade. Then they were asked to rate how much they like each same-sex child in their grade level on a scale from 1 ("don't like") to 5 ("like very much, as much as a best friend"). Children were considered to be "close friends" if at least one listed the other as a best friend, and the average of the liking ratings they gave one another was at least 4 on the 5-point scale. To ensure that one child in a friend pair did not give the other a neutral rating—a 3 paired with a 5 rating would meet Berndt's criteria—others have included as friends only pairs in which one child nominated the other as a friend and both children gave the other a 4 or 5 rating (e.g., Berndt & Das, 1987; Bukowski, Pizzamiglio, et al., 1996; Jones, 1985).

Rating scales can also be used without specific friendship nominations by identifying friends as two children who each give the other the highest liking rating. There may be some conceptual differences between how much a child likes another and whether that child is really a close friend. In addition, in direct comparisons of various methods, Bukowski, Pizzamiglio, and colleagues (1996) conclude that reciprocal liking ratings may not be as precise as friendship nominations because they are influenced by other factors, including a child's idiosyncratic use of rating scales. Nevertheless, both rating scales and nominations are appropriate strategies to assess whether a child has a reciprocated friend (Bukowski, Pizzamiglio, et al., 1996). When friendship and popularity or peer status are examined together, reliance on nomination techniques to assess both dimensions of peer relations may create shared method variance (Parker & Asher, 1993). Thus, Bukowski, Pizzamiglio, and colleagues (1996) suggest that using rating scales to measure popularity and nominations to measure friendship helps to avoid associations between friendship and popularity that are due solely to using the same measurement technique.

Nominations of friends is a useful and reliable method even among young children. Fifty years ago, McCandless and Marshall (1957) demonstrated that a picture sociometric technique is effective for identifying preschool children's friendships and correlates reasonably well with teacher nominations of children's friends. In this procedure, children are shown photographs of all of their classmates and asked to identify the children they would like to play with during a variety of activities (e.g., playing outside, playing inside, listening to stories). Each child in the class is given a preferred playmate score based on the target child's nominations—the sum of weighted scores (5 points for first choice, 4 points for second choice, etc.) across all of the interview questions—and these scores are used to identify friends.

Asking children who their friends are makes intuitive sense, but this strategy obviously will not work for preverbal children. Thus, particularly when the interest is in assessing very young children's friendships, an alternative method is needed. There are several options, and often a combination of strategies is the most effective, but the key is that friendship must be defined based on children's behavior rather than on their verbal descriptions. Observations of children's behavior with peers is one method for identifying young children's friendships. The question then becomes, What observed behaviors are indicative of friendship? Howes (1983, 1996) suggests that companionship, intimacy, and affection (central characteristics of friendship across the lifespan) can be observed among young children.

Typically, companionship is defined by proximity or by mutual preference for one another. For example, mutual preference can be observed by noting the number of social initiations by one child toward another that successfully result in an interaction (Howes, 1983). Companionship as proximity can be operationalized as two children being within a certain distance of one another during a specified number of observations. Howes (1988), for example, used a distance of 3 feet during at least 30% of the observations. George and Krantz (1981) defined "preferred partners" for preschool children as other children with whom they were most frequently engaged in mutual social participation (e.g., cooperative play). In another study using proximity or time spent together to define preschool children's friendships, proximity was defined as being within 6 feet of a particular peer for any part of each 10-second observation interval (Hartup, Laursen, Stewart, & Eastenson, 1988). A ratio of time spent in proximity with a particular peer to time spent with all peers was calculated, and mutual friends were defined as pairs of children who spent 25% or more of their time with each other. Using this strategy, "unilateral associates" were also identified for dyads in which only one of the children spent 25% of his or her time in proximity with the other.

Affection and intimacy are not used as often as companionship for defining young children's friendships. Nevertheless, these features may be readily observed and help define friendship as an affective relationship. For example, affection for one another may be assessed by observing shared affect—two children smile, laugh, or otherwise show their enjoyment of being together while engaged with one another (Howes, 1988). Observing children's response to peers' distress shows that children who are friends are much more likely to respond to one another than children who are not friends (Howes & Farver, 1987). Finally, Howes (1996) suggests that self-disclosure in the context of pretend play may be one way to observe intimacy between young friends. Nevertheless, such intimacy has not been explored as a way of determining which children are friends.

Other strategies for identifying friends include relying on parent report or teacher report. There are several drawbacks to using these informants to identify children's friends. Most importantly, children themselves are the only ones who decide whom they consider a friend. Parents are not able to observe their children's interactions at school and must use other information (e.g., who the child talks about, calls on the phone, plays with outside of school) to identify friends. Teachers, in contrast, have direct contact with children's peer interactions at school but may base their reports of friendship on academically oriented peer interactions rather than peer interactions at recess, in the lunchroom, and in other important settings where their access is more limited (Gest, 2006). The validity of teachers' reports of friendship has rarely been examined. With young children, mutual liking nominations and teacher reports of friendship agreed at a rate greater than expected by chance (Howes, 1988). Similar modest agreement between children's mutual friendship nominations and teacher reports of friendship dyads was found for school-age children, especially older elementary-age children; nevertheless, teacher reports overestimated the degree of behavioral similarity between children and their friends (Gest, 2006). Overall, then, children's mutual friendship nominations remain the gold standard for identifying friendships.

QUESTIONS IN ASSESSING THE PRESENCE OF FRIENDSHIP

Several questions arise from the procedures to identify the presence of friendships that may affect the conclusions we draw about children's participation in these relationships. Here we consider four:

1. How many nominations are children asked to make?
2. At what level must a nomination be reciprocated?
3. Is reciprocity of friendships necessary?
4. Does the quantity of friends matter?

How Many Nominations Are Children Asked to Make?

A typical number of nominations children are asked to make is three, but there is nothing magical about three. Some investigators allow children to make unlimited nominations, identifying as many peers as they want as friends. Unlimited nominations give children more opportunities to be identified as having a mutual friend. What effect the number of nominations children make has on the outcomes of particular studies is an empirical question that has not been systematically studied. There is some evidence that summary measures (e.g., average scores) across many friends gives a more complete picture of a child's friendship network, suggesting that unlimited nominations are valuable. For example, Berndt and colleagues found that a composite measure of the quality of adolescents' multiple friendships was more strongly associated with outcomes, such as school adjustment and self-esteem, than the quality of the adolescents' very best friendship (Berndt, 1996; Berndt & Keefe, 1995; Keefe & Berndt, 1996). The complexity of social networks, especially by adolescence, provides a challenge to researchers who typically limit their assessments to one or just a few friends even though most youth live in rich friendship networks.

At What Level Must a Nomination Be Reciprocated?

Some investigators distinguish between categories of friendship based on the level of reciprocation. For example, a fairly exclusive definition is when a friendship is determined only for two children who list one another first in their list of friendship nominations (Bagwell et al., 1998). Parker and Asher (1993) asked children to nominate three friends and then to select the one friend who was their "very best friend." If the named very best friend selected the target child as one of his or her friend nominations, the target child was determined to have a "very best friendship." Relationships were considered to be "best friendships" when any of a child's three nominations were reciprocated. In this study, children could have only one "very best friendship" but could have up to three "best friendships." The need to identify one specific friendship is often important when friendship quality is also assessed. As described below, self-report measures of friendship quality are typically completed about only one relationship, and the name of the specific friend is often incorporated into the quality measure.

Is Reciprocity of Friendship Nominations Necessary?

Nearly all children name friends when asked, and unless these nominations are reciprocated, it is impossible to know what is the relationship between the nominating child and the nominated friend. In some cases, the two children may indeed be friends (e.g., perhaps the friend would have named the child if given more choices). In other cases, the child may simply wish the other was his or her friend when in reality, no friendship exists. And, still in other cases, these "unilateral" nominations may simply index liking on the part of the nominating child. A number of studies have compared mutually nominated friends and pairs based on unilateral nominations, primarily to assess the importance of reciprocity. In our own work based on a meta-analysis of studies comparing reciprocal and unilateral friends, we found significant differences between these two types of pairings with reciprocal friends showing greater positive engagement toward one another (e.g., social contact, positive affect) and having more of the deeper properties of friendship in their relationship (e.g., closeness, loyalty, equality) (Newcomb & Bagwell, 1995). These findings suggest that the distinction between mutual and unilateral friends is a meaningful one at least in terms of differences in the characteristics of the relationship.

Unfortunately, the common strategy of defining friendship based on reciprocal nominations means that both friends must be participants in the assessment. To satisfy this criterion, nearly all studies limit friendship nominations to other children in the classroom or grade level. As a result, children who have close friends in the neighborhood or at another school or who are older or younger may be classified as "friendless" when they actually have a reciprocal best friend. There may also be a greater likelihood for certain children and adolescents to have friends outside their classroom (Kiesner et al., 2004). For example, aggressive children and adolescents are more likely than nonaggressive youth to have friends in their neighborhood (Bagwell & Coie, 2004; Dishion, Andrews, & Crosby, 1995). These friends are expected to have greater influence on aggressive children's behavior than peers or friends at school, but these relationships are missed if friendship nominations are restricted to school-based friends. Parker and Asher (1993) asked children to name three friends and did not restrict them to peers at school. On average, children named just under one peer who was not a schoolmate as a friend.

Does the Quantity of Friendships Matter?

Assessments of children's participation in a mutual friendship typically result in a dichotomous measure—children either have a reciprocal friend, or they do not. From an analytical perspective, this dichotomous measure has limited variability, and using it to predict hypothesized outcomes is thus sometimes difficult. For a measure with greater variability, some investigators have examined the number of reciprocal friends a child has. This number may be artificially capped if, for example, children are asked to nominate up to three peers as friends. More concerning, however, is the fact that there is limited theoretical evidence to suggest that the number of friends a child has is associated with any particular positive or negative outcome (Bukowski & Hoza, 1989). Sullivan (1953) talks primarily about a child's "best" friend but does not say that youth can have just one. In fact, most children and adolescents name several best friends (Hartup, 1993). Empirically, as well as theoretically, there is limited evidence to indicate whether the effects of friendship are cumulative, such that having more friends relates to better adjustment, or whether simply having one friend is what matters. A few recent studies suggest that the extensivity of children's friendships may be related to some components of adjustment. Having more friends is associated with less loneliness and, for boys, with less depression (Erdley et al., 2001), and children with more friends (rather than fewer) are perceived as having leadership abilities and good humor (Gest et al., 2001).

Other research suggests that the number of friendships an adolescent has may indirectly contribute to adjustment through friendship quality (Demir & Urberg, 2004). Thus, having more friendships allows for higher-quality relationships. It is also likely that individuals who are able to establish a high-quality relationship with one friend are likely to be able to establish high-quality friendships with multiple others (Demir & Urberg, 2004). These findings indicate that it may be premature to dismiss the importance of assessing the quantity of friends even though quality or simply having a friend at all may be more directly related to adjustment; instead, we should consider both the structure of the friendship network (e.g., quantity of friends) and the quality of those relationships. In the social support literature, these distinctions are conceptualized as indicators of social embeddedness versus indicators of enacted support (frequency of supportive behaviors as is typically measured in friendship quality assessments; Wolchik, Beals, & Sandler, 1989).

Summary

Assessing whether a child has friends is most often accomplished by reciprocal nominations. This strategy captures the mutuality in the relationship—the sine qua non of friendship. Overall, it is a reliable and valid measure. Concerns may arise, however, for some children for whom limiting their nominations to other children in their school class may miss the friendships that are most important to them, or may result in them being classified as friendless when they have a close, mutual friend outside of school. This concern is especially problematic if certain children, say aggressive or rejected children, are affected more than others. It is important, therefore, to test empirically the degree to which this is a problem and continue to examine the validity of other methods for identifying friendships.

ASSESSING FRIENDSHIP QUALITY

Beginning in the early 1980s, in particular, several research teams began to investigate children's perceptions of their own friendships (e.g., Berndt & Perry, 1986; Sharabany, Gershoni, & Hofman, 1981). These studies focused on identifying the features that characterize friendships in childhood and adolescence and that are distinct from relationships with other peers. In many ways, this research built on and expanded the literature on children's conceptions of friendship and expectations of friends—ideas about the relationship in general and friends in general rather than about the features of their relationship with a specific friend (e.g., Bigelow, 1977; Bigelow & La Gaipa, 1975). Although the term *friendship quality* was not consistently used until the 1990s, these studies documenting the positive and negative features of children's friendships are really the first studies of friendship quality.

What Is Friendship Quality?

At the most basic level, there is some inconsistency in the use of the term *friendship quality* throughout the literature, and it would help to establish a consistent definition of the construct. In our discussion, we use Berndt's (1996) distinctions among *friendship features, friendship quality,* and *friendship effects*. Friendship features refers to the "attributes or characteristics" of the relationship (p. 346). These include the various dimensions of friendship assessed in the measures described above—conflict, intimacy, companionship, and help, to name a few. As Berndt notes, this term is not evaluative and thus refers to both positive and negative characteristics of the relationship. Specific friendship features may further be distinguished according to whether they are relationship *processes* or *provisions* (Ladd & Kochenderfer, 1996). Processes are those friendship features that indicate interactions between friends, such as self-disclosure and conflict. Friendship features identified as provisions are those that indicate the benefits children receive from their relationship. These features include security, intimacy, and closeness. We note, however, that in the literature, friendship features are often referred to as friendship qualities.

Friendship quality, in contrast to friendship features, is evaluative in nature and suggests that some relationships are "better" than others. In this way, friendship quality tells us about the value of the relationship. The positive and negative features of friendship define the quality of the relationship (see also Berndt, 2002, for a review). For example, friendships with many positive features and few negative features are high-quality relationships, and children are likely to experience a high degree of satisfaction from these friendships. Finally, friendship effects refer to the ways in which friendships (friendship features or friendship quality) influence a child's adjustment and well-being. The hypotheses that high-quality friendships promote adaptive adjustment and that high-quality friendships provide a buffer against negative outcomes associated with other problematic peer experiences are hypotheses about the effects of friendship.

Measures of Friendship Quality

In the 1990s, friendship quality became a prominent topic of study as researchers were increasingly focused on individual differences in friendships and in finding out whether variations in friendship quality relate to differences in children's adjustment and well-being. At this time, measures were developed to define specific relationships in terms of their features and quality. These measures are all self-report measures that ask about a child's perceptions of the features of a particular friendship (usually with a best friend). Some investigators have also used these measures to ascertain the friend's perceptions of the friendship to provide two perspectives on the same relationship. Six of the most commonly used self-report measures of friendship features and quality (and adaptations of them) are described below.

Berndt's Friendship Interview

In several studies, Berndt and colleagues (e.g., Berndt & Keefe, 1995; Berndt & Perry, 1986) have assessed children's and adolescents' perceptions of the features of their relationships with friends and acquaintances. They have used several versions of a measure to index these features. In the initial version of the measure, children and adolescents responded to a structured interview followed by open-ended interview questions.

The interview questions asked respondents about the degree to which six features of friendship described their relationship with a particular peer—play/association (e.g., companionship and spending time together), prosocial behavior (e.g., sharing and helping), intimacy (e.g., self-disclosure), loyalty (e.g., dependability), attachment and self-esteem enhancement (e.g., closeness and encouragement), and conflict (e.g., arguing and fighting). Each feature included five sets of questions. Children are first asked whether a particular behavior happens (or is expected to happen) in the friendship, and following an affirmative response, they are asked how often it occurs. These responses are transformed to a 0 (not at all) to 4 (all of the time) scale to be used for analyses. In later versions, Berndt and colleagues have used a questionnaire version of this interview (Keefe & Berndt, 1996).

Interestingly, Berndt and Perry's (1986) factor analysis of the items revealed age differences in the structure of perceptions of relationship features. For children and early adolescents (second, fourth, and sixth graders), all six features loaded on one factor, with conflict items reverse scored to indicate absence of conflict. For eighth-grade adolescents, however, two factors emerged—one including most of the positive features and a second including primarily absence of conflict items. These results suggest that for adolescents (as with adults; Bagwell et al., 2005; Rook, 1984), positive and negative friendship features can coexist, but children may view positive and negative features as opposites that cannot exist in the same relationship.

Network of Relationships Inventory

One of the first widely used assessments of the quality of children's friendships was the Network of Relationships Inventory (NRI) developed by Furman and Buhrmester (1985, 1992). This measure was not intended to be a specific assessment of friendships. Rather, it was based on the theories of Sullivan (1953) and Weiss (1974) that different relationships offer different social provisions. Friendship, thus, is understood as one relationship in a child's network of social relationships that might also include parents, siblings, other family members, and teachers, for example. As a result, the items on the NRI tap social provisions and functions that might be especially likely to be found in friendships as well as those that might be more likely obtained in other relationships.

The NRI consists of 30 items with three items tapping each of seven social provisions—reliable alliance (counting on the relationship to last), nurturance (protection and care), affection (feelings of love or liking), admiration (respect and approval), instrumental help (guidance and assistance), companionship (enjoying time together), and intimacy (self-disclosure)—and each of three additional relationship features—relative power (who has more control in the relationship), conflict (arguing and disagreeing), and antagonism (bothering and annoying behavior). Respondents use a 1 (little or none) to 5 (the most) scale to indicate the degree to which each item characterizes a specific relationship, and researchers can ask about as many or as few different relationships as they choose. The original measure was developed with fifth- and sixth-grade youth but has been used successfully with children as young as age 7 (Buhrmester & Furman, 1987) and with adolescents and young adults (Furman & Buhrmester, 1992). The internal consistency of the subscales is adequate (average alpha across relationships = .80; Furman & Buhrmester, 1985). Furman and Buhrmester (1992) report that the seven social provisions subscales are highly correlated and can be combined into one index of support. Likewise, conflict and antagonism are combined into one index of negative relationship features.

Recently, Furman and Buhrmester (2009) developed a new version of the NRI to assess the attachment, caregiving, and affiliative behavioral systems across different relationships. This version of the NRI includes eight subscales: the attachment subsystem is assessed with two subscales (i.e., seeks safe haven and seeks secure base); the caregiving subsystem is assessed with two subscales (i.e., provides safe haven and provides secure base); the affiliative system is assessed with the companionship subscale from the original NRI; and negative interactions are assessed with the three subscales of conflict, antagonism, and criticism. Two summary scales can be calculated consisting of the five positive support subscales (i.e., support) and the three negative interaction subscales. Furman and Buhrmester (2009) note that the new version of the NRI, called the NRI—Behavioral Systems version, and the original NRI, called the NRI—Social Provisions version, index similar constructs at the level of the overall support and negative interactions scales, but that unique information is gained by examining the specific subscales within those overarching dimensions.

Friendship Qualities Scale

In 1994, Bukowski, Hoza, and Boivin published their Friendship Qualities Scale (FQS), and this measure has become a widely used instrument for assessing children's perceptions of the features and quality of their friendships. The FQS consists of 23 items grouped into the five broadband subscales of companionship (four items), conflict (four items), help (five items), security (five items), and closeness (five items). Help, security, and closeness may be further broken down into the narrow-band subscales of aid and protection (help), reliable alliance and transcending problems (security), and affective bond and reflected appraisal (close-ness). These five dimensions of friendship quality were chosen based on theoretical understandings of the important features that define chil-dren's relationships with friends and the goal of indexing a particular relationship with minimally overlapping subscales. The companionship scale taps children's enjoyment of and frequency of time spent with their friend. Help assesses both instrumental aid and sticking up for the friend in the context of other peers. The security subscale includes items indicat-ing that the friend is a trustworthy confidant and items indicating effec-tive conflict resolution. Closeness reflects the strong affective tie between friends as well as friends' enhancement of one another's self-esteem. Finally, the conflict subscale assesses the frequency of disagreements and arguments between friends.

The FQS was originally developed with fifth- through seventh-grade children and early adolescents. Responses are given on a 1 (not true) to 5 (really true) scale, and the score for a particular subscale is the mean score for the items on that friendship feature. The FQS is designed to assess one relationship—the relationship a child has with his or her best friend. Some items on the FQS describe both children (e.g., "My friend and I can argue a lot") and some describe only one partner in the relationship (e.g., "I can get into fights with my friend" or "My friend would help me if I needed it"). Bukowksi and colleagues (1994) report correlations between the five broad-band subscales with absolute magnitudes ranging from .13 to .61. In addition, internal consistency for the subscales is adequate (alpha range = .71 to .80), and the measure distinguishes between recip-rocated and nonreciprocated friendships and between relationships that are stable and not stable over a 6-month period.

Friendship Quality Questionnaire

At the same time that Bukowski and colleagues developed the FQS, Parker and Asher (1993) were working on a similar measure—the Friendship Quality Questionnaire (FQQ). Some of the items on the FQQ were based on an earlier version of Bukowski and colleagues' measure. The measure was originally developed with third- through sixth-grade children, but the FQQ has been adapted and used with adolescents and young adults as well (e.g., Bohnert, Aikins, & Edidin, 2007; French, Bae, Pidada, & Lee, 2006). The FQQ assesses six dimensions of friendship quality. Vali-dation and caring (10 items) indexes a child's subjective feeling about the degree to which the friend feels affection toward the child and enhances the child's self-esteem. Intimate exchange (six items) includes items about talking together about personal matters such as problems and secrets. The items on the companionship and recreation subscale (five items) assess the amount of time friends spend together in their free time in and outside of school and their enjoyment of being together. Help and guidance (nine items) includes items about the instrumental help friends provide one another as well as the more intangible help of providing good ideas. Conflict and betrayal (seven items) is the only subscale assessing negative aspects of the relationship and considers the frequency of minor disagreements and fights as well as one item about failing to keep promises. Finally, a separate subscale called conflict resolution (three items) indexes the degree to which friends easily overcome the arguments and disagreements they do have.

Children respond to the FQQ about one specific friend, and Parker and Asher (1993) recommend customizing the instrument for each child by inserting the friend's name in each item. Responses are given on a 0 (not at all true) to 4 (really true) scale, and subscale scores represent the mean score for the items loading on that subscale. The questionnaire is designed to be administered to children in a group setting, such as a school classroom. Parker and Asher report good internal consistency for the subscales (alpha range = .73 to .90), and the absolute magnitude of the correlations between subscales ranges from .16 to .75.

The original intent of the FQQ was to assess features of children's *relationships* with friends. Nevertheless, interest in how friends' perceptions of the same relationship may differ and in how one individual in a relationship may contribute differently to the overall relationship than the other has led some researchers to revise the wording of some of the FQQ items (e.g., Rose & Asher, 1999). On the original measure, items are worded such that some assess what the friend does to or for the target child, and others are worded to assess what the friends do together in the relationship. For example, in the help and guidance subscale, two items include "helps me so I can get done quicker" and "gives advice with figuring things out." These items suggest ways that the friend assists the target child. Yet, additional items include "help each other with schoolwork a lot" and "do special favors for each other," and these items assume both friends help one another. Thus, they do not specify whether the friend does these things for the target child or the target child does them for the friend. These differences are subtle and may not matter in many cases, but in friendships that are unequal or perhaps in low-quality relationships, the different contributions of the two children may be significant. In addition, revising the items slightly allows researchers to decide whether they are most interested in a child's report of his or her friend's behavior or a friend's report of a target child's behavior.

Other adaptations of this friendship quality measure have also been used in the literature. Grotpeter and Crick (1996) incorporated many of the scales and items of the FQQ and additional items from Bukowski and colleagues' (1994) FQS in their Friendship Qualities Measure (FQM). The FQM was designed to capture especially the relationship features and quality of aggressive children's friendships. Thus, additional subscales were added to focus specifically on aggression. These included subscales tapping relational aggression within the friendship, overt aggression within the friendship, the degree to which the friends engage in relational aggression together, the degree to which the friends engage in overt aggression together, and the exclusivity of the relationship.

In addition, Grotpeter and Crick (1996) hypothesized that the effect of particular friendship features on children's satisfaction with the relationship and general well-being would depend in part on the importance of that dimension for the individual child. In other words, one child might not place much importance on the degree to which her friend sticks up for her to others, but it might matter a great deal to her that her friend sits with her at lunch. To this end, Grotpeter and Crick developed the Importance of Friendship Qualities Measure (IFQM). Items on this measure ask respondents to indicate how upset they would be if a particular positive quality did not exist (e.g., companionship) or a particular negative feature did exist (e.g., relational aggression) in the relationship.

The FQM contains 43 items comprising 14 subscales, and the IFQM contains 33 items consisting of 11 subscales. There are three more subscales on the FQM because the exclusivity, intimate exchange, and conflict subscales are included twice—once to indicate what the target child receives from the friend and once to indicate what the friend receives from the target child (e.g., "I can tell my friend secrets" vs. "My friend can tell me secrets"). A 5-point response scale is used for both measures, and subscale scores represent the average score for items on that dimension. After combining the two conflict subscales and the two exclusivity subscales, adequate though somewhat low internal consistencies were found for the 12 FQM subscales and the 11 IFQM subscales. Alpha values ranged from .61 to .87.

McGill Friendship Questionnaires

Unlike the various measures described above, the McGill Friendship Questionnaires were developed for use with older adolescents (Mendelson & Aboud, 1999). Two instruments are used to tap positive feelings toward the friend and the functions a friend is perceived to fulfill. The affection measure includes a subscale about positive feelings for a friend (nine items) and a subscale about satisfaction with the relationship (seven items). Respondents use a 9-point scale to indicate how much they agree with each statement. The second questionnaire assesses a friend's functions and includes six specific functions with five items indexing each one—stimulating companionship (e.g., doing fun things together), help (e.g., offering guidance and instrumental assistance), intimacy (e.g., being sensitive to the other), reliable alliance (e.g., being loyal and dependable), self-validation (e.g., offering encouragement and promoting a sense of well-being), and emotional security (e.g., offering comfort and support in difficult situations). A 9-point scale is used for respondents to indicate how often the friend fulfills each function. A factor analysis supported the structure of the friendship functions assessment with the exception of the emotional security subscale. Nevertheless, internal consistencies were high for all subscales on both measures (alpha range = .84 to .96). Evidence for the validity of the McGill Questionnaires was found by positive correlations between the subscales (except emotional security) and the duration of the friendship and by positive correlations between a measure of self-esteem in relationships and the subscales. Finally, satisfaction and positive feelings toward the friend were associated with the degree to which the friend fulfilled the positive friendship functions. Interestingly, the McGill Questionnaires are focused only on the positive aspects of friendships and do not include any measure of negative friendship features. Nevertheless, they provide a measure that is appropriate to use with older adolescents and one of the only ones specifically developed for and with adolescents rather than children.

Friendship Features Interview for Young Children

None of the measures described above were specifically designed for young children; thus, Ladd, Kochenderfer, and Coleman (1996) developed an assessment of friendship features with kindergarten-age children. The measure was based on the existing measures for older children and was empirically derived from a larger battery of items that included the friendship features of companionship, validation, aid, self-disclosure, exclusivity, and conflict. These friendship processes were expected to predict young children's satisfaction with their friendship and the stability of the relationship. Factor analysis did not support the companionship factor, and the final measure included items loading on five subscales of friendship features—validation (three items about receiving support from the friend), aid (four items about emotional and instrumental help), disclosing negative affect (two items about sharing personal negative feelings), exclusivity (four items about the friendship being mutually selective), and conflict (four items about negative and angry behavior)—and two additional subscales indexing satisfaction with the relationship and the friend's influence on children's affect about school.

Children were individually interviewed, and their friend's name was inserted into each question. Responses to each item were given as 0 (no),

1 (sometimes), or 2 (yes). Internal consistencies were adequate (alpha range = .63 to .81), and the subscales were generally moderately correlated with one another (absolute value range = .08 to .50). Additional support for the distinctiveness of the features assessed comes from evidence that different features were associated with different outcomes. For example, validation, exclusivity, and conflict predicted children's satisfaction with their friendship; validation and conflict were also associated with friendship stability; and other features predicted various aspects of school adjustment.

QUESTIONS IN ASSESSING FRIENDSHIP QUALITY

There are a number of questions—both theoretical and methodological—to consider when assessing friendship quality. Here we discuss three:

1. How many friendship features are there?
2. What are the theoretically important negative features of friendship?
3. Are we assessing perceptions or reality or both?

How Many Friendship Features Are There?

An ongoing controversy in the literature on friendship features and quality concerns just how many dimensions there are. Parker and Asher (1993) identify six; Bukowski and colleagues (1994) propose five; other measures include still different numbers of features. Yet, some research suggests that there may be only two—a positive dimension and a negative dimension—and these two are not highly correlated. Thus, for example, friendships may have many positive features and many negative features. Evidence for this view comes primarily from factor analytic studies of measures like those described above. In addition, in some studies, many of the distinct features of friendship are positively correlated to such a degree that they might not represent truly unique features. As such, the discriminant validity of multiple features is questionable (Berndt, 1996). For example, Furman (1996) reanalyzed data provided by both Parker and Asher and Bukowski and colleagues from their respective instruments and found that although the reported five- and six-factor solutions fit the data, a two-factor solution was also appropriate. In the two-factor solution, the positive items loaded on one factor, and the conflict items loaded on the second. These two factors accounted for 35% (vs. 54%) of the variance in the

Bukowski and colleagues (1994) data and 45% (vs. 58%) of the variance in the Parker and Asher data.

This question about the number of features on which friendships differ is important not only at the methodological level but also at the conceptual level. For example, there may be developmental differences in children's ability to discriminate among various positive features of their friendships as well as variations in the specific positive features that are important at different developmental periods. Using only a global measure of positive friendship features would make it impossible to identify these potentially important developmental trends. For example, the importance of intimacy as a critical friendship feature increases dramatically in adolescence (Berndt, 1982; Sharabany et al., 1981), yet companionship is a particularly important feature of high-quality relationships among younger children (Howes, 1983). In addition, when considering the effects of friendship, specific features may be associated with specific outcomes—a finding that would be difficult to ascertain with only global measures of positive and negative features.

In our own work, positive friendship features provided a buffer against girls' feelings of anxiety and depression associated with being victimized by peers (Schmidt & Bagwell, 2007). However, the various positive features we assessed did not function in the same way. Only the positive features of help and security provided such a buffer, and, in fact, closeness was associated with increased internalizing distress for girls who were victimized by peers. Researchers must decide, then, what is the appropriate level of analysis for their particular question—is it at the level of global dimensions of friendship features, or is it important to examine specifically the various specific positive or negative features. Furman (1996) cautions that when interpreting findings, we must be cognizant of the fact that differences at the level of global features may actually reflect differences among only a few specific dimensions. Likewise, if we find similar effects for many specific features, we may really be tapping into an overall effect for a global positive (or negative) dimension.

What Are the Negative Features of Friendship?

Early investigations of children's friendships were biased toward the positive outcomes and functions of these relationships. In part due to the theoretical conceptualizations, such as Sullivan (1953), that guided early research and that focused on the benefits of having friends, negative features and potential downsides of some relationships were largely ignored. Having friends was assumed to mean having high-quality friendships. Thus, limited attention was given to negative features of friendship. The measures of friendship quality described above generally include only conflict as a negative feature; the McGill Friendship Questionnaire, for example, includes no negative features. Indeed, conflict is a key dimension along which friendships differ. As we learn more about the vicissitudes of friendship, however, it will be important to explore other negative dimensions of friendship and their effects. For example, given the central nature of reciprocity and equality as foundations of friendship (Hartup, 1996a; Sullivan, 1953; Youniss, 1980), inequality has been included in some measures as a negative friendship feature. In the NRI, a subscale assessing the balance of power in the relationship gets at this concern about equality. Interestingly, though, factor analyses of the NRI subscales have consistently found that the relative power subscale loads on a separate factor and not with the other negative features.

Specific questions about aggression (both overt and relational) within the friendship, such as those included in Grotpeter and Crick's (1996) version of the FQQ, more specifically assess this particular form of conflict. Rivalry is another dimension of children's relationships that may influence the quality of the friendship (Berndt & Keefe, 1995). Specifically, rivalry suggests competition that is not necessarily healthy—boasting or bragging about one's superiority, or frequently trying to "one up" or outperform the friend, for example. Another potentially important negative dimension of friendship that has not been included in measures of friendship quality to date is the degree of negative influence friends may have on one another. Specifically, the ways in which one friend may entice another to engage in rule-breaking talk and behavior or other negative behavior is an aspect of friendship that has received extensive attention recently (e.g., Dishion, Spracklen, Andrews, & Patterson, 1996; Granic & Dishion, 2003) but has not yet been assessed on friendship quality measures. Finally, friendship-related jealousy can lead to loneliness and depression (Lavallee & Parker, 2009; Parker, Kruse, & Aikins, 2010) and should be considered as a negative feature of relationships, even though proneness to jealousy may be an individual characteristic that children bring to their friendships.

What Do Friendship Quality Measures Actually Measure?

There is a question about just what it is that self-report measures of friendship quality assess. At the most basic level, they are designed to assess a child's *perceptions* of his or her relationship with a best friend. For any given friendship, it is unknown, however, how closely these perceptions match the actual interactions and behaviors of the friends. It is reasonable to expect that some children's perceptions will be more accurate than others. One way of addressing this question is to match observations of friends' interactions with their perceptions of the relationship. For some features of friendship this is inherently easier to do than for others. Companionship and overt prosocial behaviors may be somewhat easy to observe. Intimacy and self-disclosure, for example, are not clearly overt behaviors that would be subject to observations by external observers in natural settings. Likewise, subtle forms of conflict and relational aggression, for example, are likely to occur outside the purview of even the most astute observers. Below are some illustrative examples of different conclusions about friendship quality due to differences in reporters.

Observations versus Self-Reports

In one example of a lab-based study comparing children's perceptions and outsiders' observations of friends' behaviors in contrived settings, Brendgen, Markiewicz, Doyle, and Bukowski (2001) asked adolescents and their friends to engage in several short discussion tasks and correlated observations of interactions during these discussions with the adolescents' ratings of friendship quality. Interestingly, both positive and negative features as assessed with the FQS were associated with specific behaviors the target adolescents demonstrated when talking with their friend. Positive affect and responsiveness were related to higher ratings of positive friendship quality, whereas observed critical behavior, negative affect, and conflict were associated with more negative perceptions of the relationship. In contrast, only perceptions of negative friendship quality mapped onto the behaviors adolescents received from their friend during the discussion tasks (the more criticism they received from their partner and the more conflict initiated by their partner). As Brendgen and colleagues discuss, this may not be surprising given that negative interactions with friends are unexpected and may be more salient than positive interactions, which are assumed to define a friendship. In studies of older adults, for example, it is the absence of negative and contentious relationships rather than the presence of supportive relationships that is most clearly linked with psychological well-being (Pagel, Erdly, & Becker, 1987; Rook, 1984). Phillipsen (1999) also found that children's perceptions of conflict in a friendship were associated with less positive, coordinated, and sensitive interactions as observed in a laboratory task.

In our own research, we included both observations and self-reports of friendship features and quality in a lab-based study of aggressive boys and their best friends (Bagwell & Coie, 2004). Based on self-report of friendship quality, aggressive and nonaggressive boys did not differ in their perceptions of the quality of their relationship and also did not rate their friendship differently than their friends. In contrast, however, when observers rated the quality of the boys' relationship based on the boys' open-ended responses to questions about their friendships, aggressive boys' friendships were rated as lower in quality. Furthermore, based on observations of their interactions during several tasks in the lab, nonaggressive boys were perceived by observers as more positively engaged and as showing more reciprocity in their interactions than aggressive boys. This study revealed substantial differences between the aggressive boys' own perspectives of their friendship (which were notably positive) and outside observers' ratings of the features of their interactions. One possible explanation is that observer ratings cannot account for the subjective impact of particular experiences within the friendship. Children may perceive similar benefits and satisfaction from different objective features of their relationships. If this is the case, self-report measures of friendship quality would be identical whereas observer ratings of friends' behavior would distinguish them.

Do Friends Agree?

In addition to the question of how children's perceptions match actual behavior is the question of whether two friends' perceptions of the same relationship are concordant. In other words, do friends have a shared perspective on their relationship? Some research suggests that often they do not and that discrepancies are particularly strong for certain youth—aggressive or depressed children and those who are rejected by peers, for example. Even among children, adolescents, and young adults not selected for potential problems in peer relations, concordances between friends are generally moderate (e.g., among children, rs range from .21 for conflict to .64 for companionship—Parker & Asher, 1993; among adolescents, $r = .54$ for positive features and $r = .34$ for negative features—Furman & Buhrmester, 2009; among young adults, rs range from .30 for antagonism to .54 for companionship—Bagwell et al., 2005). As these data suggest, friends tend to agree about some features of their relationship more than they do about others. Little, Brendgen, Wanner, and Krappmann (1999) suggest that agreement is likely to be high for behaviors and interactions that are easily observed, such as the frequency of sitting together at lunch or visiting one another outside of school. However, features of friendship that are more influenced by subjective interpretations are likely to show more limited agreement. Indeed, in the examples above, companionship, which reflects observable behaviors, tended to show better agreement than conflict or antagonism, features that are more highly subjective in their interpretation.

In a series of investigations, Brendgen and colleagues have addressed the question of friends' shared perspectives for aggressive, depressed, and rejected youth. The correlation between rejected children's perspective on positive friendship features, such as closeness and fun, and their friends' perspective was essentially zero and significantly lower than the correlation between average or popular children and their friends (Brendgen, Little, & Krappmann, 2000). Interestingly, the pattern of low correlations between rejected children and their friends was due to rejected children themselves reporting positive features of the relationship at the same level as average and popular children. Yet, rejected children's friends perceived their relationships to be less close and more conflictual than the rejected children themselves (and as compared to average and popular children's friends). Thus, there was a clear lack of mutuality in the friendships of rejected children in terms of their thoughts and feelings about the relationship (Brendgen, Little, & Krappmann, 2000). Aggressive children also show this same discrepancy. Although aggressive children view the quality of their best friendships as no different than nonaggressive children, aggressive children's friends rate the relationship lower in quality than the friends of nonaggressive children (Brendgen, Vitaro, Turgeon, & Poulin, 2002). Likewise, aggressive and antisocial adolescent boys showed no agreement with their friends on assessments of the quality of their relationship, whereas nonantisocial boys and their friends demonstrated more of a shared perspective on their friendship quality (Poulin, Dishion, & Haas, 1999). In contrast, children with elevated levels of depression view the quality of their friendships less positively than do their friends (Brendgen et al., 2002). Interestingly, children who overestimated the quality of their friendship were more likely to have that friendship continue over the course of the school year, suggesting that these positive illusions might help children maintain the relationship, such as by encouraging them to express this positive view to the friend—showing enjoyment at being together, helping and supporting the friend, or seeking out interactions with the friend, for example (Brendgen, Vitaro, Turgeon, Poulin, & Wanner, 2004).

Do Different Perceptions Matter?

Even if it were possible to clearly map observations of friendship features to children's perceptions of those features, it is not clear which is more important—children's perceptions or a reality as defined by others. Likewise, perhaps more important than documenting differences in friends' perceptions is discovering whether these differences actually matter—for the children or for the relationship. We argue that they potentially matter a great deal. The way children perceive their relationship with a friend is likely to affect their behavior toward the friend and others and thus to influence the nature and course of the friendship (Brendgen et al.,

2004; Furman, 1996). With children who are depressed, for example, the degree to which they think they are accepted by peers predicts their adjustment and well-being better than their actual peer acceptance or rejection (Hymel, Rubin, Rowden, & LeMare, 1990; Kistner, Balthazor, Risi, & Burton, 1999; Panak & Garber, 1992). Similarly, if children expect negative interactions with a friend, they may be more likely to behave in ways that elicit conflict or may be more sensitive to negative interactions. A significant discrepancy between friends' perceptions may simply reflect actual differences in children's experiences of the same relationship. However, it may also be an indication of larger problems within the relationship, such as problems with interpersonal understanding (Brendgen, Little, & Krappmann, 2000). In addition, particularly for the child who has a much more positive view of the relationship, such a discordance may lead to unfulfilled expectations or a very one-sided relationship—expecting the friend to provide support in a time of crisis and being disappointed or angry when that support is not available, for example. Thus, perceptions that are really wishful thinking about how a child wants the relationship to be (rather than how it really is) could be problematic.

How Do Differences Arise?

Why might some children perceive the features and quality of their best friendships so differently than either the friend or outside observers? In the case of aggressive or rejected children, there is some evidence that they have biased or inflated perceptions of their friendship. Due to their unfavorable characteristics and negative styles of interaction, aggressive or rejected children may never have experienced the quality of friendship experienced by others, and their perceptions of their current best friendship may be limited by a lack of experience with anything better. A related explanation is that rejected or aggressive children demonstrate styles of interaction with their friends that they may perceive as appropriate and fun (e.g., high rates of confrontation, "joking" behavior they see as enjoyable) but might be viewed by their friends as immature and problematic (Brendgen, Little, & Krappman, 2000).

We know that aggressive children experience multiple difficulties in encoding and interpreting cues in social interactions (Crick & Dodge, 1994). Perhaps these social cognitive biases also operate in their interpretation and evaluation of close social relationships like friendships. Recent research on children who are rejected by the general peer group has identified subgroups of low-accepted children. Comparisons of these subgroups indicate that aggressive–rejected children show less loneliness and social dissatisfaction than submissive–rejected children and, in fact, do not differ from average-status children in their reports of loneliness and concern about social relationships (Boivin, Thomassin, & Alain, 1989; Parkhurst & Asher, 1992). Furthermore, aggressive–rejected children tend to overestimate their social competence and social status in the peer group, are not likely to refer themselves for help with peer relations, and make self-protective misjudgments when evaluating peers' negative feelings toward them (Asher, Zellis, Parker, & Bruene, 1991; Hymel, Woody, & Bowker, 1993; Zakriski & Coie, 1996). Taken together, there is much evidence indicating that aggressive–rejected children have distorted perceptions of social situations and their own relationships. Parker and Asher (1993) compared low-, average-, and high-accepted children's reports of the quality of their best friendship and found the greatest heterogeneity within the low-accepted group. They suggested that subgroup differences may account for this within-group variability. Thus, aggressive and rejected children are likely to display distorted perceptions of their relationships, and these biases appear to emerge in their perception of the quality of their friendships.

There are mixed interpretations about the degree to which a positive illusory bias (i.e., overestimation of competence) is helpful or detrimental to well-being. On the one hand, some research suggests that mild positively biased perceptions are associated with mental health and promote adaptive functioning (e.g., Taylor & Brown, 1988). These positive illusions may serve a self-protective function and help individuals cope with setbacks. Alternatively, in the context of peer relations, they may give children the confidence to approach others and may in turn facilitate the development and maintenance of relationships with peers (Brendgen et al., 2004; Rabiner & Coie, 1989). In support of this hypothesis, children's overestimation of their friendship quality (relative to their friend's perceptions) increased the odds that they would be nominated as a friend by that same child several months later (Brendgen et al., 2004).

On the other hand, to the extent that accurate self-appraisals are important for mental health (e.g., Colvin, Block, & Funder, 1995), inflated perceptions of competence might be problematic. This perspective is supported by research linking the positive illusory bias with aggression (e.g., Baumeister, Smart, & Boden, 1996) and findings that children with attention-deficit/hyperactivity disorder (ADHD) show more extreme overestimations of competence than children without ADHD, particularly in the domains in which they have the most skill deficits (e.g., Hoza, Pelham, Dobbs, Owens, & Pillow, 2002; Hoza et al., 2004). As Hoza and colleagues (2004) suggest, such misperceptions may interfere with treatment if children are not willing to admit a problem and are thus not motivated to change.

Summary

Taken together, these findings highlight the subjective and distinctly individual nature of the friendship experience. The take-home message, then, is that whenever possible, friendship quality should be assessed from multiple perspectives—the child, the friend, and outside observers. As discussed above, there are a number of carefully developed and reliable self-report assessments of friendship quality. These questionnaires are easy to administer with individual children or in large group settings. They focus on particular relationships and tell us about the relative amount of both global dimensions (e.g., positive) and more specific friendship features. Nevertheless, there is much room for the development of other measures of friendship quality—particularly assessments based on observations and assessments that more fully capture negative features of friendship in addition to conflict.

ASSESSING THE CHARACTERISTICS OF FRIENDS

Assessing the characteristics or identity of children's friends answers the question, What are a child's friends like? This dimension of friendship is particularly relevant when examining the effects of friendships with particular peers. The assumption here is that friends' attitudes and behaviors influence one another. For example, does having aggressive or antisocial friends promote a child's own antisocial behavior? Do friendships with prosocial, academically oriented peers foster positive adjustment? To what degree are friends similar to one another? These questions all tap into the identity of children's friends.

In terms of assessment, there are two general methods for examining the characteristics of a child's friends. The first strategy involves asking children to respond to questions about what their friends are like. This is typically accomplished by asking a child how many of his or her friends have certain characteristics. For example, how many of your friends (e.g., none, some, many, all) smoke cigarettes? Alternatively, children may be asked to identify a particular friend by name, such as their best friend, and then respond to questions about that specific friend's behaviors. The second strategy involves researchers matching children to their friends (such as via reciprocal nominations) and using information gathered from multiple sources (e.g., self-, peer, or teacher report) to specify the characteristics of children's friends. Asking children about their friends is a much easier method than is gathering information on the friends from other sources.

The implications of using each of these methods are unclear. One concern is whether children and adolescents are accurate reporters of their friends' behavior and characteristics. Estimates of similarity between children and their friends based on children's reports of their friends' behavior may exaggerate similarity as children assume that their friends are more like them than they really are (Wilcox & Udry, 1986). This may be particularly true when children and adolescents are asked about anti-social behavior and believe or want to suggest that "everyone is doing it." Berndt and Keefe (1995) directly tested the accuracy of adolescents' perceptions of their friends' involvement in school and disruptive behavior in school. Correlations between adolescents' reports of their own behavior and their reports of their friends' behavior were much stronger than correlations between adolescents' reports of their friends' behavior and their friends' own self-reports. In other words, adolescents perceived themselves to be similar to their friends in their school involvement and disruptive behavior, but those perceptions were not completely accurate. In general, adolescents also perceived themselves to be more similar to their friends than they actually were based on comparisons of either students' self-reports and their friends' self-reports or on teacher reports of both adolescents' behavior. Swenson and Rose (2009) also evaluated whether friends' reports of youths' internalizing and externalizing symptoms are accurate or biased. Accuracy was apparent when friends' reports were predicted by youths' own reports. Bias was apparent when friends' reports were predicted by friends' own adjustment. Overall, accuracy effects for internalizing and externalizing symptoms emerged, but the bias effects were stronger than the accuracy effects.

Selection and Socialization

The characteristics or identity of children's friends has been studied less completely than either the presence or quality of friendship. This dimension of friendship is most often studied in the context of antisocial and other negative behaviors as an indication of the influence of friends on one another—topics that are discussed further in Chapter 5. More commonly, researchers have examined the degree to which two friends are similar to one another by simply correlating measures of friends' behaviors, attitudes, adjustment, and other characteristics. One problem, however, with using correlations to assess similarity between friends is that these measures do not yield an unbiased assessment of the degree to which friends influence one another because similarity results from at least two processes. First, children seek out others who are similar to them when they form friendships (i.e., selection effects). According to the similarity–attraction hypothesis, individuals are attracted to others whose attitudes, personal characteristics, and behaviors are similar to their own, and friendships are thus likely to develop (Byrne & Nelson, 1965). Similarity can also be conceptualized as a reinforcing agent (Lott & Lott, 1974), and we are attracted to others who provide us with positive reinforcement. Second, as their relationship continues, friends mutually influence one another and become more similar over time (i.e., socialization effects).

Correlations cannot, however, distinguish between selection and socialization effects. One way to isolate friends' influence on one another is to examine whether one child's characteristics at one point in time predict changes in his or her friends' characteristics over time. For example, adolescents' perceptions of their friends' school involvement and disruption in the fall were associated with changes in their own involvement and disruption from fall to spring, especially for girls, suggesting that perceptions of friends' characteristics have an effect on adolescents' own school adjustment and behavior (Berndt & Keefe, 1995). In our own research, we have attempted to separate selection and socialization effects using a longitudinal design (Newcomb et al., 1999). We had assessments of children in six different elementary schools before they moved to a single middle school the following year. Thus, we could examine similarity between children who did not yet know one another but who would eventually become friends the following year (i.e., selection effects). Indeed, interpersonal similarity was an antecedent to the development of a friendship. Children who would become reciprocal friends in sixth grade were more similar to their future friend the year before they met than to a randomly selected classmate in terms of their prominence in the classroom and their social competence. Socialization effects were also evaluated by examining what happened over the course of the school year to reciprocal friends who were not similar to one another in their social reputations in the fall of sixth grade. Those dissimilar friendship pairs whose relationship continued (i.e., they were reciprocal friends in both fall and spring of the school year) became more similar in their aggression and competence. In contrast, for the dissimilar children whose relationship did not continue, there was no change in their degree of similarity in aggression and social competence from fall to spring. Taken together, these findings show the importance of both selection and socialization as determinants of friends' similarity to one another. Said another way, by selecting certain children as friends, children select different socialization opportunities.

Summary

The characteristics or identity of children's friends is a rarely studied dimension of friendship. Assessing similarity between friends is one way to index friends' characteristics, and indeed friends tend to be similar to one another. The field is wide open, however, for the development of new strategies for assessing similarity beyond simple correlations. In addition, preliminary evidence suggests that identifying who children's friends are and then relying on independent information about those friends' characteristics yields better information than asking children to report on what their friends are like. Unfortunately, this is more complicated for researchers. The choice of strategy here has significant implications for the conclusions that might be drawn about how similar friends are. Interest in the characteristics of friends embraces the view that not all friendships are alike and that who children's friends are in part determines how the relationship affects the child. It is implied, then, that friends influence one another. We are just beginning to develop process-oriented measures to assess influence, and ethnographic observations may be particularly helpful in generating hypotheses and suggesting processes that warrant further study.

ASSESSING CHILD CHARACTERISTICS
AND THE CONTEXT OF FRIENDSHIP

As shown in Figure 2.1, the individual characteristics of the child and the context of the friendship are relevant dimensions for assessing children's experience in friendships. Specific methods of assessment for these components of the model in Figure 2.1 are beyond the scope of this chapter. They include all measures designed to assess individual children (e.g., behavior, attitudes, skills and competencies, emotions, clinical symptoms) as well as measures to assess peer status and social networks. Below we briefly discuss why these dimensions are included in the model.

At first blush, it may seem inappropriate to examine characteristics of individual children as a central component in assessing friendships given their inherently dyadic nature. Nevertheless, examining the characteristics of the children and adolescents who participate in friendships recognizes individual differences in the experience of friendship. As discussed further in Chapters 5 and 6, characteristics that children bring with them to the friendship table (e.g., aggression, withdrawal, social competence, emotion regulation skills) have implications for their ability to form and maintain friendships, the quality of their relationships, the characteristics of the children they select as friends, and the significance of the relationship for their own development. In addition, there are significant gender and age differences in friendships that should not be overlooked in a broader assessment of children's friendship experience.

There are multiple ways to define the context within which a particular friendship exists. Figure 2.1 includes four—the larger social networks in which the friendship is embedded, the degree to which the friends are accepted versus rejected by the larger peer group, other support systems (such as family relationships) in which the children are involved, and the cultural context (discussed in Chapter 7). Several of these are consistent with different levels of Bronfenbrenner's (1979) ecological systems model. Assessment of these contextual features may provide insight into the importance of a particular relationship for the children involved. In addition, appreciation for the multidimensional nature of children's peer relationships suggests that friendship may influence and be influenced by phenomena at other levels of the peer system, such as children's acceptance or rejection in the peer group and their broader social networks. Although we do not detail here the many ways to measure individual child characteristics and aspects of the larger context in which friendships occur, we recognize the importance of including them in a thorough assessment of children's friendship experience.

ASSESSING INTERACTIONS WITH FRIENDS

The final dimension included in Figure 2.1 is children's interactions with their friends. Often, but not always, this dimension is examined as a dependent variable with one or more of the other domains as the independent variable(s)—for example, how do children's characteristics or the quality of the relationship or the characteristics of a friend or the cultural context affect friendship interactions? How do boys' interactions with friends differ from girls' interactions? How do aggressive children versus nonaggressive children interact with friends? Do popular children differ from rejected children in their friendship interactions?

A common research design for investigating children's interactions with friends and especially for examining what might be unique about how children behave with friends is comparing dyads of friends and dyads of nonfriends (e.g., acquaintances and familiar classmates who are not friends, strangers, even disliked peers). A decade ago, we summarized this literature comparing friends and nonfriends with a meta-analysis (Newcomb & Bagwell, 1995). At that time, there were approximately 80 studies using this friend versus nonfriend design, and more have been completed since then. From a methodological perspective, what is interesting about these studies is that they have used a variety of strategies to document interactions and characteristics of friends and nonfriends. Whether using a friend versus nonfriend design or any other design to examine children's behavior with their friends and friendship processes, researchers have used observational methods, self- and friend reports on questionnaires and interviews with children and their peers, and even reports from parents, teachers, or others.

Observational Assessments

Observational assessments are frequently used in comparisons of friends versus nonfriends. In fact, approximately 63% of the variables included in our meta-analyses were assessed with observational methods (Newcomb & Bagwell, 1995). One of the first decisions when using observational methodologies is whether to observe children and their friends in a natural setting or a laboratory setting. Developmental psychologists have often gravitated toward laboratory observations whereas research from sociological and anthropological perspectives is much more likely to rely on ethnographic studies in naturalistic settings.

Ethnographic Studies

Several recent excellent examples of ethnographies of children's peer relations are Corsaro's observations in preschools in the United States and Italy (2003), Adler and Adler's (1998) study of preadolescent peer relations, Eder's (1995) lunchtime observations of middle school students, and Thorne's (1993) observations of boys and girls in elementary school. Ethnographic approaches to studying friendship and peer relations begin from the premise that the researcher must become a part of the lives of the children they study—"going native" as Corsaro (2003, p. 8) describes. A primary goal is to develop an insider's view on children's worlds. A key to ethnographic approaches is that the researcher develops a relationship with the children under study. Ethnographers get to know their participants closely, and even as they are trying to study the children's friendships and peer relations, they enter into a type of relationship that they might even label as a friendship (e.g., Corsaro, 2003). This aspect of ethnographic research is captured in Graue and Walsh's description, "The researcher is not a fly on the wall or a frog in the pocket. The researcher is there. She cannot be otherwise. She is in the mix" (1998, p. 91).

Typically, ethnography involves participant observation, and there are a variety of roles the researcher can assume. Fine and Sandstrom (1988) suggest that the roles vary along two dimensions: the amount of positive contact between the researcher and the children being observed, and the degree of authority the researcher has over the children being observed. Examples of roles include leaders (such as teachers, coaches, or camp counselors), outside observers, or friend. In the role of friend, the researcher aims to interact with those he or she studies in "the most trusted way possible" (p. 17). Obviously, an adult will never be completely accepted by children as a peer (Corsaro, 2003; James, Jenks, & Prout, 1998). At the same time, by taking on the role of an atypical adult—one who does not try to control interactions or place demands on children as teachers, parents, and other adults usually do—and letting children react to him or her as opposed to initiating interactions, researchers can gain special status among the children they study and have access to peer interactions and settings that most adults would not. Alternatively, the longitudinal study of preadolescent peer relations conducted by Adler and Adler (1998) involved especially close ties between researcher and research participants. They used a "parent as researcher" strategy, and their own children as well as their children's friends, acquaintances, and classmates were intimately involved in their research. An advantage of this method is that the researcher does not have to create an artificial role in which to enter the peer culture. The role of parent is obviously a naturally occurring one that provides access to children in a variety of settings and over an extended period of time.

Despite the strengths of ethnographic study of children's peer relations, this approach raises a number of ethical concerns—what is the researcher's responsibility when observing potentially harmful situations or when possessing knowledge about children's rule-breaking behavior? How should the research be described to the children and informed consent received? How should a researcher negotiate the power differential between him- or herself and the children being observed? What are the limits of confidentiality? These and other ethical questions arise as well in lab-based experimental research but are particularly salient when ethnographers hope to develop a friendship with the children they study. A thorough discussion of these questions is beyond the scope of this chapter, but interested readers are referred to thoughtful and careful discussions by Adler and Adler (1998) and Fine and Sandstrom (1988).

The qualitative nature of the data generated is perhaps the most significant difference between ethnographic studies and laboratory studies that usually generate quantitative data. With careful field notes and even some videotaping or audio recording of children's interactions, researchers document children's friendship interactions and processes that occur within the peer group as part of broader overarching goals, such as learning "what was it like to be a child in the school" (Corsaro, 2003, p. 15), studying "the nature of these children's lives" (Adler & Adler, 1998, p. 194), or discovering "how children made friends in school" (Rizzo, 1989, p. 12). Researchers who use ethnography to study peer relations argue that it is particularly well suited for theoretical perspectives that emphasize ways in which children take an active role in their socialization and create a dynamic peer culture (Corsaro & Molinari, 2000). In addition, ethnographic approaches are typically designed to focus on friendship processes rather than outcomes (Corsaro, 2003), and they may emphasize generating hypotheses rather than testing them (Rizzo, 1989).

Structured Observations

Of course, more structured observational assessments can also take place in naturalistic settings (e.g., Hartup et al., 1988; Howes, 1983). More typically, though, structured observations occur in laboratory assessments in which friends engage in free play or are given particular tasks to accomplish, and their behavior is coded using a priori coding schemes. Two studies conducted by Hartup and colleagues (Hartup, French, Laursen, Johnston, & Ogawa, 1993; Hartup et al., 1988) illustrate some of the advantages and disadvantages of structured observations in naturalistic versus laboratory-based settings. Both studies compared conflict and the process of conflict management between friends and nonfriends. In the first, conflicts were coded from narrative accounts of children's interactions in their preschool classrooms. In the second, pairs of third- and fourth-grade children played a board game together after each child was taught slightly different rules to the game. Conflicts were coded from videotapes of these game-playing episodes. Playing a board game together is an activity that friends might do regularly, yet the situation was set up so that conflict would likely arise. Thus, researchers exercised some control over ensuring that the children would be presented with multiple opportunities to engage in conflict. In this "closed-field" setting (i.e., children do not choose interaction partners, activities, or duration of interaction), conflict was more frequent among friends than among nonfriends. In contrast, in the "open-field" setting of a preschool classroom where children can choose their interaction partners and can leave a particular activity at will, the frequency of conflicts did not differ between friends and nonfriends.

The results of these two studies are not directly comparable because the age of the friends varied significantly (preschool vs. middle childhood). Nevertheless, the findings suggest that constraints of the social setting and the context of conflict may directly affect this social process between friends. When disagreements do not put their continued interaction at risk, children may feel more free to disagree with friends whom they know better and with whom they are more emotionally secure than with other peers (Hartup et al., 1993). In open-field settings, however, a primary social goal may be to continue the interaction with the friend; thus, disagreements should be minimized. From a methodological perspective, then, the choice of observational strategy affects conclusions that are drawn about this friendship process. This example illustrates quite well the point that multiple assessment strategies should be used and conclusions based on a compilation of findings across methodologies.

Observations in naturalistic settings have the advantage of being more, well, natural. They are the only way we can capture friends' interactions as they really occur. Laboratory observations provide a degree of control and allow researchers to isolate particular behaviors of interest or to vary systematically conditions for the children's interactions. Damon (1977) eloquently summarized the importance of both types of observational settings: "[Experimental or laboratory techniques] offer us a means of encouraging children to engage in an activity of theoretical interest to us, without waiting around for days for something to happen (and then never being certain what did happen)" (p. 54). Nevertheless, naturalistic observation is valuable because "real life is 'rough around the edges' in a way that is lost by the structures necessarily imposed by the laboratory" (p. 54).

Observations of Negative Behaviors

Certain behaviors with friends are clearly amenable to multiple kinds of observation—in naturalistic settings, in laboratory settings, ethnographic observations, and structured observations with coding schemes. Overt prosocial behaviors, such as sharing and cooperation, positive and negative affect, and communication strategies are examples of behaviors between friends that have been studied effectively using all of these methods. What about behaviors that are not so positive—aggressive or antisocial behavior, discussions about taboo topics, and other behaviors that are not usually condoned by adults? Can these be readily observed? There is plenty of evidence that the answer to this question is a resounding yes. Ethnographers discuss witnessing bullying and social exclusion (Adler & Adler, 1998); swearing, gossiping, and insulting along with a few instances of more severe verbal and physical harassment (Eder, 1995); and various behaviors that defied school rules (Corsaro, 2003).

In lab studies, work by Dishion and colleagues provides an excellent example of ways in which structured observations yield valid information about antisocial behavior. Dishion and colleagues brought pairs of early adolescent friends to the lab to engage in several videotaped interactions (called the Peer Interaction Task). In a 25-minute session, friends discussed five topics for approximately 5 minutes each. They first planned an activity together and then talked about four problems—one each boy was having with his parents and one each boy was having getting along with peers. These conversations have been examined using several structured coding schemes. The Topic Code (Poe, Dishion, Griesler, & Andrews, 1990) codes the conversations into two topic categories and two types of reaction. Deviant or rule-breaking talk includes verbalizations and gestures that violate conventional norms or rules. Normative talk includes all verbal and nonverbal behavior that is not considered rule-breaking talk. The two codes for interpersonal reactions include "laugh" (e.g., positive affective reactions, including laughter, and non-verbal positive reactions such as smiles and "high fives") and "pause" (e.g., three or more sections of silence).

A number of variables can be derived from these four categories, such as the average duration of an episode of deviant talk (Dishion & Owen, 2002) or the rate per minute of deviant or normative talk (e.g., Dishion, Capaldi, Spracklen, & Li, 1995; Dishion et al., 1996). In addition, sequential scores capture the process of friends' interactions—for example, the degree to which rule-breaking talk versus normative talk is followed by the reinforcing response of laughter (Dishion et al., 1996). In more recent studies, Dishion and colleagues have created a deviant friendship process construct that includes the duration of rule-breaking talk, a rating scale assessing coders' impressions of friends' talk about drugs, a rating scale assessing interviewers' impressions of friends' support of one another's antisocial behavior, and friends' reports of the amount of time they spend together (Dishion, Nelson, Winter, & Bullock, 2004; Dishion & Owen, 2002; Patterson, Dishion, & Yoerger, 2000). Remarkably, this construct of deviant friendship processes, based largely on only 25 minutes of conversations in an unfamiliar lab setting, accounts for escalating drug use in adolescence and adulthood (Dishion, Capaldi, et al., 1995; Dishion & Owen, 2002); increased levels of delinquency, including new types of antisocial behavior (Dishion et al., 1996; Patterson et al., 2000); and more extreme violence according to self-reports and police records (Dishion, Eddy, Haas, Li, & Spracklen, 1997).

A promising measure that truly captures the temporally based process of deviancy training in friendships was developed by Granic and Dishion (2003). The measure is the slope of the duration of rule-break talk bouts across time within the conversation. This slope measure indicates whether dyads' successive rule-break bouts become shorter or longer in duration over the course of their conversation. Dyads with a strong positive slope show a pattern of deviant talk that might indicate an "absorbing state" whereby the friends are repeatedly drawn to these topics, become absorbed in this type of conversation, and have trouble moving on to other topics. This measure shows much potential; even after controlling for current antisocial behavior, family coercion, and association with deviant peers, it predicted conflicts with authority figures and drug abuse 3 years later.

Beyond Observations

Aside from observational methodologies, there are no specific assessment strategies that have been used more than others. A number of researchers have conducted lab-based or other experimental studies that present children with hypothetical situations and assess differences between how children respond with or to friends versus nonfriends. One of the advantages of these designs is that they do not require that both members of the friendship dyad participate in the study. Rather, researchers identify the target child's friend (or nonfriend), and that child is referred to throughout the study without necessarily being present. Another advantage of these lab-based studies is that the experimenter maintains a good deal of control over the variables and can isolate very specific situations to which children respond. Some examples of the variety of behaviors that have been studied using these designs include emotional responsiveness to the plight of a friend or nonfriend as presented in a puppet show (Costin & Jones, 1992), allocation of resources to friends versus acquaintances (Knight & Chao, 1991), disclosure to a friend or nonfriend when making an audiotape for the peer (Rotenberg & Sliz, 1988), perceptions of friends' versus nonfriends' intentions in stories (Hendey & Butter, 1981), and strategies and goals children have when giving and seeking help to or from a friend (Rose & Asher, 2004).

Asking children about their relationships with their friends and about what they do with friends and how they spend time with them is a fairly straightforward strategy for assessing children's interactions with friends. Often, studies relying on children's self-report assess the features of their relationships, and in turn are studies of friendship quality. For example, Frankel (1990) interviewed girls about support and stress in their relationships with reciprocal versus unilateral best friends. Gershman, Hayes, and colleagues (Gershman & Hayes, 1983; Hayes, Gershman, & Bolin, 1980) interviewed preschool children about why they like certain peers and identified particular common features of reciprocal friendships. As discussed above, Berndt and Perry (1986) interviewed children about the support and conflict in their relationships with friends and acquaintances and found that friends were perceived to be more supportive than were acquaintances.

Summary

Interactions and behaviors with friends can be assessed using a variety of methods and techniques. And, in fact, the assessment strategy that is chosen may have implications for the conclusions that are drawn. The Newcomb and Bagwell (1995) meta-analysis comparing friends and nonfriends showed that "relationship properties" including equality, closeness, loyalty, similarity, dominance, and mutual liking were assessed using both observational and nonobservational methodologies. Nevertheless, the differences between friends and nonfriends were significantly greater when nonobservational methodologies, such as interviews and hypothetical situations, were used than when assessed with direct observations, and this difference was particularly strong for the intimate characteristics of friendships (closeness, mutual liking, and loyalty). This difference in findings based on choice of assessment technique may reflect children's exaggerated perceptions about these aspects of their friendships or may indicate that researchers are simply not very good at observing these intimate characteristics of friends in their interactions. In any case, the fact remains that we need to be aware of how the ways in which we generate and collect data on children's friendships affects what we learn about these relationships.

CONCLUSIONS

As Figure 2.1 makes clear, the question *How do we measure children's friendships?* does not lend itself to a simple answer. Rather, there are at least six key dimensions from which to take a look—whether a child has a friend, the quality of the relationship, the characteristics of that friend, the characteristics of the child, the context of the friendship, and the child's interactions with that friend. In terms of assessment, we have very good methods and techniques for assessing many of these dimensions. Using reciprocal nominations to identify school-based friendships is reliable and valid, for example. There are well-established methods for assessing some aspects of the context of friendship—peer status, in particular. There are a variety of self-report measures for friendship quality that provide easy-to-administer reliable and valid snapshots of the quality of a particular relationship. Systematic observation and ethnography provide important strategies for examining children's interactions with their friends. The characteristics of friends seem to be measured most effectively by combining an assessment of who a child's friends are with information about the characteristics of those friends from other sources. And though they are not discussed in this chapter, developmental psychology and child clinical psychology provide countless measures of individual child characteristics.

Future Research Directions

Nevertheless, as the previous discussion has highlighted, there are a number of areas where improvements in our assessment techniques and ways of studying friendships will serve to advance our knowledge about the developmental significance of friendship. Six are discussed below.

1. As the remainder of this book shows, we know much about the nature of children's friendships—what makes them different from other peer relations, what many of the important features of friendship are, how they differ at different ages, and how they are associated with various aspects of adjustment. We know comparatively little, however, about the important processes that occur within children's interactions with friends that are responsible for their uniqueness and their influence on children's development. In part, what goes on between friends is a mystery because we lack techniques and tools that adequately measure friendship processes. Notable exceptions include Gottman's (1983) classic study of how children form friendships and recent work on the processes of deviancy training (Dishion & Owen, 2002) and corumination (Rose, 2002; Rose, Carlson, & Waller, 2007). Developing process-oriented measures is critical.

2. There is a rich body of ethnographic research on peer culture in childhood and adolescence, yet this work is not well integrated with research on friendship using quantitative approaches. Careful integration of ethnographic methods with experimental designs, questionnaire-based studies, and other quantitative methods has great potential for illuminating key friendship processes and contributing to theory development.

3. With the long-standing assumption that friendships contribute to positive adjustment, the potential negative aspects of friendship were not systematically considered until fairly recently. Even when negative features are studied, for example, in assessments of friendship quality, often conflict is the only dimension included. With increased attention to individual differences in friendship and a focus on its multidimensional nature, we need to develop better ways to identify and assess the aspects of children's friendship experience that are not positive. This requires attention to features other than conflict—for example, rivalry, inequality, deviancy training, jealousy, and social aggression between friends.

4. The assessment of friendship quality has relied almost exclusively on children's and adolescents' self-reports. This makes sense—only children themselves can tell us their perceptions of the positive and negative features in their relationships. Yet, the degree to which these perceptions match behaviors between the friends and any objective indicators of reality is not clear. A few studies have examined how reports of friendship quality map onto observations of friends' interactions. Additional research along these lines is needed and may encourage the development of other methods to assess friendship quality.

5. Similarity is an important determinant and outcome of friendship and provides one way to assess the characteristics of children's friends.

Nevertheless, our understanding of how the characteristics of children's friends affects the child requires moving beyond assessment of similarity. Other ways to measure friendship characteristics are needed. Likewise, as suggested above, new methods to assess friendship processes will contribute to our understanding of how friends' characteristics affect a child.

6. Finally, we anticipate that the significant advances in our understanding of friendship and its importance in the near future are likely to come from research that simultaneously considers several of the dimensions depicted in Figure 2.1 and that focuses on the intersections between these dimensions. In all of these endeavors, careful consideration of the ways in which the method we choose to study friendship affects what we learn about the relationship is essential.

PART II

THE NORMATIVE EXPERIENCE OF FRIENDSHIP

Chapter 3

The Developmental Significance
of Friendship in Childhood

Why do you like Charlie?
    Because he's my friend.

What makes him your friend?
    He likes trucks.
        —Truck-loving 3-year-old Noah talking with his mother

Hi. I'm Joey. Do you want to be my friend?
        —Four-year-old Joey approaching his classmate
            Will on the first day of school

He helps me on homework and we talk about stuff that's very
private and we don't tell no one. ... With other kids, it's not
like this [puts two fingers together to indicate closeness]. You
know, we sometimes argue a lot, but we have fun and we laugh
together. ... We have lots of fun and laugh at each other so it
makes it lots of fun. And we can tell each other stuff.
        —Ten-year-old Josh describing
            what he likes about his best friend

How are 3-year-old Noah's and 10-year-old Josh's relationships with their
friends similar and different? How do their friendships both reflect their
level of social, emotional, and cognitive development and contribute to
their development? Will it matter if Joey is unsuccessful in establishing
a friendship? In this chapter, we take a developmental perspective to the
topic of friendship and consider friendships from their earliest beginnings

65

to preadolescence. Our goal is to answer the question: What is the developmental significance of friendship in childhood? In other words, how does friendship contribute to children's social, emotional, and cognitive development and psychosocial adjustment?

The perspective we take is threefold. First, we emphasize that friendships are normative. That is, most children have friends although, of course, there are numerous individual differences in the experience of friendships. Despite these differences, we can draw conclusions about friendships that hold true for most children within and across the developmental periods from early childhood through preadolescence.

Second, we take a functional and contextual view of friendship. In other words, we examine the functions that friendships serve both in children's daily lives and in providing a context to help children achieve various tasks of development that are particularly important at different ages. We make a distinction between "development" and "adjustment." By that we mean that when considering the role of friendship in social, emotional, and cognitive *development,* we examine how friendship contributes to the changes children undergo in these domains over time. For example, achieving emotional competence is an important developmental task that unfolds over time and involves expressing emotion, understanding emotion, and regulating emotion. In contrast, when we consider the contribution of friendship to psychosocial *adjustment,* we are interested in how friendship influences children's socioemotional well-being—how they are doing at a particular time in terms of adapting to their current situation. For example, friends are expected to help one another cope with stress and thus serve as important resources in promoting positive psychosocial adjustment.

Third, a critical task in specifying the developmental significance of friendships is that we must show how friendships are special relationships with unique contributions that go beyond the importance of having a group of same-age peers (e.g., classmates, team members, neighbors). In the sections that follow, we first consider what we know about the normative development of friendships. Then, we evaluate the developmental significance of friendship for social, emotional, and cognitive development and for psychosocial adjustment.

FRIENDSHIP AS A NORMATIVE EXPERIENCE IN CHILDHOOD

From a developmental perspective, childhood friendships are a normative experience. Most children have friends, and the origins and development of friendship from early childhood through adolescence proceeds in a consistent way for most children. From an evolutionary perspective, humans are social beings who live in groups because of the resources groups provide for survival and reproduction. One primary benefit of living in groups is that they provide numerous "potential friends" (Buss, 2005, p. 581) who can offer rich mutually beneficial social exchanges. The motivation for friendship may have evolutionary roots, including as a solution to the dilemma that individuals may not receive help when they need it the most because they are the least able to reciprocate (Tooby & Cosmides, 1996). Friends, however, may provide help and support in just those kinds of situations. Such an evolutionary perspective helps us understand the normative nature of friendships.

In addition, psychologists generally agree about the core elements of friendship. It is a mutual relationship between two children that is based on a strong affective tie. In other words, friends like each other a lot. Although different researchers carve up the primary features of friendship differently, there is agreement that friendships are based on reciprocity and involve having fun together, sharing feelings of closeness and intimacy, and providing one another support. In addition, most friends experience conflict from time to time. We discuss each of these characteristics in more detail later in the chapter.

The characteristics of friendships change as children develop, and particular functions of friendship ebb and flow, yet friendships are important developmental resources in all phases of life from childhood to older adulthood (Hartup & Stevens, 1997). In this chapter, we focus largely on young children's dependence on friends to be fun and reliable playmates and older children's tendency to look to friends as sources of support during school transitions. Chapter 4 focuses on the fact that adolescents spend much time confiding in friends who are helpful in negotiating a more complex social world. Here we briefly consider two questions about friendship as a normative experience across childhood: When do friendships begin? and What are the characteristics of children's friendships?

The Beginnings of Friendship

The Toddler Years

There are two important issues regarding very young children's friendships. One is when true friendships emerge. The other is whether the earliest friendships are developmentally important in the same way as later friendships might be. The emergence of friendships is determined in part by children's capabilities—at what age do children have the social, emotional, and cognitive abilities required to have a friendship? When friendships emerge is also dictated by children's social context. Specifically, a necessary but not sufficient criterion for establishing friendships is that children spend time in the company of same-age peers so that there is an opportunity for friendships to develop. For children in day care, these opportunities are available from a young age, but many other children do not spend significant amounts of time with peers until they are enrolled in some kind of formal schooling, such as preschool. Thus, even though it may be possible for friendships to form as toddlers, many children simply do not have the opportunity to do so.

How might we identify the earliest friendships? For school-age children, it is relatively easy to identify friendships—just ask about friends, and they will quickly and readily list their friends and describe their relationships in great detail. However, if given the opportunity to be with agemates, most children develop friendships well before they begin school. Even preschool children often speak concretely, yet eloquently, about their friends, and they clearly recognize friendship as a special relationship. The question then is whether children even younger than preschool age establish and participate in friendships. The existing research clearly suggests that toddlers and even infants can exhibit preferences for some peers over others (for a review, see Dunn, 2004), but are these *preferences* really friendships? Does preference for another peer suggest the existence of a relationship based on mutuality and affection that includes companionship, support, intimacy and/or other characteristics of friendships?

Obviously, we cannot ask preverbal toddlers about their friends. Therefore, we cannot establish the existence of a friendship through reciprocal nominations (i.e., Sarah names Sue as a friend, and Sue names Sarah as a friend), which are the gold standard for identifying friendships among older children. Instead, we must look to other methods for identifying friendships among young children. Observing young children's interactions with peers is the most common strategy. Across a number of studies, Howes identified three criteria for friendship based on observations of young children in peer groups (Howes, 1983, 1988, 1996; Howes & Lee, 2006). These criteria include (1) preference for another child as indexed by proximity during much of the observation period, (2) a social partnership that takes the form of engaging in reciprocal play, and (3) a shared positive affect that suggests an affective component to the relationship. Howes suggests that shared positive affect best distinguishes toddler "friendships" from other playmates (Howes, 1983). Using these criteria, Howes (1987) reported that about half of the toddlers in one of her studies were part of a reciprocated friendship and that these relationships were generally stable over a 1-year period.

Other researchers are more conservative in applying the label "friends" to toddlers. Although toddlers show more positive affect and more often initiate interactions with familiar peers than with strangers, one friendship researcher suggests that toddlers may simply be differentiating between familiar and unfamiliar peers (Furman, 1982). Nevertheless, it is clear that the building blocks for friendship are established in toddlerhood. These include preference for particular peers and directing interactions toward preferred others, sustained and reciprocal play, expression of positive affect and enjoyment, helping and sharing, and creating shared meaning from "ritual activities" such as playing with the same toys in the same way day after day or always sitting next to one another at snack time (Howes, 1996; Howes & Lee, 2006; Lewis, Young, Brooks, & Michalson, 1975; Vandell & Mueller, 1980; Whaley & Rubenstein, 1994). However as Dunn (2004) notes, shared activities can be very brief, positive affect can rapidly give way to anger, and sharing may be predicated on the whim of the moment.

One way of reconciling these views about whether or not friendship begins in toddlerhood is by acknowledging that toddlers *can* form friendships and that *some* do. In fact, many articles and chapters on the topic begin with compelling anecdotal descriptions of very young children whose relationship contains elements of friendship commonly observed among older youth and even adults—including providing mutual comfort and support, spending most of their time together, showing strong attachment to one another, and experiencing distress when apart. The relationships of toddlerhood, however, may not be as typical or normative as they are for older children in that there are many toddlers who simply do not have opportunities to form relationships with same-age peers outside the family. Likewise, they may not be developmentally significant in the same ways that they are for older children; having or not having a "friendship" in toddlerhood may not be associated with adaptive adjustment and functioning. Nevertheless, we expect that early friendships are most important for providing a context for learning and practicing important social skills—sharing and cooperating, taking turns, and enjoying activities with another. In some instances, preferred familiar peers may provide comfort and support, such as when children are upset when being left at day care in the morning.

Although these preferential relationships may be advantageous to children, we do not yet have evidence to indicate that they provide independent contributions to social, emotional, or cognitive development beyond that obtained in relationships with parents or siblings or even other peers. Thus, the question of the developmental significance of friendships in toddlerhood has not been fully addressed in existing research. Longitudinal studies of the developmental implications of having or not having preferential early peer relationships are needed.

For young children to establish friendships, they must be in settings that provide exposure to the same peers on a regular basis, such as in day care centers or other child care settings (Howes & Lee, 2006). Despite the growing numbers of children in child care settings that provide a context in which a friendship *could* develop, many children do not have such opportunities in toddlerhood. Instead, they spend their time primarily with parents or other caregivers and siblings and interact with potential "friends" on an irregular or infrequent basis. Having friends may be uniquely important only to children who spend much of their time in environments where they are surrounded by peers (e.g., day care settings; Laursen & Mooney, 2005). Given this simple fact, it is difficult to imagine that there is anything developmentally *necessary* about a relationship that many children simply do not have.

The Preschool Years

Over the preschool period (roughly ages 3–5 years), friends come to occupy a more important place in children's social world. Spending any amount of time around preschool children quickly leads one to the conclusions that most preschoolers have friends and that their friends are highly valued. Friendship at this age typically revolves around play. Preschoolers' expectations for friends are not as mature or complex as older children's. Rather, they focus on enjoying common interests and activities together (Bigelow, 1977; Sebanc, 2003). Friends are people who are fun to play with and who like to play the same things; thus, both play and similarity are important for choosing friends in the first place and then spending time with them (Lindsey, 2002). As a result, friendships provide preschool children someone with whom to "test out" various behaviors and emotions while at play.

Estimates of the number of preschool children who have friends vary depending on the way friendship is measured, but clearly *most* preschoolers have a friend. For example, across several studies, at least two-thirds of preschoolers had friends when friendship was assessed by mutual nominations (Lindsey, 2002; Sanderson & Siegal, 1995; Sebanc, 2003), three-fourths to four-fifths had friends based on observations of time spent together (Hinde, Titmus, Easton, & Tamplin, 1985), and all preschoolers had a friend when asked to invite a friend to participate in a study with them (Slomkowski & Killen, 1992). Preschool friendships are generally not as stable as those of older children, yet they are not all fleeting either. Some last for at least a year, and many even longer (Howes, 1988; Park, Lay, & Ramsay, 1993).

In one of the most extensive and important observational studies of preschoolers' interactions with peers, Gottman (1983) identified six processes that occur within preschool friendships, primarily during play, and that likely contribute to two children establishing a friendship:

(1) understanding of each other's communication and openness to clarification, when necessary; (2) willingness to ask and answer questions; (3) engagement in common activities with discussion of similarities and differences in play; (4) sharing of feelings; (5) extension and elaboration of each other's play; and (6) ability to resolve conflict. Although Gottman identified these processes as critical for successfully establishing a friendship, they are also involved in maintaining a friendship over time. Furthermore, they reflect both conditions for and outcomes of friendship. In other words, as Gottman identified, preschool children who have the social, emotional, and cognitive skills to manage these processes effectively are more likely to establish a friendship. And, preschoolers are frequently presented with opportunities to further hone these skills with their friends. For example, Corsaro (2003, pp. 38–40) describes the elaborate and extensive work that preschoolers engage in to maintain play and contact with friends once they have initiated interactions, including keeping other children from joining in. He describes two children who have initiated a coordinated play episode involving animals in a zoo. They quickly reject the bids of another child to join their play because the third child is not their friend today. Corsaro interprets these actions as the two girls carefully protecting the shared interaction and "friendship" they have established at the moment.

In many ways, preschool is a time in which children's friendships gain substance. Preschool children are able to show that they care about one another by saying so directly and by demonstrating that they understand how their own behavior matters to their friends. In fact, they use the fact that they are friends with a particular child as a reason for their behavior ("I'm sharing the red crayon with Julie because she's my friend"). Some of the basic components of friendships that older children value are present in the relationships of preschool children. Preschoolers recognize that a friend is someone who is fun to be with, someone you really like and who likes you equally, someone who helps you. Likewise, preschool children's friendships vary along some of the same dimensions as do older children's friendships. In one study, teachers were able to describe reliably four features of preschool children's friendships—support, conflict, exclusivity/intimacy, and asymmetry (Sebanc, 2003). These are the key features that also emerge for older children's friendships. The fact that different friendships can be distinguished by the relative amounts of these characteristics suggests that friendships among preschoolers are more complex than they are often given credit for.

Nevertheless, we need to be careful not to overlook the significant developmental changes that occur in friendships from preschool through childhood. There are a number of aspects of preschool children's friendships that look very different from older children's relationships. Other examples from Corsaro's (2003) observations in preschool classrooms show how preschool children use the idea of friendship to control others ("You can't be my friend unless ... "). Comments like "you're not my friend today" are commonly heard in preschool classrooms and are partly what convey the impression that preschool friendships are fleeting. For preschool children, the term *friends* often refers simply to whomever they happen to be playing with at a particular time. Similarly, parents and teachers of preschool children often use the term *friends* to refer to all classmates. "We don't hit our friends." "Can you pass out the napkins to all of your friends?" "Be sure to share the scissors with your friends." These comments demonstrate deliberate attempts to teach social skills and how to get along with others by invoking friendship.

There are very few studies of young children's friendships that provide evidence for the developmental significance of particular friendships that form in preschool, yet we have several glimpses that these relationships are important and may be influential in promoting skills and competencies that foster positive friendships in middle childhood. Over a 1-year period, friends' play interactions become more coordinated and positive (Park et al., 1993). These changes are likely due both to age-related increases in children's own social skills and changes in the quality of the relationship because of the friends' history of shared interactions. An even longer-term study followed children over 5 years and showed that forming close friendships at age 4 predicted having a high-quality relationship with a best friend at age 9 (Howes, Hamilton, & Philipsen, 1998). Another way of considering the question of the developmental significance of preschoolers' friendships is to compare children who have friends with those who do not. Lindsey (2002) reported that preschool children with at least one mutual friendship were more socially competent and better liked by other peers than preschoolers without a mutual friend. Taken together, the results of these studies suggest that there is some continuity over time in children's friendships that begin in preschool, and having these friendships is likely associated with various aspects of social competence both concurrently and over time.

Overall, then, friendships may develop for some children in toddlerhood, provided they have opportunities for developing them. Regardless, important social skills and competencies emerge in toddlerhood and these contribute to later friendship development (e.g., initiating and sustaining reciprocal play, expressing positive affect, and helping and sharing). Across the preschool period, participating in friendships clearly becomes the norm, and the rich peer culture that emerges in preschool classrooms fosters friendship creation and maintenance.

Expectations and Characteristics of Friendship

Understanding the normative experience of friendship also involves knowing how children think about friendship—what they expect from friends and what they believe their friendships *should* look like—as well as what friendships *really* look like. Not surprisingly, children's beliefs about friendship change with age. In an early study of children's conceptions of friendship, Bigelow and La Gaipa (1975) simply asked children in first through eighth grades to write an essay about what they expected of their best friends that they did not expect from other acquaintances. First, there were age differences in children's expectations. Even at the youngest ages, children noted companionship (i.e., enjoying common activities, spending time together, and playing). Then from the fifth grade on, there were expectations of loyalty and commitment, genuineness, intimacy, and sharing similar values. Notably, there were no age differences in the beliefs that friends like one another, share, and make one another feel good about themselves. Of course, these findings depend on children's ability to verbalize their expectations for friends, something that improves from first to eighth grade; thus, the data do not provide unequivocal evidence of developmental progressions in friendship expectations per se.

However, other scholars have found some similarities in age trends. Berndt (1986) examined children's descriptions of their best friendships in response to the question "How do you know that someone is your best friend?" Kindergarten, third-grade, and sixth-grade children all described playing together and spending time with friends as important. The two younger groups were less likely than early adolescents to describe intimacy and trust in best friendships. In contrast, the younger children were more likely than early adolescents to describe definitional aspects of friendship (e.g., someone who knows you or likes you). Taken together, these findings underscore two important points: (1) as children mature, their conceptions of friendship change, but (2) regardless of age, children *expect* their friendships to have positive features.

Given these expectations for friendship, what do friendships *really* look like? Without a doubt, this is the question about friendship that has received the most empirical attention, and it has been answered most frequently by comparing pairs of children who are friends and pairs of children who are not friends ("nonfriends"). Nonfriends include acquaintances (e.g., classmates who neither strongly like nor dislike one another), strangers, and disliked peers (e.g., children who both dislike the other). A meta-analysis of 80 studies completed over a decade ago identified four key areas in which friend's relationships differ from those of nonfriends (Newcomb & Bagwell, 1995). Friends, as compared to acquaintances, demonstrate (1) greater positive engagement, including cooperation and positive affect; (2) greater resolution of conflict; (3) better performance on task-related activities; and (4) more of the "deeper" properties of relationships such as similarity, equality, closeness, and loyalty. The difference between friends and acquaintances was small for most areas, with the exceptions of mutual liking, closeness, and loyalty, which showed medium-sized effects (e.g., Newcomb & Bagwell, 1995; Simpkins & Parke, 2002a). Notably, similar findings exist across a wide range of studies from the 1930s to the 1990s and across methodologies and sources of information (e.g., interviews, hypothetical situations, direct observations). This diversity in historical period and methodology provide confidence that the findings are meaningful.

The meta-analysis also confirmed and extended our understanding of age differences in comparisons of friends. Across preschool, childhood, and early adolescence, observations and children's own reports revealed that friends were more positively engaged than were acquaintances. Friends showed more positive affect, shared and cooperated, and demonstrated enjoyment and companionship more than nonfriends at all of the studied ages. Although the deeper properties of the relationship did not distinguish between preschool friends and acquaintances, friends' relationships in childhood and early adolescence were characterized by considerably more equality, closeness, and loyalty than nonfriend relationships. These findings about age differences in the characteristics of children's actual friendships parallel their understanding of what friendships are all about as we discuss above.

Summary

In brief, this is what we know about the normative experience of friendship in childhood. Friendships develop early in life. For some toddlers who spend time with peers regularly, relationships are characterized by preference, enjoyment, and frequent interactions. Preschool friendships—some built on earlier foundations and some that are new—show increased coordination, warmth, and supportiveness, most particularly in play. Fortunately, most preschoolers have friends, and these relationships tend to be increasingly stable. Throughout the school-age years, friendships become increasingly characterized by helping, loyalty, and commitment. These changes are reflected both in what children believe about and expect from friends and in what children's friendships really look like (i.e., the characteristics of friendships).

SOCIAL DEVELOPMENT

One of the most obvious ways in which friendships contribute to children's development is that they provide a context for learning and practicing social skills and competencies. To be sure, establishing and maintaining friendships require interpersonal skills, but it is also true that children hone and develop their social competence in interactions with friends. We have identified three components of children's friendships that contribute in important ways to social competence—companionship, intimacy, and conflict. Each of these friendship features shows a specific developmental trajectory, and together, they capture the essence of friendship.

Companionship

Companionship is the aspect of friendship that involves spending time together, enjoying one another's company, and engaging in collaborative activities. It is the earliest manifestation of friendship, yet it is an aspect of friendship that is mentioned at nearly every age as a centrally important feature of the relationship (Bigelow, 1977; Buhrmester & Furman, 1987). In fact, friendship has been defined for young children simply as the relative amount of time they are in physical proximity to one another compared to other peers (e.g., Hartup et al., 1988; Howes, 1988); this proximity measure reflects companionship between two children.

Companionship clearly changes with development, and two major changes over the course of the first several years of life contribute most significantly to advances in children's ability to engage in companionship. These include the development of language and the emergence and growth of more sophisticated play, especially social pretend or fantasy play. By 18 months, children often play with peers by engaging in similar activities, imitating the other, and laughing with delight (Eckerman, 1993; Howes & Matheson, 1992). By 24–30 months, children are able to cooperate in ways impossible merely 6 months earlier. They communicate about their pretend actions and even offer direction to one another's activities or otherwise contribute to the joint activity—"Drive the truck to the garage" "I'm making spaghetti for dinner" (e.g., Dunn, 1988; Ross & Lollis, 1989). These kinds of comments demonstrate increasing integration and coordination between the two children as they play. Pretend play continues to increase in complexity throughout the preschool years.

In middle childhood, companionship takes on new dimensions. The key component—spending enjoyable time together—is the same, but now companionship involves sharing specific interests and initiating time together across a variety of settings. The two friends who spend hours playing with, sharing, and trading their baseball cards; the friends who decide to play on the same soccer team together; the friends who tear through the neighborhood on their bikes; and the friends who always sit together at lunch and work together on school assignments all demonstrate the richness of companionship. Companionship is also evident when friends simply spend time together talking. Achieving companionship in middle childhood requires more than simply being able to play with another. It requires being able to suggest and initiate activities, to engage in the give-and-take that comes with pursuing activities with a friend, and to recognize the kinds of activities that would be fun for the friend, too (Asher, Parker, & Walker, 1996). Children who are particularly effective at these behaviors are likely to have an easier time making and maintaining friendships that include high levels of companionship. At the same time, friendship affords children a context in which to sharpen the kinds of social competencies that involve reciprocity, cooperation, and integration.

In sum, one of the key functions of friendship is providing companionship. To be sure, classmates and other peers are also sources of companionship (Furman & Robbins, 1985), yet we contend that the experience of companionship with friends is special. Friends know each other better, are more frequent companions, engage in more sophisticated play, and have more in common than other peers. In addition, their relationships are characterized by strong affective ties. Overall, the sense of companionship children obtain from friends differs from that received from group activities, or from being accepted or well liked by others.

Intimacy

There are many images of intimacy between friends: images of friends giggling hysterically about private jokes no one else would understand, sharing fears and worries and secret crushes, throwing their arms around each other in greeting as if the 3 hours they have been apart were 3 years, and constructing elaborate games and rituals with rules only they know. The growth of intimacy and changes in the way that intimacy is expressed between friends are among the most significant developmental changes in friendship from early childhood to adolescence. Here we discuss three central issues concerning the role of intimacy between friends in social development: the definition of intimacy, developmental changes in intimacy, and the significance of intimacy for social development.

Definitions and Theoretical Perspectives on Intimacy

As discussed in Chapter 1, Sullivan (1953), one of the most authoritative voices in the early studies of friendship, suggested that the need for interpersonal intimacy arises between the ages of 9 and 12 years. This is the developmental period Sullivan labeled preadolescence, and he viewed the development of same-sex friendships as the singular accomplishment of this period. Friendships develop specifically to satisfy intimacy needs. In Sullivan's conceptualization, self-disclosure is one manifestation of intimacy, but intimacy encompasses much more than sharing secrets and confiding in one another. According to Sullivan, intimacy is broadly defined as the outcome of a collaborative, affectively based relationship that is grounded in reciprocal caring, closeness, and involvement between equals. In more recent empirical studies, researchers embrace the multidimensional nature of intimacy, yet different components of intimacy are often measured in different studies (e.g., Bauminger, Finzi-Dottan, Chason, & Har-Even, 2008; Buhrmester, 1990; Sanderson, Rahm, & Beigbeder, 2005; Shulman, Laursen, Kalman, & Karpovsky, 1997). The consistency across studies is that self-disclosure is almost always included. This is because self-disclosure is often considered the sine qua non of an intimate friendship, and self-disclosure is typically viewed as an important process through which feelings of closeness and commitment between friends develops (Bauminger et al., 2008; Buhrmester & Prager, 1995; Laursen, 1993).

Distinctions can also be made between friends' intimate behaviors, such as self-disclosure or sharing activities, and the emotion-based components of intimacy, such as strong feelings of connection and shared affect between friends (McNelles & Connolly, 1999; Radmacher & Azmitia, 2006). According to Selman's (1980; Selman & Shultz, 1990) cognitive developmental model, the behavioral experiences of intimacy between friends change with age, but the feelings of affective connection are relatively stable with development. McNelles and Connolly (1999) tested the assumption that intimate behaviors necessarily engender feelings of closeness and connection between friends. They found that self-disclosure increased throughout adolescence and that this behavior indeed predicted friends' shared intimate affect. Gender plays an important role here, too, because self-disclosure is the primary pathway to intimacy and emotional closeness for girls, but both shared activities and self-disclosure lead to feelings of closeness for boys (Camarena, Sarigiani, & Petersen, 1990; McNelles & Connolly, 1999).

Manifestations of Intimacy at Different Ages

The fact that intimacy is a cornerstone of friendships by adolescence raises several questions: How does intimacy develop between friends at different ages, and when does intimacy become so important? Can intimacy, as defined by self-disclosure, be a part of relationships between

young children when they have neither the language and cognitive abilities nor the social and emotional competencies required for complex collaborative relationships?

YOUNG CHILDREN'S FRIENDSHIPS

Some degree of intimacy reflected in self-disclosure might be apparent in
young children's pretend play. Preschoolers often enact situations that
involve fear and anxiety in their make-believe cooperative play (Howes,
Droege, & Phillipsen, 1992; Paley, 2004; Parker & Gottman, 1989).
Moreover, Corsaro (2003) describes recurring themes involving danger,
loss, and death in preschoolers' spontaneous fantasy play. Nevertheless,
in the absence of empirical age-related comparisons, we simply do not
know whether these preschool pretend play themes represent the varied
forms of self-disclosure observed among older children and adolescents
(e.g., the confession of fear to a close friend).

The primary issue here is one of interpretation. It is useful to distinguish between "rich" versus "lean" interpretations of young children's
friendships and social behavior. This same distinction has been used by
Brownell and Kopp (2007) in the context of understanding young children's emotional competence. Rich interpretations of young children's
friendships would suggest that these early displays of disclosure and collaborative play reflect intimacy in the same way that older children's sharing of secrets and confiding in one another demonstrate intimacy. More
lean interpretations suggest that what we may be observing are some
elemental forms of self-disclosure/intimacy that occur years before the
development of more mature forms of intimacy. This line of reasoning
follows recent findings in cognitive development that show some elemental aspects of executive functions appearing as early as age 2 years (Carlson, 2003, 2005; Hughes, 2002; Hughes & Ensor, 2007), yet these early
skills do not fully represent the more mature manifestations of 4-year-
olds' executive function skills.

What the existing data do tell us is that young children's play differs between friends, familiar peers, and unfamiliar agemates. Three-
and 4-year-olds are more socially competent and engage in more cog-
nitively mature play with a familiar peer than with a newly introduced
child (Doyle, Connolly, & Rivest, 1980). Preschoolers who are friends
show more cohesion in their pretend play than pairs of classmates who
are not friends (Howes, Matheson, & Wu, 1992). There is also more
self-disclosure between friends than nonfriends (Howes, Matheson, &
Wu, 1992). Importantly, this self-disclosure is not necessarily intimate.
However, sharing any information about the self, even as mundane as
telling a peer about a favorite color or favorite food, may be a precur-

sor to the more intimate self-disclosure that characterizes older children and their friends. Also in line with this reasoning, some early beginnings of more mature intimacy may be seen in preschoolers' development of a joint understanding of their social play through negotiation with one another (Goncu, 1993; Howe, Petrakos, Rinaldi, & LeFebvre, 2005). This collaboration occurs through verbal and nonverbal exchanges as friends suggest ideas for play, build on one another's ideas, coordinate their perspectives, and create mutually agreed upon interactions and understandings. These comments are consistent with Dunn's (2004) recent book on friendships, with a subtitle of *The Beginnings of Intimacy*. Again, there is an intimation that a foundation for intimacy and the ongoing "*practice* with intimacy" is a part of young children's relationships.

OLDER CHILDREN'S FRIENDSHIPS

Several lines of research converge to suggest that it is during preadolescence and early adolescence that friendships become more intimate. Asking children about their beliefs about friendships in general indicates that intimacy emerges as a salient expectation of friendship in early adolescence (Berndt, 1986; Bigelow & LaGaipa, 1975; Selman, 1980). Older children and adolescents expect friends to trust one another, to confide in one another, to share feelings, ideas, and concerns with one another, and to feel emotionally close. Even across very different cultural contexts, these age trends hold. Adolescents refer to trust and feelings of intimacy more frequently than younger children when describing what makes people friends (Gummerum & Keller, 2008). In addition, most studies find that self-disclosure and mutual support from friends become more frequent in adolescence (e.g., Buhrmester & Furman, 1987; Gottman & Mettetal, 1986; McNelles & Connolly, 1999; Sharabany et al., 1981). And, sharing ideas and feelings with a friend who provides security and support becomes an increasingly important dimension along which adolescents organize and maintain their friendships (Hartup, 1993; Shulman et al., 1997).

Yet, a few studies find no difference in reports of intimacy between preadolescents and adolescents. Buhrmester (1990) found that youth in fifth or sixth grade and youth in eighth or ninth grade reported similar levels of intimacy in their best friendships. In addition, across seventh, eighth, and ninth grades, there were no age differences in adolescents' perceptions of intimacy with their best friends (Bauminger et al., 2008). However, there is evidence of a more complex association between age and intimacy. Age differences depend on the particular aspect of intimacy in question. For example, in one study, older adolescents were more likely to engage in self-disclosure with friends than younger adolescents, and greater self-disclosure was in turn predictive of greater feelings of intimacy. In addition, it seems that certain aspects of intimacy, such as trust, emotional closeness, and preferring to spend time with the particular friend are established *prior* to preadolescence and remain stable from that period on (Buhrmester, 1990; Sharabany et al., 1981).

Significance of Intimacy between Friends

There is little empirical evidence evaluating the hypothesis that intimacy becomes more important for social and emotional adjustment as children get older. This is surprising given that it is a key assertion of Sullivan's (1953) theory. Asking the question of whether the *importance* of intimacy increases with age relates directly to the developmental significance of intimacy. In the one direct test of this question, Buhrmester (1990) found that adolescents' reports of intimacy in their friendships were more strongly associated with higher sociability, lower internalizing distress, and higher self-esteem in adolescence than in preadolescence. These findings suggest that in adolescence, but not earlier, intimacy between friends is integrally related to social competence and well-being. Individual differences also play a role in the significance of intimacy for social development. For example, some adolescents approach friendship with intimacy goals and motives, but others pursue friendships with more individually oriented, agentic goals. Those with a stronger focus on intimacy goals more often give and receive social support, more often engage in self-disclosure with friends, and more constructively resolve conflicts than adolescents with weaker intimacy goals (Sanderson et al., 2005). Thus, adolescents' friendship goals are associated with particular patterns of interaction that in turn determine the context the relationship provides for social development (e.g., practicing self-disclosure and carefully managing conflicts).

Further specification of how intimacy contributes to social development awaits additional research in at least three areas. First, we need additional studies that isolate intimacy as a feature of friendships and consider how it is associated with social competence. Second, it is crucial to ask whether different aspects of intimacy are significant at different ages, and if the importance of intimacy per se changes as children develop. As an example: Do self-disclosure and emotional closeness show different developmental trajectories such that they are more or less important at different ages? Third, longitudinal studies are needed to better understand the correlates of intimacy among friends and the associated short- and long-term implications of establishing and maintaining intimacy.

Conflict

Developmental Trends

Disagreements, disputes, and conflict are inevitable when friends interact, and friendships provide excellent opportunities to develop and practice skills in conflict management. There are clear developmental trends in the kinds of conflicts children have with peers and in the strategies they use to resolve them. Object disputes—conflicts over who has the red truck, who gets to put the baby doll to bed, or who rides the tricycle with the bell—are frequent among toddlers and preschoolers, and physical aggression is a common outcome of these disputes. In fact, in observations of play sessions, 1-year-olds spent 16% and 2-year-olds spent 27% of their time in conflict over toys (Caplan, Vespo, Pedersen, & Hay, 1991), and for 3- to 5-year-olds approximately 40% of conflicts involved disputes over toys (Hartup et al., 1988), which may relate to increasing awareness of self and personal possessions.

Preschoolers' conflict with peers continues to be frequent, yet much of this conflict does not involve aggression or angry emotion and is brief (Laursen & Hartup, 1989). In general, trajectories of physical aggression—hitting and pushing and similar behaviors—indicate that approximately half of children engage in physical aggression occasionally in toddlerhood, and levels of physical aggression decrease to infrequent by preadolescence (Cote, Vaillancourt, LeBlanc, Nagin, & Tremblay, 2006). By later childhood and adolescence, object disputes are seldom the source of conflict among friends, and aggression is rarely the resolution strategy. Instead, conflicts typically involve disagreements about interpersonal issues, and they are often settled by negotiation or simply by disengagement (Laursen, 1993).

The "Meaning" of Conflict between Friends

Disagreements and conflict may hinder the establishment of a friendship by indicating a lack of compatibility or common ground between children (Gottman, 1983; Hartup, 1992a), and too much conflict may threaten existing friendships. Nevertheless, there are positive outcomes of conflict between friends as well. As two friends disagree over whose turn it is to "go first" in a game, for example, they are confronted directly with the fact that others see the world differently, that their own perspective might be misleading, and that perhaps their friend's happiness is a worthwhile goal as well. Conflict can promote social understanding by providing opportunities for advances in communication, perspective taking, and realization that others' behaviors and goals matter (Dunn, 2004; Laursen & Hafen, 2010; Shantz, 1987). Perspective taking is a critical ability for effective conflict management. In a recent study using hypothetical situations, children heard a story in which a friend behaved unkindly (Tsethlikai, 2010). Those who heard a second story explaining the situation from the friend's perspective integrated the new information in their own memory and interpretation of the situation.

In addition, as children's social-cognitive abilities improve, their skills in managing conflicts and using negotiation (e.g., "I'll go first this time, and you go first next time") rather than coercion (e.g., "It's my turn to go first or I'm not playing!") improve (Laursen, Finkelstein, & Betts, 2001). Children themselves recognize that conflicts can be learning opportunities. Children as young as 7 years readily describe lessons they learn from conflicts with peers and friends, typically lessons about appropriate behavior (things they should or should not do such as "not to say mean things") but also about conflict ("It would be better just to walk away") and friendship ("Friends don't like when I don't share") (Shantz, 1993). Older children recognize that some conflicts actually make a friendship stronger once they are resolved (e.g., Selman, 1980).

Acknowledging the potential positive outcomes of conflict between friends raises the question of whether there are skills and competencies fostered in managing conflicts with *friends* that are not gained as readily in conflicts with other classmates and peers. Studies comparing conflicts with friends and with nonfriends provide some evidence to answer this question. Although it is important to note that just because friends and nonfriends differ does not necessarily mean that friendships are an *essential* context for developing these skills. A number of comparisons of friends and nonfriends from various age groups reveal that children engage in similar amounts of conflict with friends and peers (Laursen, Hartup, & Koplas, 1996; Newcomb & Bagwell, 1995). However, there is an important difference in the way conflict is managed and resolved. Among friends, in general, there is a more rapid move from coercion to negotiation as the preferred mode of conflict resolution. Moreover, children are more likely to resolve conflicts with acquaintances with coercion rather than negotiating or disengaging; however, they are likely to use both negotiation *and* coercion with friends (Laursen et al., 2001). In considering whether conflict between friends has positive or negative effects on individual adjustment, Laursen and Hafen (2010) suggest we need to take into account the quality of the relationship—detrimental outcomes are more likely in low-quality relationships—and the type of conflict—constructive versus coercive. Thus, there are numerous moderator variables to consider.

The Setting as a Moderator of Conflict

CLOSED-FIELD SETTINGS

Moderators of the link between friendship and conflict include the setting in which conflict occurs and the age of the children involved. With respect to setting, a closed-field situation such as a laboratory context prevents children from making choices about interactions. In one study, 9- and 10-year-old friends engaged in more frequent and longer conflicts than nonfriends. Children may feel more secure with friends than with others, and the sense of security provides less prohibition for disagreements with friends than with acquaintances (Hartup et al., 1993).

However, the age of the friends seems to matter as well in determining the frequency of friends' conflicts compared to conflicts with other peers. In another closed-field setting, children and adolescents participated in a competitive task with a close friend or a former friend. To "win" the game, the youth needed to complete more of a coloring task than their partner, but the task required use of a particular item that had to be shared (Berndt et al., 1986). Elementary school children shared *less* with friends than nonfriends, but adolescents shared *more* with friends (Berndt, 1981b; Berndt et al., 1986). Berndt and colleagues (1986) suggest that children are more competitive with friends because they do not want to feel inferior to a friend. By adolescence, however, friends are motivated to achieve equality, which they view as a defining characteristic of friendship, despite being part of a competition (Berndt, Perry, & Miller, 1988). Still other studies show that even in closed-field settings, school-age friends are concerned with effective conflict management and spend more time negotiating and compromising than do nonfriends (Fonzi, Schneider, Tani, & Tomada, 1997; Tomada, Schneider, & Fonzi, 2002).

OPEN-FIELD SETTINGS

Classrooms and playground settings are examples of open-field settings that involve numerous available partners for interactions. If an interaction in an open-field setting is not going well, a child can easily terminate it and find someone else to play with. However, there is strong motivation for friends to maintain their interactions in these settings and, thus, conflict management is critical.

In a study of preschoolers engaged in free play in their classroom, characteristics of conflicts differed significantly between friends and nonfriends (Hartup et al., 1988). Mutual friends engaged in fewer affectively intense conflicts, but there were striking differences in the resolution of conflicts. Friends, compared to peers, were more likely to disengage from conflict (rather than firmly holding their position), as if aiming to reach an equitable solution so they could continue their interaction (Hartup et al., 1988). These findings likely represent key elements of friendships: they are voluntary and interdependent relationships that involve social and emotional investments. There is little to be gained by winning a conflict but losing a friend.

In sum, there is no doubt that conflict is a central feature of friendship from preschool through adolescence. The very nature of the relationship involves a dialectic between agreements (e.g., positive interactions) and disagreements or conflict (Hartup, 1992a; Rawlins, 1992). What is not yet clear from research to date is if, when, and how conflicts between friends contribute to social development. That conflict can contribute in positive ways to social development is a compelling hypothesis that awaits rigorous evaluation. Still there are hints that conflicts among friends provide unique opportunities to learn the "delicate art of negotiation and conciliation" (Laursen, 1993, p. 52). We also need to understand the distinction between situations in which conflict harms friendships and when it is beneficial (e.g., providing opportunities to enhance social competence). Seemingly relevant factors would include the study of characteristics of conflict (underlying reason, intensity), frequency of conflicts, characteristics of friends (goals, strategies, negotiation skills), and characteristics of setting (open- vs. closed-field settings).

Summary

We contend that friendship provides optimal contexts for social development because of the ongoing experiences of companionship, intimacy, and conflict. Companionship clearly exists in many peer relationships aside from best friendships. By middle childhood, for example, children often have many peers with whom they interact, and they may seek different types of companionship from different ones—"my soccer friends" versus "my school friends" versus "my church friends." In part, these different companions represent the nonoverlapping settings and activities in which children spend their time, and in part, they represent the fact that children often turn to specific peers for specific types of companionship and social interaction. Overall, the companionship offered by a best friend is qualitatively different from companionship with other peers due to stronger affective bonds, the amount of time spent together, and the emotional closeness within the relationship. In terms of social development, the companionship of friends appears to promote social competencies that are a byproduct of satisfying and effective interpersonal interactions (e.g., offering and receiving help, sharing and cooperating, and maintaining a sense of reciprocity and equality).

Intimacy is viewed by children themselves and by researchers who study friendship as a defining feature of the relationship. Even though the earliest manifestations of intimacy may be seen in the play of very young children, intimacy continues to develop and blossom between friends in childhood and into adolescence. Surprisingly, there is limited evidence about significant increases in friends' intimacy as children reach preadolescence and early adolescence. Also, definitional issues are yet to be untangled. Researchers have used the term *intimacy* to describe a range of behaviors and characteristics between friends: sometimes it refers only to self-disclosure and sometimes to a broader construct that includes closeness, nurturance, and trust. It is not clear, though, how the experience of friends' intimacy contributes to developmental growth.

Lastly, turning to research on conflict between friends indicates that disagreement is common and, in concert with cooperation and agreement, allows children to discover common ground between them (Hartup, 1992a). An ongoing friendship thus provides a context for practicing conflict management skills and for learning effective strategies of handling disagreement that allows the relationship to continue and flourish. Although there are a number of empirical studies of conflict between friends, it is difficult to draw firm conclusions about the role of this conflict in promoting social competence because the answer to so many of the relevant questions is "It depends." As noted earlier, conflict between friends depends on the settings in which the conflict occurs and the age of the children. Further research that evaluates these and other variables simultaneously is needed. Currently, conclusions require piecing together the findings of studies that consider single variables—for example, comparisons of friends and nonfriends in either a closed-field or an open-field setting.

Overall, the primary contribution of friendship to social development is in providing opportunities for practicing and further developing the social skills and competencies that are necessary for positive interpersonal interactions. However, this is something of a catch-22 because some level of skills in companionship, intimacy, and conflict management are needed to establish a good friendship in the first place, yet over time, advances in these areas contribute to positive social development and social competence. What is not yet clear is the degree to which the experience of friendship renders it a unique context for social development.

EMOTIONAL DEVELOPMENT

A great deal of emotional learning takes place during the first decade of life. Children's environments are filled with rich emotional information that is communicated to them by others (Mayer & Beltz, 1998) through a process often referred to as the "socialization of emotions" (see Denham, Bassett, & Wyatt, 2007). In early childhood, especially, caregivers are the primary source of emotion information and feedback, through both intentional/direct socialization processes (e.g., showing approval or disapproval for an emotional display) and unintentional/indirect socialization processes (e.g., passively model-ing emotional behavior; Bugental & Goodnow, 1998; Cole & Tan, 2007; Denham et al., 2007). For example, an infant receives impor-tant emotional information when her mother deliberately models an expression in front of her or when her mother engages emotionally with others simply in her presence. Saarni (1999) contends that an important developmental task for children is to become emotionally competent through understanding the *interpersonal* consequences of emotion and subsequently using that information to determine their own emotional behavior. Peers and friends certainly play a valu-able role in the process of becoming emotionally competent, but an important question is whether friends provide *unique* opportunities for achieving emotional competence.

Friendships certainly have the *potential* to provide unique contexts for emotional development. As early as the toddler years, children develop distinct ways of interacting with different social partners (Ross & Lollis, 1989; Saarni, 2008), and they continue throughout childhood to play dif-ferently with "friends" than with acquaintances or nonfriends (Howes, Droege, & Matheson, 1994; Simpkins & Parke, 2002a). In fact, an ear-lier meta-analysis (Newcomb & Bagwell, 1995) and more recent research (Simpkins & Parke, 2002a) demonstrate that school-age friends tend to engage in more positive behaviors and more sophisticated play than do nonfriends. Thus, friendships provide children with different opportuni-ties for emotional learning than other relationships do. Unlike parents or siblings or even larger peer groups, friends are chosen for particular reasons and are optional (see Herrera & Dunn, 1997). This means that valued friendships require maintenance, and without it, the friendship will end (Asher & Rose, 1997; Benenson & Christakos, 2003; Shantz & Hobart, 1989).

In the following sections, we examine more specifically the extent to which friendship is related to and, more importantly, might help children achieve emotional competence. We use Saarni's (1990) con-ceptualization of emotional competence as a framework for consider-ing the role of friendship in three areas of emotional development. Friendships (1) offer a context for learning appropriate emotional expression and response, (2) contribute to the development of emo-tion knowledge, and (3) provide opportunities to improve emotion regulation skills.

Emotional Expression

Developmental Trends

Drawing upon the rich history of developmental research on emotion, we have a relatively good understanding of how emotional competence in the area of emotional expression changes during childhood. Although definitions of various emotions, the methods employed to study emotional behavior, and the contexts in which emotions are examined differ in studies of emotional expressivity in the beginning of life, there is evidence that infants have the capability of expressing a range of emotions (for multiple theories on the development of facial expressions in infancy, see Camras & Fatani, 2008). For example, infants express positive emotions such as joy and surprise, and they typically express more positive than negative emotions (Bennett, Bendersky, & Lewis, 2002). Although there is disagreement about whether discrete negative emotions are expressed in the first year of life (see Camras et al., 2007), some researchers have identified infants' abilities to express fear (e.g., Bennett, Bendersky, & Lewis, 2002; Nagy et al., 2001) as well as anger and sadness (Bennett et al., 2002; Bennett, Bendersky, & Lewis, 2004). Others have identified negative emotions but report that, at the end of the first year of life, distinctions cannot be drawn between some negative emotions, such as anger and fear (Camras et al., 2007).

Building on the emotional repertoires established in infancy, emotional expression becomes better developed throughout childhood. During toddlerhood, the expression of emotion becomes more sophisticated as the toddler is able to combine sensorimotor and cognitive abilities (see Mascolo & Fischer, 2002). The anger from the first year of life can be newly expressed, for instance, in the form of a temper tantrum during the second year of life. Later, preschoolers demonstrate that they are capable of expressing vivid emotions, both through increasing language abilities and nonverbal cues (Denham, 1998). During the preschool years, the expression of more complex emotions is clearly tied to children's sense of self and is evaluative in nature as children become increasingly aware of those who observe their behavior (Harter & Whitesell, 1989). The elementary school years bring additional exposure to emotions through the family but also through teachers in the school setting. Studies show that children's emotional expression often mimics both parental expressiveness (e.g., Snyder, Stoolmiller, Wilson, & Yamamoto, 2003) and that of the child's teacher (e.g., Demorat, 1999).

The Role of Friends in Emotional Expression

How do friendships fit into the process of emotional development? From research on friendship, we know how friendships change developmen-

tally and how these changes unfold with advances in emotional competence. Toddlers have preferred playmates, preschoolers have reciprocated
friends with whom they enjoy playing, and school-age children have
increasingly intimate friendships. Research to date is clear that emotional
expression, whether initiated by the child or displayed in response to
another child's emotional expression, contributes to the formation and
nature of social relationships (e.g., Denham et al., 2003). Overwhelmingly, however, research on links between emotional expression and
social relationships tells us more about social competence in the larger
peer group (e.g., peer-rated likeability, teacher-rated social competence)
than about social competence with friends (e.g., friendship formation
and friendship quality).

One line of research that considers the uniqueness of emotional
behavior within the context of friendship compares emotional expression with friends, peers, and mothers. Children's choices with regard to
the expression of emotion are tied to the likelihood of receiving support
for the expression of that emotion. School-age children are more willing
to show negative emotions to parents than to friends (Zeman & Garber, 1996), and school-age children view their mothers as better sources
of support when feeling angry (Zeman & Shipman, 1996). Not surprisingly, though, children expect peers to be more accepting of aggressive
expressions than parents (Shipman, Zeman, Nesin, & Fitzgerald, 2003).
Shipman and colleagues (2003) suggest that friends give each other more
freedom to express mild aggression as long as it is not directed at the
friend and thus does not directly impact the friendship. Collectively,
this research suggests that children learn that it is socially and culturally
acceptable to show different emotional behaviors with different social
partners (Saarni, 1999). Importantly, although research does not explain
the process through which friendships cultivate emotional competence
(Shipman et al., 2003), it does suggest that friends are unique social partners in the process.

A second line of research has focused on how positive and negative emotional expressions may facilitate or interfere with social relationships. For example, much of the work by Denham and colleagues over
the past two decades suggests that more positive emotional expression is
related to being more well liked by peers, and may even facilitate friendships (e.g., Denham et al., 2003; Denham, McKinley, Couchoud, & Holt,
1990; Denham, Renwick, & Holt, 1991; see also Hubbard, 2001). In
contrast, negative affect may cause difficulties for children in their peer
playgroups (Denham et al., 2001). This is not surprising; as Denham
and colleagues (2003) note, " 'feeling good' in many situations not only
'greases the cog' of ongoing social interaction, but also makes it easier for
a child to enter the peer world in the first place" (p. 251).

Research at the intersection of emotional expression and peer relations is limited to date. Based on Zeman and his colleagues' work with school-age children, we know that there are certain "rules of emotion" that apply to different social partners (Zeman & Garber, 1996; Zeman & Shipman, 1996). Additionally, based on Denham and her colleagues' work with preschool-age children, we know that positive emotionality and positive social relationships are connected (Denham et al., 1990, 2003). What we do not know, however, is whether children who are fortunate to have high-quality friendships "create" more positive affect *together,* or whether children who are positive draw others to them (including high-quality friendships) because of their positive affect. Together, this area of research suggests that meaningful links exist between emotional expressivity and friendship but additional research is greatly needed to fully understand the importance of friendship for emotional competence.

Emotion Knowledge

Developmental Trends

With increasing age and experience, children become better not only at appropriate emotional expression but also at *understanding* emotions. Early in life, the increase in emotion understanding is largely because parents talk about the antecedents and consequences of emotions and carry on conversations rich in emotion language with their children (Denham, Zoller, & Couchoud, 1994; Garner, Dunsmore, & Southam-Gerrow, 2008). For example, a preschooler who watches a movie with a scary theme is often soothed by a parent who discusses what frightened the child and why. Similarly, a school-age child who deals with sadness over the loss of a pet usually has a parent who discusses the emotional experience. All of these conversations serve as important lessons on emotion— what emotions mean; why we experience them; and how we can best deal with them (for a discussion of how negative parental expression can interfere with emotion knowledge, see Denham et al., 2007).

How does emotion knowledge unfold developmentally? Emotion knowledge increases substantially from preschool to middle childhood. For example, during the preschool years, children become proficient in understanding the causes of primary emotions (e.g., happy, sad), and then become better at understanding the causes and consequences of more complex emotions (e.g., guilt, envy) during the school-age years (Denham, 1998; Saarni, Mumme, & Campos, 1998). Preschoolers also learn that current emotions can be related to past events. For example, someone can become scared thinking of a scary movie that they saw in the past (Lagattuta & Wellman, 2001). Two key markers of advancement in school-age children are learning that people can experience more than one emotion at a time (e.g., happy to get a present but disappointed about what it is) and that the same event does not result in the same emotional reaction for everyone (e.g., a roller coaster may be exciting or scary) (Denham & Weissberg, 2004).

The Role of Friends in Emotion Knowledge

Do friends contribute to advances in children's increasing emotion knowledge? Intuition says that any social interaction has the potential to contribute to emotion knowledge, and empirical evidence suggests two general conclusions. First, children learn that emotion understanding—recognizing their peers' emotions and talking about their own emotions—contributes in positive ways to their relationships. Second, there is a bidirectional relationship between emotional understanding and friendship. That is, improving emotional understanding influences the nature of interactions with friends, and interaction with friends provides important opportunities to build greater competence in emotion understanding.

Specific empirical findings show that the ability to understand a friend's thoughts and feelings helps children coordinate their play successfully. For example, 3-year-olds' understanding of others' feelings, thoughts, and beliefs predicted coordinated play with friends 7 months later (Slomkowski & Dunn, 1996) and frequency of pretend play episodes with friends 3 years later (Maguire & Dunn, 1997). Furthermore, 6-year-olds who engaged in more complex play with friends at the beginning of the school year were better able to understand others' mixed emotions (feeling happy and sad at the same time) at the end of the school year. Additionally, there is evidence that children with more stable friendships show increased emotion knowledge by the end of the first semester of kindergarten (Dunsmore & Karn, 2004). Clearly, better emotion understanding is associated with social competence, more cooperative pretend play, better peer relations, and more positive interactions with friends (e.g., Dunn & Cutting, 1999; Oppenheim, Nir, Warren, & Emde, 1997).

There is clearly recognition among many researchers that interaction with friends and peers provides a unique emotional life for a child. Interactions with peers may "inspir[e] new conceptualizations of emotion by the child" (Gordon, 1989, p. 328) and provide children with the opportunity to acquire, learn, and understand emotional language (Saarni, 2007). Asher and Rose (1997) indicate that among school-age children, the need for equity within friendships, as well as friends' roles in helping one another, being trustworthy and reliable, managing conflict, and recognizing that friendships are part of a larger peer network provide children with important opportunities to gain knowledge and understanding about emotions. Nevertheless, the vast majority of research describes mother–child relationship contexts, only occasionally peer–child relationship contexts, and very rarely friend–child relationship contexts (Davies, Forman, Rasi, & Stevens, 2002; Katz & Woodin, 2002). We are left then with a shortage of empirical studies that demonstrate the unique contribution of friendship to the development of emotion understanding. Two important questions that warrant empirical attention are To what degree do children demonstrate emotion understanding with their friends? Does emotion understanding becomes more sophisticated as a result of friends' interactions? The studies above indicate that the preliminary answers to these two questions are "a great deal" and "most definitely," respectively.

Emotion Regulation

Definitions and Developmental Trends

A relatively new addition to the emotions literature is a focus on emotion regulation. Although now widely studied, there is still a lack of consensus about how to conceptualize the term—for example, does emotion regulation refer to how emotions regulate something else, or to how emotions themselves are regulated (Gross, 2008)? Also, do we regulate our own emotions (an intrinsic process) or do we regulate others' emotions (an extrinsic process) (Gross & Thompson, 2007; for in-depth discussions of the conceptual issues surrounding emotional regulation, see Bridges, Denham, & Ganiban, 2004; Campos, Frankel, & Camras, 2004; Cole, Martin, & Dennis, 2004; Gross & Thompson, 2007). Some definitions of emotion regulation are broad: "systematic changes associated with activated emotions" (Cole et al., 2004, p. 32) and others are narrow: "the process of initiating, avoiding, inhibiting, maintaining, or modulating the occurrence, form, intensity, or duration of internal feeling states ... in the service of accomplishing affect-related biological or social adaptation or achieving individual goals" (Eisenberg & Spinrad, 2004, p. 338). For our purposes, we use a definition of emotion regulation that allows room for the contributions of peer processes: "extrinsic and intrinsic processes responsible for monitoring, evaluating, and modifying emotional reactions, especially their intensive and temporal features, to accomplish one's goals" (Thompson, 1994, pp. 27–28).

Our overview of emotion regulation skills begins in the second year of life. Toddlerhood has been described as "the beginning of most ... important developmental progressions" in emotion regulation (Thompson & Goodvin, 2007, p. 324). Emotion regulation strategies of the toddler include redirecting attention, soothing oneself, seeking comfort, and withdrawing when coping with emotions, and these strategies increasingly help the child in social situations with peers and adults. For example, a toddler will close his eyes or cover his ears when he is frightened. She will suck her thumb or look for a comfort object when she is sad. What is mastered during toddlerhood will be carried forward into the preschool years, when children will continue to make great strides in emotion regulation (Denham, 1998). Importantly, parents continue to serve as important models and coaches during both toddlerhood and preschool as children establish new ways of managing feelings (Berlin & Cassidy, 2003; Denham, von Salisch, Olthof, Kochanoff, & Caverly, 2002; Spinrad, Stifter, Donelan-McCall, & Turner, 2004; Thompson & Meyer, 2007). During the preschool years, emphasis is placed on regulating negative emotions (Lagattuta & Wellman, 2002) as children's social worlds and expectations from others increase dramatically (Denham, 1998). For example, as parents focus on reacting to negative emotions, children understand the need to control negative emotions (Denham et al., 2003). This can be seen within the peer group, where preschoolers are better than younger children at restraining from crying and acting aggressively. Girls, in particular, may do this in order to conform to the societal expectation of "being nice" (Underwood, 2003). In middle childhood, children continue to become more capable of regulating their emotional expression to be consistent with social display rules (Jones, Abbey, & Cumberland, 1998), and adherence to display rules helps children avoid disapproval and maintain social harmony (e.g., Saarni, 1999). With developmental advances and additional information about emotions, emotion regulation becomes more a matter of behavioral coping strategies (e.g., trying to avoid something undesirable) and less a matter of support seeking (e.g., going to the teacher for help) (Denham et al., 2002).

The Role of Friends in Emotion Regulation

As children become increasingly social beings, emotion regulation becomes even more important for effectively navigating their social worlds (and conversely, these social exchanges are important to the development of emotion regulation). This is demonstrated as early as toddlerhood in a handful of studies that show more positive peer exchanges and behaviors indicative of social competence for children who are better at regulating their emotions (e.g., those who are less angered and frustrated with peers), either on their own or with the help of a caregiver (e.g., Calkins, Gill, Johnson, & Smith, 1999). In preschoolers as well, greater emotion regulation (e.g., less dysregulated coping strategies) is related to higher social competence with peers (Denham et al., 2003). Within friendships in middle childhood, children who use hostile strategies when dealing with conflict tend to have fewer reciprocated best friends and are more likely to argue with their best friends (Rose & Asher, 1999), suggesting that emotion regulation affects both making and keeping friends.

Different people—parents, teachers, peers, siblings, friends—all provide different opportunities for children to learn and practice emotional competence, including regulation skills. Friends provide important developmental opportunities to negotiate conflict, engage in cooperation, and promote connectedness—all opportunities for developing and honing emotion regulation skills—because they need to ensure that the relationship continues (Shantz & Hobart, 1989). Thus, the key conclusion about emotion regulation and friendship is that we have some understanding of the importance of emotion regulation in friendships, but we have a long way to go to really understand what happens within friendships to influence emotion regulation. Questions to be addressed include Do emotion regulation abilities of friends become more similar over time? What are the consequences of dysfunctional regulation within a friendship? How does emotion regulation influence peer relations versus more intimate friendships?

Summary

Overall, there are two limitations in the existing literature that preclude definitive conclusions about the role of friendship in promoting emotional competence. First, emotion researchers have explored links between emotional competence and social competence much more extensively at the level of the peer group than at the level of the dyadic friendship. Second, we have learned more about how emotional competence *influences* friendship and peer relationships than how friendships have the potential to influence emotional competence. So, we are left with the overarching empirical question: What unique role does friendship play in the development of emotional competence?

Several reviews of the socialization of emotional competence, spanning nearly 20 years, have acknowledged the absence of literature addressing this specific question. In 1989, Gordon observed, "Developmental psychology has emphasized only the mother as the socialization agent for emotions" (p. 329). He questioned whether peers might be a key agent in emotion knowledge and expressed the importance of considering socialization messages from different agents. In 2007, Denham and colleagues concluded:

> Knowing how mothers socialize emotion is very important but does not come close to telling the whole story of how emotional competence

is supported by persons in each child's environment. If developmental scientists are serious about understanding the socialization of emotion, *everyone* who is important to children as they grow *must* be considered. (p. 629)

Friends are most definitely included in this list of important people.

COGNITIVE DEVELOPMENT

It seems more obvious that friendship would serve as a context for social and emotional development than as a context for cognitive development. Indeed, there is much less evidence of links between friendship and cognitive growth than between friendship and social-emotional development. At the same time that research on friendship has largely ignored its potential contributions to cognitive development, a large body of empirical and theoretical literature on cognitive development discusses the importance of social interaction, including peer interaction and collaboration, for promoting cognitive development (for reviews of this extensive literature, see Azmitia & Perlmutter, 1989; Rogoff, 1998; Tudge & Rogoff, 1989). This interest in the social nature of cognition is not new. Both Piaget's (1926, 1932) and Vygotsky's (1978, 1986) theories place social interaction at the center of processes responsible for cognitive growth.

In Piaget's (1926, 1932) theory, an essential process for cognitive growth is the disequilibrium that results from conflicts between a child's own views and his or her peers' views. In simple terms, acknowledging these discrepancies and resolving these contradictions leads to equilibration of cognitive structures and processes at a more advanced level, thus promoting a child's cognitive growth. Unlike adult interaction, "peer interaction is uniquely relevant to cognitive development because it forces the child to coordinate his or her views with those of the companion (i.e., to restructure his or her own views) rather than to conform to them" (Hartup, 1996b, p. 219).

In Vygotsky's (1978, 1986) theory, cognition is inherently social. Cognitive development takes place within social interactions as children are encouraged by others to take part in the social world around them and in the activities that are valued in their culture. Much of the research inspired by Vygotsky is on adult–child or child–sibling interaction because these interactions involve an expert and a novice rather than two children on relatively equal footing. Nevertheless, in Vygotsky's social constructivist view, peer collaboration can also lead to cognitive growth, especially to the extent that such collaboration involves the creation of a common ground for interaction and communication as each child comes to a shared perspective on the task.

Surprisingly, though, despite extensive work on the value of peer interaction for cognitive development, very little attention has been paid to whether the affective relationship between the children influences the amount or type of cognitive growth that results from their collaboration (Hartup, 1996b). In other words, does the close relationship between friends offer any advantages for the individual children's cognitive growth above and beyond interactions they have with classmates, acquaintances, strangers, or any other peers? In this section, we answer this question by examining two important contexts for peer interaction and collaboration—play among preschool-age children and problem solving in the school setting for elementary-age children.

Preschool Children at Play

For preschoolers, play has a significant role in multiple aspects of development. Play contributes to social competence and confidence (Howes, Matheson, & Wu, 1992), self-regulation and behavior management (Haight, Black, Jacobsen, & Sheriden, 2006), and coping abilities (Priessler, 2006). Pretend play provides 3- and 4-year-olds with a way to share what is worrisome and anxiety-producing as well as what is exciting and enjoyable (Dunn, 2004). Play is an integral part of preschoolers' social relationships. When asked what they do with their friends, the majority of preschoolers (75%) indicate that they play together, and when asked why people need friends, approximately 50% respond, "to play with" (Field, Miller, & Field, 1994).

As we discussed earlier, children play differently with their friends than with other peers. The primary differences are in the frequency and complexity of friends' play. Preschoolers participate in more fantasy play with their best friends than with acquaintances (Vespo, 1991). In free play, when two friends are grouped with a third child who is not a friend, the friends engage with the nonfriend but contribute more to the pretend play than the nonfriend does (Goldstein, Field, & Healey, 1989). When preschool friends play together, their pretend play is more sustained, sophisticated, and harmonious compared to that of acquaintances (Zerwas & Brownell, 2003). We know that play with familiar peers, and especially friends, is more frequent and more complex than play with other peers. The next question is whether play with friends provides a distinct opportunity for learning and cognitive development (Lewis et al., 1975). In this section we explore how preschoolers' play with friends provides opportunities for two aspects of cognitive development that are particularly relevant for preschool-age children—the development of language and theory of mind.

Language

The synergistic association between language development and friendship is demonstrated in at least three ways in young children's play—in understanding and participating in friendship, in conflict resolution, and in the development of intimacy between friends. First, language allows children to talk about friendship, and it is important in the establishment of a peer culture and in gaining knowledge about friendship. Over the preschool period, children's play styles become increasingly sophisticated, largely because language guides play behavior and allows children to talk about friendships. In an ethnographic study of 3- to 5-year-olds, Corsaro (1985) describes how children express their understanding of friendship through language. Children use talk of friendship to gain entry into play activities, and they discuss being friends when they are playing with another child. Corsaro observed that "We're friends, right?" is used as an explanation for why children are playing together (2003, p. 43). Corsaro also observed that language is used as a means of social control ("I'm not gonna be your friend if you don't ... "), to express concern for a friend, or to indicate how much friends care about each other ("You wanna know because you're my best friend") (p. 66).

Second, language skills are important for developing more sophisticated conflict resolution strategies. As noted earlier in this chapter, conflict between friends provides special motivation and opportunity for developing conflict management skills. Conversational exchanges between friends contribute to conflict resolution and exploration of feelings during a conflict, and help create shared experiences between friends. Friends are better at resolving conflict and they tend to use more emotional terms and literate language than acquaintances do (Pellegrini, Galda, Bartini, & Charak, 1998).

Third, language during preschoolers' play aids in the development of intimacy between friends. Intimate groups of preschoolers demonstrate that they have their own language of friendship (Emihovich, 1981). Followed over a 4-month period, these preschoolers showed different patterns of communication with their friends than with other classmates. At the beginning of the school year, only friends called each other by name and engaged in elaborate regular pretend play scenarios; nonfriends made bids to join the intimate groups but were denied entry. In a study of kindergartners, Pellegrini and Galda (2001) found that friends used more intimate and emotional terms when interacting with each other than with acquaintances, suggesting that friendships promote and support the use of literate language.

Overall, then, language allows us to communicate with each other and thus promotes social relationships and exchanges. Independent of friendships specifically, as language abilities increase, children are better able to communicate their needs, feelings, and preferences. During prekindergarten, having peers with high expressive language abilities predicted increases in children's own receptive and expressive language over the course of the school year (Mashburn, Justice, Downer, & Pianta, 2009), suggesting that having peers with well-developed language skills is a valuable resource for children's own language development. Within friendships, language development enhances friends' sense of connection with one another and the development of intimacy in their relationship. In turn, friends' interactions during play can enhance their language development. Play, and we suggest that *play with friends* in particular, allows children to display language knowledge and to learn new language through listening, imitating, and practicing (Ervin-Tripp, 1986).

Theory of Mind

Theory of mind refers to children's ability to understand that mental states—thoughts, beliefs, and desires—are related to behavior and that they and others around them are mental beings with sometimes inconsistent thoughts, beliefs, and desires (Hughes & Dunn, 1997; Kavanaugh, 2006). The study of the connections between inner states and action has received increasing attention in the preschool social-cognitive development literature over the last decade. Researchers are interested in how theory of mind skills relate to social behavior. It is possible that theory of mind predicts social behavior (Jenkins & Astington, 2000), or that social behavior predicts theory of mind (Cutting & Dunn, 2006), or that the two are inextricably linked in a bidirectional way. By considering children in their various relationships, it is possible to examine whether specific relationships provide an opportunity to use and further develop theory of mind skills (Cutting & Dunn, 2006). The preschool period is of most interest because it is during this time that children begin to develop a theory of mind (Jenkins & Astington, 2000). Several recent studies show connections between theory of mind and friendship experience.

Judy Dunn and her colleagues have studied extensively how preschoolers' close relationships with mothers, siblings, and friends provide them with unique opportunities to foster social-cognitive abilities, including theory of mind. One study found that around 3 years old, children's talk of inner states is largely with their mothers. By 4 years of age, however, this talk shifts to siblings and friends, especially in the context of cooperative play (Brown, Donelan-McCall, & Dunn, 1996). In another study, Cutting and Dunn (2006) found that children in high-quality friendships engage in more shared cooperative play. In turn, more shared cooperative play is associated with better theory of mind skills. Other empirical evidence indicates that pretend play with friends is related to performance on theory of mind tasks (Hughes & Dunn, 1997), that friends' "smoothness of communication" is positively related to their theories of mind, and that friends are similar in their theory of mind abilities (Dunn & Cutting, 1999). Taken together, these studies provide evidence that friendship provides a distinct context for the use of and development of social-cognitive abilities like theory of mind.

Children are likely to select as friends others who are similar to them in theory of mind skills. Children with similar social-cognitive abilities may feel rewarded by their similar play styles and enjoyment of specific kinds of dramatic play. Additionally, friends' social understanding and mind-reading abilities may become more similar as they engage together in the kinds of play that foster theory of mind. For example, when children engage in fantasy play with friends, they must imagine the emotions, thoughts, and beliefs of the characters they develop and the characters their friends portray. This kind of play may promote both mind-reading abilities and similarity in friends' theory of mind skills.

Although the direction of causality in studies like those described above is unclear, sharing and creating narratives in play with another child, especially a friend, likely contributes to the development of theory of mind abilities (Cutting & Dunn, 1999). Yet to be explored are questions of how continuity and change in children's friendships relate to children's growing mental awareness (Hughes & Dunn, 1998). For example, do theory of mind skills displayed within friends' interactions predict later behavior? Although one study found that better-developed theory of mind and executive function at age 4 predicted fewer negative interactions in a competitive game with a friend at age 5 (Hughes, Cutting, & Dunn, 2001), more research is needed to understand the interplay of these social and cognitive factors over time.

Problem Solving and Creativity among School-Age Children

When children enter school, they face numerous new cognitive demands, and suddenly many of their waking hours are focused on academic pursuits. They do not engage in these academic endeavors alone. In their classrooms, they are surrounded by at least one teacher and as many as 30 same-age peers who are roughly at the same level of cognitive development. Educators and psychologists have studied the value of cooperative learning and peer collaboration at school, yet most studies do not differentiate between friends and nonfriends. From a practical perspective, many teachers who otherwise view peer collaboration as an important learning tool explicitly prohibit friends from working together for fear that their close relationship will interfere with their learning outcomes. The concerns are that friends will distract one another and that their off-task behavior will negate any possible cognitive or academic benefits from their collaboration (e.g., Hartup, 1996b).

We contend, though, that there are a number of reasons why friendship might provide an important context for cognitive development by promoting problem solving and creativity. First, friends know one another better than they know other peers. Therefore, they may be better able to support and offer help and assistance that fits with the friend's skills, needs, strengths, and personality. In the same way that parents often describe knowing that their child responds better to direct instruction than to subtle suggestion, friends may be better able to tailor their support to one another in ways that are especially helpful and result in better cognitive outcomes.

Second, friends have a shared history of working and playing together, and reciprocity is at the core of their relationship. This mutuality may mean that friends are better able to achieve a joint understanding of tasks than are acquaintances or unfamiliar peers. A related point is that even from a young age, children expect friends to cooperate, work together, and strive for compromise, and this may promote more effective collaboration. Indeed, a study of specific processes that make peer collaboration successful showed that achieving a shared understanding via coordinating communication and activity is an essential key to successful collaborative problem solving (Kumpulainen & Kaartinen, 2003). Friends are expected to have an easier time establishing this shared understanding than are nonfriends in part because of their history of experience generating new ideas together. For example, friends spend much of their time together thinking of fun things to do, making up games and activities, and generally creating a shared reality that is critical for successful peer collaborations (Rogoff, 1990).

Third, friends trust and rely on one another. Hartup (1996b) contends that trust functions to promote cognitive growth because information and help from a trusted friend may be accepted and acted upon more readily than information from other sources. This feeling of security may provide a sense of freedom to share opinions, disagree, and challenge one another without fear of damaging the relationship. The kinds of challenges that promote exploration of ideas and that lead to more sophisticated strategies or solutions may thus be easier to achieve with friends.

Fourth, to the extent that richer, more extensive communication can promote cognitive growth, friends may have an advantage over other peers. We know, for example, that friends communicate more with one another than nonfriends (Foot, Chapman, & Smith, 1977; Newcomb & Brady, 1982), and further that friends' communicative exchanges are more mutually oriented (Newcomb & Brady, 1982). Friends may be especially likely to engage in "transactive communication"—dialogues that demonstrate the two children are operating on one another's reasoning (Berkowitz & Gibbs, 1983, 1985; Kruger, 1992). Evidence of transactive statements include clarifications, elaborations, critiques, and justifications ("What I'm trying to say is. ..." "I'm not sure that's right because. ..." "Why do you think that's true?" "I think we may be saying the same thing because. ..."). Transactive communication demonstrates mutual engagement in a task and is likely to occur more readily in friends' than nonfriends' interactions.

These particular speculations about the developmental significance of friendship for cognitive development have rarely been tested directly, yet evidence from a few studies of friends' collaborations on scientific reasoning tasks and on creative tasks support the speculations and raise important questions requiring additional research. Azmitia and Montgomery (1993) directly compared friends' and nonfriends' collaborative problem solving in tasks that require scientific reasoning. Collaborations between friends resulted in more accurate problem solving than collaborations between nonfriends, yet the difference was only apparent on difficult tasks. When task demands require extensive mutual coordination and assistance—hallmarks of friendship—the advantages of working with friends are obvious. In tasks that do not demand mutual effort, coordination, and extensive cooperation, the special relationship between friends does not seem to confer any particular advantages for problem solving and reasoning (Azmitia & Montgomery, 1993; Newcomb & Brady, 1982). In support of the hypotheses offered above for why friends might be better problem solvers than nonfriends, Azmitia and Montgomery also found that friends are more likely to justify their problem-solving ideas spontaneously, perhaps as evidence of being more attuned to one another. In addition, friends engage in more transactive dialogues during conflicts, and in turn, transactive dialogues are associated with cognitive growth. Free and open exchange of ideas in a collaborative setting may be partly responsible for friends' better scientific reasoning.

Another type of collaborative task is one in which there is no "right" answer and no specific problem to solve but rather a creative activity in which the children must work together to produce something such as a story or a musical composition. These kinds of tasks require maintaining mutual engagement in order to create something new. In one study in which pairs of preadolescent friends and pairs of acquaintances composed a piece of music together, friends built on one another's musical ideas more frequently than nonfriends in the process of creating their musical piece, and their compositions were judged to be of higher quality than the compositions of nonfriends (Miell & MacDonald, 2000). It was friends' transactive communication—both verbally and musically— that best predicted how well their composition was rated musically.

Collaborating on writing tasks is another creative activity that is not focused on the pursuit of a single correct solution to a problem and that requires a number of different cognitive skills—generating content and structure for the narrative as well as employing accurately the mechanics of language (e.g., spelling, grammar, usage). There is some evidence that stories written collaboratively by friends are more interpersonally oriented than stories written by nonfriends and that in the process of writing, friends are more mutually engaged than are nonfriends (Hartup, 1996b). However, this study showed that even though collaboratively written stories were of higher quality than individually written ones, story quality did not depend on whether children worked with a friend or a nonfriend. Using a similar story-writing task, Strough, Swenson, and Cheng (2001) found that children who were better friends had better performance early in the task, but over time, more writing errors were found in the stories written by good friends. Taken together, these findings suggest that friendship provides some advantages for particular dimensions of children's writing and cognitive growth, but for others, collaboration with any peer is better than writing alone, and for still others, good friends may be more distracted and off-task, particularly as the amount of time they work together increases.

From the existing empirical evidence, it is too simple to suggest that collaborations between friends necessarily offer advantages for cognitive growth above and beyond collaborations between peers who are not friends. We know that the advantages are evident for difficult tasks but not easy ones (Azmitia & Montgomery, 1993) and that there are some situations in which friends' affiliation might lead to off-task behavior and interfere with problem solving (Hartup, 1996b; Strough et al., 2001). In addition, characteristics of the friends themselves might influence the outcomes of their collaborations. For example, Kutnick and Kington (2005) found that when working together on scientific reasoning tasks, girls achieved higher scores with friends than with acquaintances, but the opposite was true for boys. There are clearly other variables—characteristics of the tasks, characteristics of the settings in which friends collaborate, and characteristics of the friends and their relationship—that determine whether and to what degree friends' collaborations contribute to their cognitive development. Identifying these variables is an exciting direction for additional empirical research.

Summary

Although the number of studies considering how friendships contribute to cognitive development pales in comparison to studies investigating the role of friendship in social development, there is good evidence to suggest that children's experiences with friends promote cognitive competence. During the preschool period, play between friends provides an environment for sharing ideas both verbally and nonverbally and in both real and imaginary realms. Interactions between friends at play contribute to the development of richer literate language and to the emergence of more sophisticated theory of mind skills. Among older school-age children, collaboration between friends supports more advanced problem-solving skills, especially on difficult tasks, yet the evidence for more sophisticated collaboration on creative tasks between friends is mixed. We are left, then, with several theoretically strong hypotheses about why friendship would provide a unique context for particular aspects of cognitive development. These include the benefits of knowing a collaborative partner well and having a shared history based on cooperation, experiencing greater intimacy and trust that encourages challenges to one's own ideas, and more extensive and mutually engaged communication. Each of these hypotheses is supported with only limited empirical evidence, and the question of the developmental significance of friendship for cognitive competence is ripe for additional research.

PSYCHOSOCIAL ADJUSTMENT

To this point, we have considered how friendship contributes to normative social, emotional, and cognitive development. Our primary question, thus far, has focused on how children's relationships with their friends help or hinder their mastery of important developmental tasks in these three areas. Yet, an additional marker of the developmental significance of friendship is whether and how friends promote one another's psychosocial adjustment or maladjustment. Here, we ask, Do friends uniquely contribute to children's adaptation to their current circumstances and to their well-being over time?

In the sections that follow, we consider two indicators of psychosocial adjustment because they are linked theoretically with friendship (Hartup, 1992b; Rubin et al., 2006). The first indicator is coping. Thinking of friendship as a *coping resource* embraces two ideas. First, friends provide support for successfully managing normal transitions most children encounter (e.g., transition to school) and, second, friends can buffer children against the negative effects of non-normative problems in other relationships (e.g., parental relationships). The second indicator of psychosocial adjustment is avoiding loneliness and depression. According to Sullivan's (1953) interpersonal theory, loneliness is a direct outcome of failing to establish a close, intimate friendship, especially in preadolescence.

Coping with Stress and Transitions

If you ask a group of adults to describe a good friend, one of the first and most consistently named characteristics you will hear is support, especially during times of stress. Indeed, providing emotional support is viewed as a primary function of friends—"A friend in need is a friend indeed." The idea that friends provide instrumental support in the form of help (e.g., help with schoolwork) emerges early, by second grade in one study (Bigelow & La Gaipa, 1975). Some authors have suggested that instrumental aid (tangible help with specific tasks) is not specific to friendship because close friends and other peers both offer help in instrumental ways (Furman & Robbins, 1985). One peer may be better able to help with spelling homework and another with perfecting a baseball pitching wind-up. However, emotional support in the form of listening to another's intimate disclosure, being reliably available to offer a shoulder to lean on, offering consistent and sustained guidance, and providing a sense of being understood are functions that are attributed uniquely to friendship and not mere acquaintanceship. By early adolescence, children value emotional support from friends more than any other type of support friends might offer (Malecki & Demaray, 2003). If friends are indeed uniquely suited to and valued for their provision of emotional support, then we would expect to find that having friends helps individuals cope with various stressors in their life. Here we consider the degree to which that common assumption has been supported with empirical findings about (1) friendships as important resources during school transitions, and (2) friendships as buffers against maladjustment associated with problems in other relationships.

Support during School Transitions

School transitions are normative events that occur several times in a child's academic career—the transition to the first year of school (kindergarten for most children in the United States), the transition to middle school or junior high in early adolescence, and later, the transition to high school. School transitions are stressful for children because they are usually accompanied by new cognitive, academic, and interpersonal demands that require coping. Friends are an important source of support for children navigating these demands. In a series of studies, Ladd and colleagues (Ladd, 1990; Ladd & Kochenderfer, 1996; Ladd et al., 1996) investigated the contributions that friendships make to children's school adjustment as they transition to kindergarten at 5- to 6-years-old. Ladd and colleagues suggest that the specific demands of this first year of school include adjusting to a new environment and new teachers, meeting increased academic and cognitive demands, and fitting in with a new peer group (Ladd & Kochenderfer, 1996). They proposed a model of school adjustment suggesting that successful adjustment to school is a product of background factors (e.g., cognitive skills and family factors), children's behavior (e.g., prosocial, antisocial, and withdrawn behavior), and interpersonal relationships within the classroom (e.g., friendships) (Ladd, Buhs, & Troop, 2002).

Evidence for the unique role of friends in helping children successfully negotiate the demands of the school transition is strong. Ladd (1990) found that children who began school with more friends in their classroom were better adjusted at the beginning of the school year, perhaps because the affective ties with friends helped make school seem more familiar and inviting. As the year progressed, children who maintained their friendships had more positive attitudes about school. These stable friendships likely provided emotional support through a sense of security (Howes, 1988), the opportunity to deal with emotions such as fear, anxiety, and frustration through fantasy play (Parker & Gottman, 1989), and generally a wealth of positive, mutually oriented, and enjoyable interactions that help make school "fun" (Newcomb & Bagwell, 1995). Not surprisingly, children with friendships that provided particularly high levels of support and assistance believed that school is a supportive place (Ladd et al., 1996).

The value of friends in helping children cope with school transitions is not specific to the United States and is not confined to major school transitions as one study of Italian schoolchildren demonstrates. Unlike children in many countries, Italian schoolchildren experience a significant school transition between the years that correspond to second and third grades in the United States (Tomada, Schneider, de Domini, Greenman, & Fonzi, 2005). This transition is more subtle than most other school transitions because it does not involve a change in school building or a change in classroom peers. Nevertheless, children experience dramatic changes in academic demands and pressures, teaching and learning approaches, and evaluation of academic achievement that are known to be stressful. Children's own reports of how much they liked school decreased substantially across this transition, yet having a recipro-cal friend was associated with liking school more, regardless of whether it was a friendship that continued across the transition or was a post-transition friendship (Tomada et al., 2005). Notably, the children who benefited most from having a friend during this school transition were those children who experienced other life stress at the same time (e.g., birth of a sibling, divorce of parents, or grandparent moving in). Thus, it was the children who were most in need of support from a friend who benefited most from having a friend. Taken together, the evidence sug-gests that friendships serve as a supportive resource across stressful, yet normative, school transitions.

Friendship as a Protective Factor

The emotional support provided by a friend is also important when chil-dren cope with non-normative stressors, such as problems in other social relationships—family relationships and other peer relationships. Conven-tional wisdom, theories about the provisions of friendship (e.g., Furman & Robins, 1985; Hartup, 1996a; Weiss, 1974), and empirical findings that children who most need a friend's support benefit the most from that support (Tomada et al., 2005) converge to suggest that friendships may provide a buffer that protects children against potential assaults on their psychosocial adjustment that accompany nonoptimal family and peer relationships. There are a number of processes that could explain the potential buffering effect of friendship. Social support from friends may offer children validation of their self-worth and thus enhance their abil-ity to cope with negative feedback in other relationships—rejection from peers or parents, for example (Sullivan, 1953). Alternatively, a positive socializing influence from friends may compensate for less than optimal socialization experiences from parents or other peers (Schwartz, Dodge, Petit, Bates, & Conduct Problems Prevention Research Group, 2000). For example, friendship may offer children a "second chance" to learn skills and competencies they might have missed by being rejected from the peer group. Despite strong theoretical support, the empirical litera-ture specifically developed to address questions about the buffering role of friendship does not provide overwhelming support.

We consider two specific hypotheses about the protective role of friendship. The first hypothesis is that friendship offers protection against the stress and vulnerability children experience in less-than-optimal fam-ily environments. Three illustrative studies provide evidence to evaluate this hypothesis. Rubin and colleagues (2004) found that fifth graders who perceived their mothers as not very supportive experienced internalizing distress. However, for children with low maternal support, having a good friend provided a buffer against internalizing distress. A similar buffering role of friendship was found for young children who experienced harsh parental discipline (Criss, Pettit, Bates, Dodge, & Lapp, 2002). For second graders with few friends, harsh physical discipline was associated with more externalizing problems. Having many friends protected the children from externalizing problems even when they had a history of harsh parental discipline. In a third example study, friendless children with low adaptability and low cohesion in their families had poor self-esteem (Gauze, Bukowski, Aquan-Assee, & Sippola, 1996). However, for preadolescents with a mutual friend, there was no link between family functioning and children's social competence and self-worth, suggesting that having a friend buffered self-esteem in the face of poor family functioning.

On the one hand, these findings are compelling because they emerge across a wide age range (from early childhood through preadolescence), a wide variety of family problems (harsh discipline, low support, low cohesion), and a wide range of adjustment outcomes (internalizing problems, externalizing problems, and self-esteem). On the other hand, a closer look at both the significant and nonsignificant effects challenges a model that assumes the support and other provisions friends afford *uniquely* buffer against negative outcomes associated with family adversity. For example, in the Criss and colleagues (2002) study, acceptance in the peer group was a protective factor as well, and friendship was not a unique buffer of the link between parental discipline and externalizing problems.

A second hypothesis about friendship helping children cope with stress in other relationships centers on the possibility that friendship may provide a buffer against the negative outcomes of rejection by peers. Many children who are disliked and rejected in the larger peer group actually form a close friendship. The companionship, support, and intimacy in these friendships might protect them from negative consequences of peer rejection (e.g., loneliness, school dropout, and other adjustment difficulties). Rejected children who have a best friend may have more opportunities than those without a best friend to hone their social skills, and these skills may decrease externalizing problems (Kupersmidt, Burchinal, & Patterson, 1995).

In the few studies that have examined this buffering hypothesis directly, the findings are not consistent and are even somewhat counterintuitive. For example, over the course of third through seventh grade, peer-rejected children with low levels of conflict with their best friend were *more* likely to be aggressive, and those with lots of conflict were *less* likely to be aggressive (Kupersmidt, Burchinal, & Patterson, 1995). A similar study examining multiple aspects of peer relations as predictors of adjustment problems also found that friendship was not a buffer against externalizing or internalizing problems. Instead, having a mutual friend protected children who were *not* rejected by the peer group from internalizing problems (Hoza, Molina, Bukowksi, & Sippola, 1995).

It is premature, then, to conclude that the support, validation, and affection in friendships compensate for problems in other important social relationships, such as those with parents and peers. In some cases, they no doubt do—children and adults exclaim that they "never could have gotten through that stressful time" without a particular friend. But, the picture is more complicated. As we discuss in Chapters 5 and 6, the ability of friendships to buffer against maladjustment associated with stress in other relationships depends on the quality of the relationship and the characteristics of the friend. Children with aggressive friends, for example, may find reinforcement for increasing disruptive behaviors (Hoza et al., 1995) that exacerbates, not buffers against, externalizing problems associated with rejection. Furthermore, friendship is not the only relationship that offers protection during times of stress. Conventional wisdom, then, about this function of friendship may not be entirely wrong, but it tells an incomplete story.

Avoiding Loneliness and Depression

Loneliness involves feelings of sadness or emptiness that result from children's perceptions that their social relationships are deficient (Asher & Paquette, 2003). Loneliness is one potential outcome of failing to establish a close friendship, and a significant body of literature establishes the link between friendlessness and loneliness. Children without friends are more lonely than children with friends (e.g., Bukowski, Hoza, & Boivin, 1993; Parker & Asher, 1993; Valdivia, Schneider, Chavez, & Chen, 2005); children with more friends are less lonely than children with fewer friends (Nangle, Erdley, Newman, Mason, & Carpenter, 2003; Shin, 2007); and children with lower-quality friendships are more lonely than those with higher-quality relationships (Bukowski, Hoza, & Boivin, 1993; Chipuer, 2001; Nangle et al., 2003; Parker & Asher, 1993). Furthermore, making new friends that last relates to decreased loneliness (Parker & Seal, 1996), and losing friends predicts increased loneliness (Renshaw & Brown, 1993).

We expect that there are multiple reasons why lacking friends or lacking high-quality friendships leads to loneliness, but companionship and intimacy are likely to be especially salient. Clearly, not having friends or having few friends means that children miss out on many aspects of friendship (much more than companionship). Yet, to the extent that spending enjoyable time together is viewed as a necessary foundation of friendship, then feeling lonely is a likely outcome of lacking companionship. It is possible that lacking companionship with a friend may be more related to loneliness among younger children than among adolescents whose loneliness may stem more from lacking someone with whom to talk or share feelings and concerns rather than lacking a playmate (Asher & Paquette, 2003). Nevertheless, at least among third- through fifth-grade children, lacking companionship and lacking intimacy with a best friend are equally associated with loneliness (Parker & Asher, 1993).

Loneliness is also expected to mediate the link between friendship and depression. Depression is expected to be an outcome of poor experiences with friends only when children are unhappy with their social situation and feel lonely (Boivin, Hymel, & Bukowski, 1995). In other words, even if children are friendless or otherwise have problematic peer relations, if those experiences are not perceived as dissatisfying, they are not likely to lead to depression. A specific pathway showing loneliness as a mediator between friendship problems and depression was confirmed by Nangle and colleagues (2003). Specifically, children with few friends and/or low-quality friendships reported loneliness, and loneliness, in turn, predicted depression. Loneliness seems to be a specific result of friendship difficulties. When both friendship (having a friend or friendship quality) and peer acceptance are examined simultaneously, friendship is uniquely associated with loneliness, suggesting that regardless of whether children are liked or disliked by classmates, their friendship experience determines whether or not they are lonely (Parker & Asher, 1993). Even more compelling evidence comes from two studies that found that friendship is directly associated with less loneliness, but popularity is only indirectly associated with loneliness through its link with friendship (Bukowski, Hoza, & Boivin, 1993; Nangle et al., 2003). Thus, children who are unpopular are lonely because their unpopularity interferes with their ability to form good friendships.

Summary

The significance of friendship for psychosocial adjustment is intuitively appealing because it fits with adults' understanding of the relationship and with depictions of friendship in stories and films that romanticize the supportive nature of friendships. The research to date allows for three conclusions about the role of friends in helping one another cope with stress and ward off feelings of loneliness and depression. First, normative school transitions are potentially stressful experiences for children, and friends help children negotiate these transitions successfully. Friendships that precede the transition to school as well as new friendships that develop once school begins contribute to children's positive school adjustment. There are likely multiple processes occurring simultaneously that explain the link between friendships and school adjustment. These include emotional support and security from friends and friends making school more welcoming and fun. Research devoted to uncovering these processes is needed.

Second, despite the often-stated assumption that friends should play a protective role and buffer children against poor experiences in other domains, the evidence is not overwhelmingly supportive. Having friends protects against maladjustment associated with some family difficulties, but being accepted by peers may be an even stronger protective factor in some contexts. Likewise, a blanket statement that friendships provide a buffer for children who are rejected by peers is incorrect. For example, friendship may actually serve as a risk factor for externalizing behaviors among vulnerable children. Aggressive children with aggressive friends may reinforce one another's aggressive behavior resulting in increased behavior problems. It is essential to consider the quality of the friendship and the characteristics of children's friends in order to understand how friendship might protect against maladjustment associated with some negative peer experiences (e.g., victimization by peers) but not others (e.g., peer rejection).

Third, the strongest evidence for a specific and potentially unique role of friendship in psychosocial adjustment comes from studies of loneliness. Multiple aspects of friendship—having a friend, the number of friends, and the quality of the relationship—are associated with warding off feelings of loneliness. The protection against loneliness that friendship provides likely comes from several sources. Friendship provides an enjoyable other with whom to spend time, and it also provides someone with whom to share intimate thoughts, feelings, and concerns. Additional research specifying these and other processes that explain the link between friendship and loneliness is likely to identify moderators of the association, including characteristics of the children (age, expectations) and characteristics of the relationship (quality, stability). Young children may avoid lonely feelings by having a constant playmate, but older children may feel lonely even in the company of a friend if that friend fails to provide a sounding board for self-disclosure or a reliable source of emotional support. Asher and Paquette (2003) also suggest that friendship may protect against loneliness only when children have reasonable expectations for their friends. Children who expect that their friends will never let them down may experience disappointment and loneliness when their friends inevitably fail to live up to those expectations. Having just any friend is not expected to buffer against loneliness; having a low-quality relationship may contribute to feelings of loneliness, and having unstable relationships or moving in and out of friendships may also contribute to loneliness. These are the kinds of nuances that additional research can uncover.

CONCLUSIONS

Our understanding of the significance of friendship for social, emotional, and cognitive development and for psychosocial adjustment from early childhood through preadolescence can be viewed from a glass-half-full or a glass-half-empty perspective. Put quite simply, we know a lot about friendship in childhood, yet even some of the most basic questions about the significance of friendship continue to defy clear and consistent answers. In part this situation is because the overall question "What is the developmental significance of friendship?" includes two underlying questions. First, how and why friendship is important in childhood—that is, how the children's experiences with friends promote the acquisition of skills and competencies for adaptive social, emotional, and cognitive development. This question focuses on friendship as a *developmental advantage* such that children with friends (high-quality friends with prosocial peers as we discuss in Chapters 5 and 6) are at an advantage in terms of successfully negotiating developmental tasks and being well adjusted. Second, we can also ask whether and how friendship is a *unique* context for social, emotional, and cognitive development and for psychosocial adjustment. This question focuses on whether and in what ways friendships are *developmental necessities*—necessary for adaptive development and adjustment because of the developmental context of friendship. The skills and competencies fostered in friendship cannot be easily obtained in other ways—not with parents, siblings, or peers in general. In this concluding section, we discuss what we know about these two ways of evaluating the developmental significance of friendship, and we pose questions for continued research.

Why Is Friendship Important?

At the most basic level, friendship is important because children value it, even from a young age. Children go to great lengths to maintain friendships, and they value their friends as playmates, as sources of fun and excitement and happiness and good ideas, and as others like them to share their most intimate thoughts. One way researchers consider how and why friendship is important is by examining its specific features and considering how interactions with friends differ from interactions with other peers. A large body of research from these friend-versus-nonfriend studies converges to suggest that friendships are characterized by positive social interaction and engagement as well as properties of the relationship that include intimacy, closeness, and loyalty (Hartup, 1996a; Newcomb & Bagwell, 1995). The more deep and intimate properties of the relationship emerge over the course of childhood both in terms of what children expect from friends and in terms of what features are prominent in the relationship.

The importance of friendship for *social development* can be evaluated by the contributions that companionship, intimacy, and conflict make to social competence. Each of these three central components of children's friendships has a well-defined developmental trajectory. Companionship is the earliest evidence of friendship, and the condition that friends enjoy one another, spend time together, and engage with one another in fun and meaningful ways exists throughout childhood. Although the specific ways in which companionship is displayed between friends may change—two preschool friends play together in the block corner day after day and two preadolescent children talk extensively on the phone every evening—the importance of companionship is consistent throughout childhood. The beginnings of intimacy between friends may be observed among young children, yet the conclusion across a number of studies is that intimacy, especially intimate self-disclosure and mutual emotional support, increases in preadolescence and adolescence. Conflict, like companionship, is a common element of friendship from early childhood to preadolescence. The source of conflict changes with development, but children and preadolescents become better able to resolve conflicts with friends through negotiation and compromise as their social and cognitive competencies blossom. Companionship, intimacy, and conflict provide the backbone for understanding friendship's importance for social development. Friendship not only provides opportunities for developing and honing skills in getting along, sharing oneself with another, and managing disagreement, but maintaining a good friendship requires them.

Friends are important for *emotional development* from early childhood through adolescence in part because friendships are emotion-rich relationships. Friends share more positive affect than other peers, and negative emotion is also part of the close relationships of friends. Friends, like parents, are involved in the socialization of emotional competence. Within friendships, children learn and practice emotion display rules, and the closeness of the relationship helps promote emotional understanding. Friendships also provide an important context for developing competence in emotion regulation. Difficulty regulating emotions disrupts friends' interactions; thus, friends are motivated to control their emotional displays. Self-disclosure and other processes related to intimacy between friends provide opportunities to explore and manage difficult complex emotions (embarrassment, jealousy, disappointment).

Compared to social and emotional development, we know less about the importance of friendship for *cognitive development.* In early childhood, friends' play provides opportunities for developing language as well as more sophisticated theory of mind skills. Only a few studies of school-age children offer suggestions of friendship's role in cognitive development. Existing studies focus largely on collaboration, especially in problem solving and creative activities.

We want to understand what role friendship plays in children's lives as they develop. Asking about the advantages friendship offers children is thus one way to evaluate the developmental significance of friendship. Friendship matters to children, and folk wisdom, empirical studies, ethnographic investigations, parenting handbooks, and popular press books all demonstrate that friendship is an important part of development. We can be confident in describing the characteristics and features of children's friendships and in concluding that friendship is important; in other words, it is *developmentally significant.*

Is Friendship a Unique Developmental Context?

It is doubtful that anyone—child, parent, teacher, clinician, or researcher—would argue that friendships are not important. Nevertheless, there is more to answering the question of developmental significance than drawing the conclusion that friendships matter. What we really want to know is whether the context for social, emotional, and cognitive development provided by friendship is unique, and whether the skills, competencies, and experiences gained in friendships cannot be easily obtained elsewhere. In other words, are friendships *necessary* for social, emotional, cognitive development, and psychosocial adjustment? It is this question that is much more difficult to answer.

We know that friendship is unlike any other relationship in children's lives. There are numerous features that distinguish friendships from children's other relationships, yet there are four characteristics that appear most important for explaining the potentially unique role that friendships play in development and adjustment. Friendships are (1) voluntary, (2) reciprocal, (3) based on a strong affective tie, and (4) exist between children who are at similar developmental levels. These four characteristics help determine the developmental significance of friendship in each of the domains we discuss in this chapter—social, emotional, and cognitive development and psychosocial adjustment.

There are good reasons to expect that the developmental context of friendship is unique, but we need to identify the specific contributions friendship makes to development to indicate whether it is closer to a *necessary* developmental context rather than simply an advantageous one. Here are just a few ways that the four characteristics listed above demonstrate friendship's significance in children's lives. Unlike familial relationships, for example, being successful in friendships requires social skills related to initiating enjoyable interactions and managing the give-and-take nature of these interactions. At the same time, friendship seems to provide a unique context for developing social competence because of the time friends spend together, the affection in their relationship, and their knowledge of one another. Because friends are free to terminate the relationship at any time, care must be taken to manage disagreements. Thus, conflict with friends provides opportunities for practicing negotiation and compromise, for learning to express and regulate emotion, and for engaging in higher-level problem solving and perspective taking that might not emerge as easily in conflicts with other peers. The intimacy that exists between friends, particularly in preadolescence and adolescence, is simply not found to the same degree in other relationships; thus, to the extent that this intimacy and closeness provide important building blocks for other relationships, are responsible for friendship's positive effects on psychosocial adjustment, and/or promote competence in emotion understanding and emotion regulation, intimacy between friends is developmentally significant.

Although we have considered the role of friendship in social, emotional, and cognitive development and psychosocial adjustment separately, doing so has allowed us to add some topography to the discussion of friendship's developmental significance. It is clear that we can draw stronger conclusions in some areas than in others. We are most confident in the conclusion that friendships are uniquely associated with particular aspects of psychosocial adjustment. First, friendship is particularly important for helping children negotiate normative school transitions successfully. Early school transitions, such as the beginning of the first year of school, are particularly affected by children's relationships with old friends and with friends that develop in the new school setting. Second, for most children, friendship is incompatible with loneliness. Generally, children with friends, with more friends, and with high-quality friendships experience less loneliness, and changes in friendship—making new friends or losing friends—are associated with increases or decreases in loneliness (Parker & Seal, 1996; Renshaw & Brown, 1993). Loneliness appears to be *uniquely* associated with problems in friendship even when other indicators of acceptance or rejection by peers are considered. It may be that friendship is tied to a specific kind of loneliness—feelings of emptiness associated with lacking an intimate relationship with another—that has been referred to as emotional loneliness (Weiss, 1973) or dyadic loneliness (Hoza, Bukowski, & Beery, 2000). Feelings of loneliness also help to explain links between friendship and depression inasmuch as dissatisfying relations with friends contribute to loneliness, and loneliness, in turn, predicts symptoms of depression.

Future Research Directions

We want to be able to draw sharper, more nuanced conclusions about the developmental significance of friendship rather than sweeping statements about its importance. Several general strategies for future research will provide further evidence to assess the uniqueness of the developmental context friendship provides. Here we describe five.

1. The evidence is clear that children with friends are better off than children without friends, especially in terms of social competence and psychosocial adjustment (Hartup, 1996a; Newcomb & Bagwell, 1996; Parker, Rubin, Price, & DeRosier, 1995; Parker & Seal, 1996). Nevertheless, simply having a friend does not guarantee positive outcomes, and we need to consider the variations in the outcomes associated with having friends. To do so, it is essential to take a multidimensional perspective on friendship. In Chapters 5 and 6, we discuss two issues that help account for these variations in outcomes associated with having friends, namely, the individual characteristics of each friend and the quality of the relationship.

2. Only when other dimensions of peer relations are considered with friendship can we more clearly answer questions about the uniqueness of the friendship experience. As we discuss in Chapter 1, it is clear that friendship and peer acceptance and rejection are different yet related aspects of children's social experience. Simultaneous assessments of friendship and peer acceptance–rejection, for example, have led to the conclusion that friendship is uniquely associated with loneliness.

3. Longitudinal studies are critical. Assessing social, emotional, and cognitive competence as well as friendship relations at multiple points in time allow for testing models about change over time, including how changes in friendships relate to developmental progression in social, emotional, and cognitive development and to psychosocial adjustment.

4. We need to expand our understanding of moderator variables. The developmental significance of friendship is not likely to be captured accurately with models that assert that friendship has the same significance in all situations and for all children. With respect to age: Do manifestations of intimacy between young children and their friends serve the same functions for social and emotional development as intimacy between older children? Is intimacy between friends more important for psychosocial adjustment as children age? With respect to the contributions of

friendship to cognitive development: What other variables, besides task difficulty and the length of time friends work together determine whether or not collaboration with a friend leads to more advanced reasoning and cognitive growth?

5. There is a genuine need for collaborations among researchers in different areas. For example, emotion researchers consider the role of interpersonal relationships in the development of interpersonal competence. Yet, collaborations that make use of this knowledge and consider specifically what friendships offer children in the way of a context for the development of emotional competence is rare. The same can be said for research on cognitive development. Interactions with peers contribute to cognitive growth in the areas of problem solving and social cognitive competence such as perspective taking and theory of mind. Yet, the specific role of friends in promoting competence in these areas is rarely considered. Better coordination and collaboration between friendship researchers and researchers in emotional and cognitive development would promote better understanding of key issues and questions in each of these areas.

Chapter 4

The Developmental Significance of Friendship in Adolescence

Friendships in childhood are usually a matter of chance, whereas in adolescence they are most often a matter of choice.
—David Elkind (1993, p. 45)

Someone who is there for you when you need any kind of support. Someone who can cheer you up, or just listen to your problems. Someone who you're willing to be there for, as they are there for you. Someone who would be sad if you cried, happy if you were smiling. Someone you love, and who loves you, but not a romantic love. Someone who looks past your short-comings and takes your strong points. Someone who can tell you the truth.

A close friend is someone you can trust and who trusts you. The two of you should be able to talk about anything, even topics that make one of you uncomfortable. You can rely on a close friend to help you no matter how tough things get for you, just as your friend can rely on you. No sacrifice is too great for either of you to make for the sake of your friendship. This isn't to say you agree on everything; far from it. Simply put, if you disagree, you should either be able to respect your friend's viewpoint, or, in case of an argument, be able to work through your differences. In short, friendship is based on reciprocity.
—Two late adolescents answering the question
"What makes someone a close friend?"

116

Adolescence is a remarkable period of life with dramatic and complex changes taking place. Adolescents reach physical maturity as their bodies become those of adults. They become increasingly self-aware and independent from their parents; their social horizons expand as they come in contact with many different peers and establish more intimate relationships; and they become involved in a wide array of social contexts as they enter larger schools, take on after-school jobs, and participate in numerous extracurricular activities. Their cognitive abilities allow for more abstract and logical thinking, and they are faced with many significant choices about what to do in the present moment and how to plan for the future (e.g., "Should I drive home even though I've been drinking? What will happen if I do?"; "Is school important to me?"; "Am I going to college? If so, which one?").

Friendships play an important role in adolescence because they contribute to many of these changes, and they also reflect the social and cognitive changes that are central to this developmental period. The goal of this chapter is to evaluate the developmental significance of friendships in adolescence. In doing so, we continue with the perspective developed in Chapter 3 that friendships in adolescence are normative, that friendships serve as a context for development, and that the contributions of friendships are unique and go beyond the importance of being popular or a well-liked member of the peer group. In the sections that follow, we first consider the normative development of friendships in adolescence. Then, we evaluate the developmental significance of friendship in three domains that are central to adolescence—adolescent–parent relationships, identity development, and romantic relationships.

FRIENDSHIP AS A NORMATIVE EXPERIENCE IN ADOLESCENCE

Most adolescents have friends. When asked, most name one or two best friends as well as several other close friends (Adler & Adler, 1998). Asking a simple question to a parent of an adolescent or taking a trip to a local shopping center or movie theater leads to the conclusion that adolescents spend significant amounts of time with their friends. A recent study confirms these anecdotal observations, reporting that adolescent girls spend approximately 3 hours per day with their friends, and adolescent boys spend approximately 2.3 hours per day with their friends (Johnson, 2004). In middle adolescence, much more of this time is spent with same-sex rather than other-sex friends, and it is not until late adolescence that substantial time is spent with other-sex friends. Contact with friends in adolescence takes many forms—seeing them at school, spending time after school in organized activities or "hanging out," talking with them on the phone, and sending e-mails and text messages. A recent report from the Nielsen Company shows that adolescents sent and received an average of 80 text messages per day in a 3-month period—many of these to their friends (Hafner, 2009).

Clearly, then, friends are incredibly important to adolescents, but what exactly is the developmental significance of friendships? How do adolescents' experiences with their friends affect them as they negotiate the challenges and opportunities of adolescence and as they move into adulthood? Here we briefly consider four questions about the normative experience of friendship across adolescence: What are the characteristics of adolescents' friendships? What is the importance of similarity between friends? Do the various "levels" of friendship (best vs. close vs. casual) matter? What is the role of friendships with peers of the other sex?

Characteristics of Adolescent Friendships

Interestingly, questions about the normative experience of friendship and especially how friendships change with development from childhood to adolescence and across adolescence were some of the earliest questions asked about this relationship. As researchers worked to gain an understanding of how adolescents experience friendships and why these relationships are important, studies comparing friends versus nonfriends (e.g., acquaintances), studies asking adolescents what they expect from friends, and studies comparing friends of different ages became popular in the 1970s and 1980s. Numerous book chapters, narrative summaries, and a meta-analysis summarizing this literature then appeared in the 1990s (e.g., Berndt & Hanna, 1995; Berndt & Savin-Williams, 1993; Bukowski & Hoza, 1989; Bukowski, Newcomb, & Hartup, 1996; Hartup, 1993, 1996a; Hartup & Stevens, 1997; Ladd, 1999; Laursen, 1993; Newcomb & Bagwell, 1995; Rubin, Bukowski, & Parker, 1998). The bulk of empirical research in the last decade has moved away from the normative experience of friendship at different ages and has focused instead on individual differences in adolescents' friendships, especially related to friendship quality and the characteristics of friends (topics we address in Chapters 5 and 6). Nevertheless, our task here is to describe what we know about most adolescents' friendships, especially their characteristics and features.

According to Sullivan (1953), the need for interpersonal intimacy (including closeness, empathy, love, and security) emerges during preadolescence and is best fulfilled by same-sex friends. Theory and several seminal empirical works suggest that age 12 is considered a critical time in friendship development; it is when friendship becomes more sophisticated and can be most easily distinguished from popularity and group acceptance (Bigelow, 1977; Bigelow & La Gaipa, 1980; Sullivan, 1953; Youniss, 1980).

As we discuss in Chapter 3, developmental trends are apparent both in what youth expect from friendships in general and in what characteristics are present in their actual relationships with friends. Adolescents include loyalty, intimacy, authenticity, and empathic understanding in their descriptions of sought-after qualities of friends more so than do children (Berndt, 1986; Clark & Bittle, 1992). In terms of both friendship *expectations* and friends' *interactions,* the increase in level of intimacy from childhood to adolescence is considered the "strongest evidence for the hypothesis that friendships become more supportive relationships during adolescence" (Berndt, 1989, p. 311). In real numbers, one study found an 18% increase in the number of boys and girls who talked to their friends about problems from early to middle adolescence and a 12% increase for boys and a 5% increase for girls in the number who said that their friend understood them best (Crockett, Losoff, & Petersen, 1984). Indeed, self-disclosure and emotional closeness are the aspects of intimacy that show the most dramatic increases with age (Sharabany, Gershoni, & Hofman, 1981).

In addition, several features of friendship take on new meaning or may be first truly understood and appreciated during adolescence. These include reciprocity (i.e., expectations of intimacy, common interests), commitment (i.e., loyalty and trust), and egalitarianism (i.e., shared power; Hartup, 1993). More than three decades of work provide support for these age-related changes in friendship (e.g., Bigelow & La Gaipa, 1975; Crockett et al., 1984; Mendelson & Aboud, 1999). Overall, the increases in the "deeper" components of friendship including intimacy, loyalty, and emotional support seem to happen gradually rather than emerging spontaneously or out of the blue (Berndt, 2004; Furman & Buhrmester, 1992).

In fact, comparisons of the characteristics of friendships in childhood and adolescence suggest both similarities and differences. On the one hand, there are some characteristics of friendship that are similar across developmental stages. For example, in both middle childhood and adolescence, there is an understanding that friendship requires mutual liking and assistance and involves frequent interaction (see Berndt & Perry, 1990). Children from second grade through early adolescence similarly cite talking, laughing, and smiling as part of their friendship activities. Companionship is thus a valued feature and provision of friendship throughout childhood and adolescence. When asked to make judgments about whether two hypothetical youth would be friends, both children and adolescents rate those who are intimate as most likely to be friends followed by those who are supportive and those who are similar. Intimacy is an especially important determinant of friendship for adolescents and for girls (Bukowski & Kramer, 1986).

On the other hand, when we look more closely, these displays of intimacy in adolescence are more sophisticated, and they may serve different functions in adolescence. For example, interactions with friends in adolescence can make important contributions to identity development (e.g., a sense of mattering and belonging) (Cotterell, 2007). Attachment displays (including laughing, being uniquely comfortable with one another, and engaging in physical contact) and talking (sharing hopes, fears, and sources of joy, as well as talking and gossiping) in adolescent friendships make them unique contexts for sharing oneself with another person of the same developmental level and age (e.g., Gottman & Mettetal, 1986).

So far, we have compared and contrasted characteristics of friendship between childhood and adolescence. Doing so may wrongly imply that there is a major shift at some magical moment between childhood and adolescence and that friendships change very little from that point forward. Instead, important developmental trends associated with friendship are uncovered by looking at friendship within and across the various *stages of adolescence*. There is evidence that from early (approximately ages 10–14) to middle (approximately ages 15–17) to late adolescence (approximately 18 and older), expectations of friends increase, number of conflicts and levels of exclusivity decrease, empathy and sharing increase, and attachment levels and intimacy remain stable or increase (Claes, 1992). A more recent study confirmed these ideas with an examination of behaviors associated with intimacy in adolescents from ninth grade through eleventh grade (McNelles & Connolly, 1999). During this period of time, sustained intimate affect was decreasingly related to activity-based behaviors but increasingly related to discussion of topics and personal disclosure. In a longitudinal study following adolescents from ages 12 to 16 and ages 16 to 20, support from a best friend showed a curvilinear pattern of development with an increase especially from early to late adolescence and no differences between boys and girls in this pattern. In contrast, negative features of friendship started higher and generally decreased for boys across adolescence but remained stable for girls (De Goede, Branje, & Meeus, 2009). Thus, observed changes in friendship features do not simply stop with the onset of adolescence, and by late adolescence, descriptions like the ones that open this chapter are common. By late adolescence, youth have a sophisticated and nuanced set of expectations about friends and experiences with friends that include constructs of intimacy, closeness, loyalty and trust, reliability, and resolution of conflict.

Unfortunately, most of these conclusions are built on cross-sectional studies comparing children and adolescents at different ages (e.g., Furman & Buhrmester, 1992) rather than longitudinal studies that trace the development of friendships across adolescence. Furthermore, despite the fact that much of the present-day research has moved away from evaluations of the normative development of friendship, the field would be well served by carefully designed (especially longitudinal) investigations of normative changes in friends' interactions across adolescence and how those changes relate to the successful negotiation of other developmental tasks (e.g., autonomy, identity development, romantic relationships). Additionally, our current understanding of friendships is based on self-reports. Naturalistic observation of children and adolescents, for example, would give us additional perspectives on the nature of these friendships and the dynamics between friends and within friendship networks.

Similarity between Friends

There has been considerable discussion about the extent to which adolescent friends are similar to one another. As we discuss in Chapter 2, a question that falls within the realm of this discussion is whether friendships are created on the basis of similarity (i.e., selection effects), or whether friends become more similar over time due to their influence on one another (i.e., socialization effects). Here we explore the extent to which relationship formation is based on similarity and the degree to which friends influence one another, and thus, become more similar over time.

Forming Friendships

To begin, similarity often is the basis for forming friendships in adolescence. Hartup (1996a) describes two simultaneous processes through which the selection of friends takes place: (1) similarity and attraction at the dyadic level (e.g., two adolescents become friends because they are similar and it "feels right"), and (2) assortative processes that occur at the larger social network level (e.g., two adolescents sit next to each other in their advanced English class, begin to share lecture notes, and often discuss homework assignments, and their friendship builds from their shared academic engagement) (see also Dishion, Patterson, & Griesler, 1994). This latter example illustrates that adolescents often choose their friends from within a "restricted range" of choices that exist in their available social environment (Hartup, 1996b). This tendency for similarity between friends is due at least in part to the fact that the groups from which adolescents choose their friends are relatively homogeneous—their school, their neighborhood, their community sports teams and activity groups—and the result is a tendency for friends to be similar in sociodemographic factors, age, race, and sex.

Friendship selection is also based on similarity at the "behavioral level" (Epstein, 1983), such as personal characteristics (e.g., antisocial, shy) and interests (e.g., sports, music) (Hartup, 1996a) and prosocial behavior (e.g., helpful, cooperative) (Güroğlu, van Lieshout, Haselager, & Scholte, 2007). Friends tend to have a relatively long list of similarities. Adolescent friends, for example, tend to be similar on attitudes, aspirations, and achievement as they relate to school, and on attitudes and behaviors related to smoking, drinking, drug use, and dating. Socializing with similar others contributes to equity and reciprocity, as well as to emotional support and consensual support (Berscheid & Walster, 1969). Another indication that similarity drives selection of friends comes from findings that "about to be friends" are similar prior to the formation of their relationship (Newcomb et al., 1999; Urberg, Değirmencioğlu, & Tolson, 1998).

Friends' Influence

Peer influence or "peer contagion" is a second explanation for similarity between adolescent friends. Similarity between friends may occur because friends become more similar as their relationship continues. During adolescence, this process of mutual socialization and influence occurs in particular areas of life, such as social behavior, school achievement, and attitudes (Berndt, 1999; Berndt & Murphy, 2002). Friends' influence on one another has been considered most often in the area of deviant behavior, especially in the areas of sexual behavior, drug use, and delinquency. For example, adolescent friends tend to have similar attitudes about sexual behavior (DiIorio et al., 2001), and adolescents who have been sexually active are more likely to have friends who also have engaged in some form of sexual activity (Billy, Rodgers, & Udry, 1984; Billy & Udry, 1985; Prinstein, Meade, & Cohen, 2003). We discuss the issue of similarity in antisocial and deviant behavior more thoroughly in Chapter 5.

Selection and Socialization

Collectively, the evidence for the source of friends' similarity suggests that both selection and socialization processes are responsible (Güroğlu et al., 2007). Several classic and more recent examples provide demonstrations. Kandel's (1978) often-cited study of similarity between adolescent friends on marijuana use, involvement in delinquency, educational aspirations, and political views found that the effects of socialization and selection were about equal, with socialization effects being strongest for marijuana use. More recently, Popp, Laursen, Kerr, Stattin, and Burk (2008) found evidence for both selection and socialization effects on alcohol use, and interestingly, once the friendship ended, similarity decreased. Similarly, Billy and Udry (1985) reported that similarity in sexual behavior is a result of both influence and selection. The specific selection process at work is that of "acquisition" (i.e., similarity in newly formed friendships) rather than "deselection" (i.e., ending a friendship with a dissimilar peer). In contrast, a recent study of friends' influence on adolescents' depression showed the importance not only of selection and socialization (especially for out-of-school friends) but also of deselection (Van Zalk, Kerr, Branje, Stattin, & Meeus, 2010). Specifically, adolescents selected friends with similar levels of depression; friends seemed to increase one another's depression levels; and relationships were likely to end if adolescents and their friends did not have similar levels of depression symptoms. Overall, it is likely that there is a temporal relationship between these various sources of similarity. Specifically, similarity is important first in the selection of friends, and then subsequently, similarity in interests and attitudes lead the adolescents down common pathways (Urberg, 1999).

The power of selection and socialization effects may also change over the course of childhood and adolescence. Here are two examples. Véronneau and colleagues investigated a transactional model involving reciprocal influences between peer experiences, including friends' academic achievement and youths' own academic achievement from childhood through early adolescence. Beginning in the first grade and continuing through seventh grade, teachers rated students' overall academic achievement, and an average rating of achievement for students' four nominated best friends was also calculated. From grades 4 through 7, students' higher achievement predicted selecting friends with higher academic achievement the next year, and the link between own achievement and friends' achievement grew stronger over time. However, there was not evidence of socialization effects because friends' achievement was not associated with changes in participants' achievement at any grade (Véronneau, Vitaro, Brendgen, Dishion, & Tremblay, 2010). In a large sample of juvenile offenders followed over time, selection effects on antisocial behavior were limited to middle adolescence (ages 14–15), but socialization effects continued into later adolescence (ages 15–20). By young adulthood (ages 21–22), however, friends' delinquency was unrelated to young adults' own antisocial behavior (Monahan, Steinberg, & Cauffman, 2009).

In sum, similarity is a cause and an effect of friendship formation. Similarity in behaviors exists between two adolescents prior to the formation of a relationship and tends to increase as the relationship continues over time. Nevertheless, it is difficult to tease apart these two sources of similarity, and the simple finding that there is a high correlation between Friend A and Friend B on Behavior X cannot be attributed solely to the fact that friends influence one another (Berndt, 1999). New statistical models, such as the one reported by Knecht and colleagues will help tease apart the effects of one process while controlling for the other (Knecht, Snijders, Baerveldt, Steglich, & Raub, 2010). To be sure, some adolescents may choose friends who complement them in some way, such as bullies and assistants (Güroğlu et al., 2007; Salmivalli, Lagerspetz, Bjorkqvist, Kaukiainen, & Osterman, 1996), yet the bottom line for most adolescent friends is that similarity is a key feature of their relationship.

Levels of Friendship

The structure of peer groups changes in adolescence with an emphasis on multiple levels or layers of peer relationships—"my friend" (i.e., a dyadic relationship with a best or close friend) and "my friends" (i.e., a larger network of relationships that includes multiple reciprocal dyadic relationships and friends of friends) (e.g., Adler & Adler, 1998; Hartup, 1993; Hartup & Stevens, 1997). Even within dyadic friendships, adolescents easily distinguish between best friends, close friends, "just" friends, and then others in their larger peer networks (Adler & Adler, 1998; Berndt, 1996; Berndt & Hoyle, 1985; Furman & Bierman, 1984). Some adolescents also make distinctions between friends associated with different activities or groups—my baseball friends versus my Girl Scouts friends. In trying to understand the significance of friendship in adolescence, there is value in considering these "levels" of friendship because not all friendships are necessarily equal. La Gaipa (1979) presents a helpful visual depiction of these levels using concentric circles, where there is a large group of acquaintances encompassing a smaller circle of friends, which includes a smaller circle of more intimate friends. This early conceptualization of multiple "levels" of friendship has been confirmed in more recent studies. Adolescents, compared to younger children, differentiate more between types of friendships, particularly between best friends and other friends (Berndt, 1996; Furman & Bierman, 1984; Selman, 1981).

In one sample, it was estimated that children nominate approximately double the number of peers as close friends than adolescents do (i.e., "kids you know very well, spend a lot of time with in and out of school, and who you talk to about things that happen in your life"), and 76% of preadolescents and 70% of adolescents have reciprocated "close friends" (Buhrmester, 1990). Another study estimated one or two "best friends" and several "close" or "good" friends (Crockett et al., 1984).

In early adolescence, there appears to be a peak in the number of close friends—approximately four to six—which is followed by a decrease in middle and late adolescence (e.g., Cairns, Leung, Buchanan, & Cairns, 1995; Savin-Williams & Berndt, 1990).

These various levels of friendship are possible in adolescence as the social environment changes during and after the transition to adolescence. Youth have greater freedom to choose their associates and have access to more and different peers because of their increased mobility and involvement in more groups and activities; greater independence in adolescence is associated with less parent–child time and more peer time; the organization of the school also influences the developmental processes for friendship during adolescence (e.g., Berndt, Hawkins, & Jiao, 1999). Transition to a junior high, middle, or senior high school that is typically organized differently than elementary schools presents new challenges and opportunities to the individual (Isakson & Jarvis, 1999). Upper-level schools often force the adolescent to adapt to larger and less personal school environments (Simmons, Carlton-Ford, & Blyth, 1987). Students often switch classrooms and classmates frequently throughout their school day, and are thus exposed to a larger peer network than they were in elementary school (Karweit & Hansell, 1983). Importantly, there is evidence that having and keeping friends through the transition contributes to a more successful transition (e.g., Aikins, Bierman, & Parker, 2005; Berndt et al., 1999). In adolescence, friendships also move off of the playground and out of the classroom to more social environments, requiring more initiative in making and keeping different kinds of friends (e.g., Hardy, Bukowski, & Sippola, 2002; Parker & Gottman, 1989). One possibility is that friends at various levels satisfy different needs for adolescents. For example, best friends are most likely to satisfy intimacy and support needs. Other friends may satisfy needs for companionship or simply be characterized by their emergence in particular social niches ("baseball friends" or "camp friends") (Adler & Adler, 1998).

How do these various levels of friendship differ, and what are their developmental contributions? Berndt (1986) found that closer friends provide more positive ratings of their friendships, particularly on prosocial behavior, intimacy, and similarity; closer friends also fight with and tease each other more than those who do not consider themselves "close" friends. Close friendships have been characterized by sharing intimate feelings, which is what most distinguishes close friendships from "common" friendships (Oden, Hertzberger, Mangaine, & Wheeler, 1984). It is also important to note that asymmetries exist in friendships, even among the closest of friends. Berndt (1996) reported that seventh graders rate their "very best friends" high in positive features and low in negative features, even in situations where those rated as "very best friends" rated them only as their second or third "closest" friend. In contrast, the friends' ratings were less positive and more negative if they rated the friend as "second" or "third" closest friend. Thus, close friendships may be more significant to one friend than another.

Overall, it appears that the degree of closeness in a friendship is related to how much the adolescent both gives and gets from the relationship. One difficulty in this area of literature is that definitions of various levels of friendship are not universal. Some studies may use the term *intimate friend* and mean *best friend,* and other studies may refer to degree of "closeness" on a continuum. Additionally, some studies consider reciprocity a criterion for friendship, but other studies do not. The fact that adolescents have many friends and various levels of friends within their social network presents a challenge to researchers. Clearly the effects of these multiple friends matter, and their effects may be unique. Social network analyses, which are beyond the scope of this book, provide one strategy for taking into account the multiple relationships adolescents have (see, e.g., Ojanen, Sijtsema, Hawley, & Little, 2010; Rodkin & Hanish, 2007; Rubin, Bukowski, & Laursen, 2009). Therefore, although we can confidently say that different levels of friendship exist in adolescence and that adolescents' experiences at each level are unique, we cannot make global statements about each level of friendship. A meta-analysis of these studies would provide a better picture of the specific functions and qualities of different levels of friendship. This would lead to more universal terminology and thus better understanding of the various friendships adolescents have.

Other-Sex Friends

Our understanding of friendship is overwhelmingly based on same-sex rather than other-sex friendships because other-sex friendships generally do not become common or acceptable until middle or late adolescence. Even then, same-sex friends predominate. In middle and late adolescence, youth spend more time with same-sex friends on a daily basis and report that they have known them longer than their other-sex friends (Johnson, 2004; Richards, Crowe, Larson, & Swarr, 1998), even though the number of other-sex friends increases from middle to late adolescence (Blyth et al., 1982). It is not until college age that other-sex friends occupy as much or more time as same-sex friends (Johnson, 2004).

Other-sex friends have largely been ignored in considerations of the developmental significance of friendship and have been viewed as not important, except perhaps in providing access to potential romantic partners. Nevertheless, the level of intimacy experienced in other-sex friendships increases as adolescents age (Berndt, 1982; Buhrmester & Furman,

1987; Camarena et al., 1990; Karweit & Hansell, 1983; Sharabany et al., 1981; cf. Lempers & Clark-Lempers, 1993), and other-sex friendships may even eclipse same-sex friendships in cohesion and closeness by late adolescence (Johnson, 2004).

Despite the increasing importance of other-sex friendships across adolescence, same-sex friendships remain highly valued. For example, commitment to the relationship remains higher for same-sex than other-sex friendships across early, middle, and late adolescence (Johnson, 2004). In their study of sixth through twelfth graders, Lempers and Clark-Lempers (1993) found that adolescents' ratings of all positive dimensions of their relationships—such as satisfaction, intimacy, affection, and companionship—were equal to or higher for same-sex friendships than other-sex friendships across all seven grade levels.

Comparing ratings of same-sex and other-sex friendships in adolescence naturally pits the two types of relationships against each other and begs the question "Which is more important?" Yet an alternative is to think of them as parallel relationships that are both important and may have unique implications for well-being. This perspective is demonstrated by Bukowski, Sippola, and Hoza (1999) who showed that same-sex and other-sex friendships *both* contribute to developmental outcomes. One caveat that should be noted here is that much of the literature uses the term *other-sex friendships,* but that likely includes both romantic and nonromantic other-sex friends. With this in mind, two findings of the Bukowski study are particularly compelling. First, the early adolescents who were most likely to be involved in close other-sex friendships were those who were either very popular or very unpopular with same-sex peers. Youth who were popular with same-sex peers were also popular with other-sex peers, leading to more other-sex friends, and youth who were unpopular with same-sex peers tended to nominate many other-sex peers as friends. This finding represents both continuity and discontinuity between same-sex and other-sex friendships—continuity for popular adolescents whose social competence allows them to easily make friends with boys *and* girls and discontinuity for unpopular adolescents who may be successful in one type of friendship but not the other (although determining how "successful" warrants additional research). Second, for boys without a same-sex friend, having a friendship with a girl was related to higher self-worth. Thus, other-sex friendships served a "backup" function, compensating for the lack of same-sex friendships. In contrast, for girls who did not have a same-sex friend, having a friendship with a boy was associated with poor social competence. The work on adolescent other-sex friendships can be understood developmentally by considering the results of studies with younger participants (and thus include other-sex friends who are not romantic partners). One study of third and fourth

graders showed that those who reported mostly other-sex friends demonstrated lower social skills, but fewer sex-role stereotypes (Kovacs, Parker,
& Hoffman, 1996). Importantly, for those children who had same-sex
friends and then secondarily reported other-sex friends, social adjustment
was as high as for those with only same-sex friends. These results indicate
that other-sex friendships serve different functions at different ages, and
perhaps more importantly, they demonstrate that there is variability in
other-sex friendships. Additional research should look more closely at
these within-group differences.

As these findings illustrate, a discussion about the significance of
other-sex friendships in adolescence must attend to gender differences.
Most studies demonstrate robust differences between boys and girls
in their participation in and perception of other-sex friendships. Girls
tend to prefer same-sex friends over other-sex friends more than boys
do (Bukowski et al., 1999), and they name more same-sex and other-sex
friends than boys do (Blyth et al., 1982). Even so, within other-sex friendships, adolescent girls report more positive features, such as sensitivity,
giving, sharing, affection, intimacy, companionship, and emotional closeness, than boys do (Lempers & Clark-Lempers, 1993; Sharabany et al.,
1981), and they experience greater increases in intimacy and companionship with age than boys do (Buhrmester & Furman, 1987; Sharabany et
al., 1981). Other-sex relationships may also include friends who are (or
may be) romantic relationships, muddying the water a bit unless clear
distinctions are made between nonromantic other-sex friendships and
other-sex romantic relationships (e.g., Johnson, 2004, explicitly excluded
romantic partners as other-sex friends, whereas Bukowski et al., 1999,
used the term *other-sex friend* more broadly). For example, boys rate
romantic friends as more supportive than same-sex friends, but girls rate
same-sex friends as more supportive than romantic friends (Furman &
Buhrmester, 1992). By middle adolescence, girls report greater intimacy
with same-sex friends than with other-sex friends or boyfriends, but boys
rate same-sex friends and girlfriends as equally intimate (and more intimate than other-sex friendships) (Buhrmester & Furman, 1987). Finally,
it may be that there are greater differences between other-sex friendships
for boys and girls in terms of rewards gained from the relationship, especially when compared to same-sex friendships and romantic relationships
(i.e., for girls, the relationships contribute to self-development, and for
boys, they help with the development of romantic relationships) (Hand
& Furman, 2009).

We are left with the question, What functions do other-sex friends
play in adolescence? The answer seems to be that they can serve different functions for different adolescents. At least some of the functions of

other-sex friends are these: Theoretically, other-sex friendships serve as additional contexts for self-exploration and identity development (Erikson, 1968), and empirically, we understand that these friendship experiences must be integrated with same-sex friendship experiences (Lempers & Clark-Lempers, 1993). Much like same-sex friends, other-sex friends serve as sources of companionship and intimacy, particularly among older adolescents. For some adolescents, other-sex friendships may compensate for the lack of high-quality same-sex friendships (Bukowski et al., 1999). Finally, other-sex friendships may be an important precursor to romantic relationships (Dunphy, 1963). Hand and Furman (2009) evaluated opposite-sex and same-sex friendships from the perspective of social exchange theory, evaluating the rewards and costs of these different relationships. They asked twelfth-grade students what they liked and disliked about these various types of relationships. The rewards of opposite-sex friendships included learning about the opposite sex, perspective taking, and a connection to meeting other opposite-sex friends and potential romantic partners. Some of the costs included confusion about the relationship and a lack of intimacy and compatibility. Hand and Furman, however, did not find support for the idea that opposite-sex friendships are "unrealized romantic relationships" (p. 281). Instead, they are a valued relationship with distinct rewards and costs compared to same-sex friendships and romantic relationships.

With very few exceptions, our knowledge base of other-sex friendships comes from studies comparing adolescents' perceptions of various features of relationships with same-sex and other-sex friends. The next step is to investigate more clearly the proposed functions of other-sex friends in two ways. First, substantial work needs to be done on the associations between adolescents' experience and friendship quality within both same-sex and other-sex friends and their psychosocial adjustment. For example, why do unpopular youth name other-sex peers as friends? Why do other-sex friendships serve as a buffer against decreases in feelings of well-being for boys without a same-sex friend but not for girls? What accounts for the increases in intimacy with other-sex friends across adolescence? Questions such as these can provide us with a fuller understanding of the developmental nature and meaning of friendship. Longitudinal research, ideally, would more closely examine the shift from same-sex to other-sex friendships, giving us a more complete picture of the social, emotional, and cognitive processes that underlie this important transition. Additionally, longitudinal research of this nature would allow us to examine various pathways and associated outcomes (e.g., early shift to other-sex friends vs. late shift to other-sex friends).

Other-Race/Ethnicity Friendships

Just as psychological research overwhelmingly focuses on same-sex friendships, most, too, includes middle-class children and adolescents of the racial/ethnic majority group (Graham, Taylor, & Ho, 2009). Among the numerous reasons for a relative lack of research on racial/ethnic minorities' friendships are (1) when cross-race friendships are present in samples, they are often not differentiated from same-race/ethnicity friendships and, thus, are not specifically examined (Kawabata & Crick, 2008); and (2) research questions about racial/ethnic minority groups center on family relationships and dynamics more often than friendships and peer relations (Smokowski, Bacallao, & Buchanan, 2009). Notwithstanding these considerations, here we briefly discuss the two primary research questions asked about friendship and race/ethnicity: (1) What is the racial/ethnic make-up of friendships? and (2) What are the benefits of in-group and out-group ethnic friendships (Riegle-Crumb & Callahan, 2009)? We limit our focus to studies that include Hispanic and black youth, with European American youth most often serving as the comparison group (see Graham et al., 2009, for a more comprehensive review of race and ethnicity in peer relations research).

With regard to the first question—What is the racial/ethnic make-up of friendships?—previous research overwhelmingly indicates that youth of all races/ethnicities are more likely to befriend others who are of the same race/ethnicity as themselves (e.g., Graham & Cohen, 1997; Hamm, 2000; Hamm, Brown, & Heck, 2005; Kawabata & Crick, 2008; Way & Chen, 2000). There are mixed findings as to whether this trend is on the rise (e.g., Schofield & Eurich-Fulcer, 2004) or not (e.g., Aboud, Mendelson, & Purdy, 2003); nevertheless, the answer to the question of whether similarity in race/ethnicity is sought after in friendships is a clear "yes." In fact, in one study on "cross-race friendship potential," when presented with cards that depicted black and white characters, white youth were less likely to judge a black character as a potential friend (McGlothlin, Killen, & Edmonds, 2005). This result was not found for a sample of black youth in a related study (Margie, Killen, Sinno, & McGlothlin, 2005); in other words, these children did not see less potential for friendship with other-race/ethnicity characters. These findings confirm earlier research on friendship preferences (e.g., Clark & Ayers, 1992; Levy, 2000). Finally, there is evidence that same-race/ethnicity friendships are generally sought more with increasing age; however, same-sex/cross-race/ethnicity friendships may increase with age for boys (but not for girls) due to their larger social networks (Graham & Cohen, 1997; Graham, Cohen, Zbikowski, & Secrist, 1998). Nevertheless, we must be cautious when we consider the magnitude of racial/ethnic preferences for friendships, as Graham's research demonstrates that same-*sex* preferences are still stronger than same-race/ethnicity preferences (Graham & Cohen, 1997).

With regard to the second question, demonstrating the complexity of research on race/ethnicity and friendship, there is evidence for potential benefits of cross-race/ethnicity friendships as well as in-group friendships. Cross-race/ethnicity friendships for minorities are associated with more positive outcomes. For instance, they are associated with higher academic success (LaFromboise, Coleman, & Gerton, 1993) and better social adjustment, such as leadership skills (Kawabata & Crick, 2008). However, other studies have found the opposite trend (e.g., Riegle-Crumb & Callahan, 2009; Spencer, Noll, Stoltzfus, & Harpalani, 2001). As an illustration, Riegle-Crumb and Callahan (2009) found that in-group friendships were beneficial to academic achievement for Hispanic adolescents. An important point here is that, regardless of who specifically befriends whom, youth benefit when there is a critical mass of same-race/ethnicity peers in the school context (Benner & Graham, 2007). Otherwise, youth have a harder time fitting in and finding their place within the social culture.

In sum, the research on friendships of racial/ethnic minority youth is complex. In some instances minority youth benefit from having outgroup or other-race/ethnicity friendships, and in other cases, they do not. Confounding variables such as family structure, neighborhood, socioeconomic status (Kawabata & Crick, 2008), generational status, availability of other race/ethnicity peers, regional differences (e.g., minorities are more likely to attend school in the South where one-third of students are Hispanic; Riegle-Crumb & Callahan, 2009), and language (e.g., Suarez-Orozco & Suarez-Orozco, 2001) all have the potential to influence friendship formation as well as the relationship between friendship and various outcome variables, such as academic achievement and social adjustment. As an illustration of the importance of taking into account many of these variables and the complexity of this research, Riegle-Crumb and Callahan (2009) considered ethnicity, gender, and generational differences in friendships and found that, when parent education was taken into account, girls showed a positive effect of having more *third-plus generation* friendships, but boys' higher academic achievement was associated with both *immigrant and third-plus generation* friendships. The authors suggest that girls may be closer to their families and, thus, acquire their cultural identity from family, whereas boys may find their cultural identity through their friends.

Given the growing number of ethnic minority children and adolescents in the United States, additional research regarding race/ethnicity and friendship is warranted. Additionally, it is important that this research consider both the unique characteristics within and across racial/ethnic groups.

THREE IMPORTANT TASKS OF ADOLESCENCE

The differences in friendships from childhood to adolescence reflect in part some of the important developmental tasks of adolescence. As Buhrmester notes, "The central features and interactional qualities of friendship change in tandem with the issues and concerns that are at the forefront of individual development" (1996, p. 165). Adolescents' friendships both contribute to and are affected by the ways in which an adolescent successfully manages these tasks. Here we discuss three tasks that are central to individual development in adolescence and represent both the challenges and opportunities of this development period: (1) balancing relationships with parents and peers, (2) establishing an identity, and (3) developing romantic relationships.

Balancing Relationships with Parents and Friends

At a very basic level, the period of adolescence brings with it a change in the relative amount of time youth spend with important others. There is a decrease in the amount of time spent with parents, with a corresponding increase in the amount of time spent with friends (Larson, Richards, Moneta, Holmbeck, & Duckett, 1996; Richards et al., 1998). Despite this shift in the amount of time spent with friends and parents, we are careful not to imply that suddenly peers and friends take on larger-than-life significance that completely overshadows the importance of parents. This is the view of adolescence often highlighted by television shows, movies, and the mainstream media. Instead, there is usually a balance between the influence of peers and the influence of parents in the lives of adolescents (Collins & Steinberg, 2006; Parke et al., 2002), with each relationship addressing different issues of concern for the adolescent (Wang, Peterson, & Morphey, 2007). Furthermore, over the course of adolescence, both friendships and parental relationships become more differentiated (Brown & Klute, 2003). That is, adolescents maintain their established relationships within their family but they begin to expand their relationships outside of the family in unique and meaningful contexts that did not exist in the same way during the childhood years.

Clearly, some of the central tasks of adolescence include individuation, gaining increased autonomy, and renegotiating relationships with parents. Despite the influence of the psychoanalytic perspective that dominated views on adolescence until fairly recently, this realignment of family relationships does not have to include "detachment" and does not have to occur amidst storm and stress. In fact, it usually doesn't. Temporary "perturbations" between parents and adolescents are more common than major upheavals (Steinberg, 1990; Zimmer-Gembeck & Collins, 2003; for a review, see Collins & Steinberg, 2006). As a result, important questions to ask about balancing relationships with parents and friends in adolescence include How can we characterize closeness in adolescent–parent as compared to adolescent–friend relationships? What are the developmental pathways of attachment to parents and friends during adolescence? How do parents and friends contribute uniquely and jointly to adolescent adjustment? Do friends replace parents in roles once held by parents, or does adolescence present a new set of challenges for which the adolescent seeks out close friends for support? Our goal in this section is to identify the unique functions of friendship for the adolescent as compared to parental relationships in the areas of closeness, attachment, and adjustment.

Closeness with Friends and with Parents

Parent–adolescent relationships illustrate how the study of close relationships and "closeness" within relationships can take on many forms. For instance, researchers may assume two people are close because of the nature of their *relationship* (e.g., friends or parent–child) or because of the nature of the *interaction* between the two people (e.g., intimacy, understanding, and affection) (see Repinski & Zook, 2005, for a review of conceptual issues in the study of "closeness"). Adolescents' relationships with their parents and their friends are assumed to be close—by definition and as a result of the interactions that occur between them.

Closeness may be characterized by interdependence (frequency of interaction, diversity of activities, strength of influence), emotional tone (degree to which people experience positive and negative emotions with the partner), and subjective opinion (how close they characterize the relationship to be) (Berscheid, Snyder, & Omoto, 1989; Repinski & Zook, 2005). In their study of adolescents in grades 7, 9, and 11, Repinski and Zook (2005) examined differences in adolescents' relationships with their parents and friends in these three areas and found unique roles of parents and friends in providing closeness. Based on interdependence, closeness was highest with mothers compared to fathers and friends, but based on emotional tone and subjective opinion, there was more closeness with friends than with parents. Thus, adolescents seem to maintain frequent interactions with their mothers even as friends take on increasing emotional connections and subjective feelings of closeness. Repinski and Zook suggest that the high regard for friends reflects the normative

process of increased autonomy during adolescence or the increased conflict between mothers and adolescents. In general, conflict tends to be
more angry with parents than friends during adolescence (see Laursen &
Collins, 1994, for a review).

Emotional support is a form of closeness that comes from multiple
sources throughout adolescence. In a longitudinal study of Dutch children and adolescents from 9 to 18 years, Bokhorst, Sumter, and Westenberg (2010) found that parents and friends were perceived as equally
supportive from ages 9 to 15, and it was not until 16 to 18 that emotional
support from friends exceeded emotional support from parents. Intimacy
is another indicator of closeness, and intimacy with both parents and
friends is quite high in adolescence. In contrast to earlier "storm and
stress" models of adolescent relationships with parents (e.g., Freud, 1958),
more recent conceptualizations of this period suggest that the majority
of adolescent–parent relationships are high-quality, close relationships
in which parents still have influence over their children's decisions (e.g.,
Bengtson, Biblarz, & Roberts, 2002). In general, Bengtson and colleagues
(2002) concluded that adolescents viewed their friends as more influential for making choices with short-term consequences (e.g., music preferences), but parents were more influential for choices that had longer-term
consequences (e.g., educational success and school involvement, alcohol
and cigarette use). These findings support the argument advanced above
that parents and friends exert influence in different domains, in different
ways, and under different circumstances (see Kandel, 1996, for a review
of relative influence with regard to substance abuse).

One conclusion about the closeness to parents versus friends is that
the relationships in adolescence may differ in the nature of their "closeness" but both parents and friends more often reinforce and support one
another than exist at odds (Parke et al., 2002). In addition, the links
between perceptions of closeness and perceptions of support from parents
and peers may be reciprocal. In a longitudinal study across adolescence,
perceived support from parents systematically predicted support from
peers, especially in early to mid-adolescence, and support from friends
over time predicted support from parents from early to late adolescence
(De Goede, Branje, Delsing, & Meeus, 2009). In many cases, parents and
friends have similar directions of influence on adolescents (e.g., Kandel,
1986, 1996). It seems to be most valuable to consider under what circumstances and in what areas of life adolescents turn to their friends and their
parents rather than pitting these two relationships against one another
and assuming that if one relationship is valued, the other cannot be as
well. Although we focus on closeness, the question of influence inevitably
arises. To this end, Kandel's (1978, 1986, 1996) extensive work on substance abuse can guide our understanding of parent and friend influence.

Her work clearly shows both how parents and how peers differentially influence the adolescent and how they can have similar influences on adolescents.

Attachment to Parents and to Friends

A second way of examining the nature of adolescent friendships in comparison to relationships with parents is by using an attachment framework. Although there is a body of literature that demonstrates that early attachment with parents predicts later psychosocial adjustment and attachment with peers (see Chapter 5; see also Allen & Land, 1999), our interest here is in answering the following question: What is the relative importance of attachment to parents and to friends in adolescence?

Although research suggests that children turn to parents in times of need and adults turn to a spouse, partner, or friend, it is less clear to whom adolescents turn (see Nomaguchi, 2008). It can be argued from an attachment standpoint that until late adolescence and early adulthood, adolescents should still use parents as their primary attachment figures (as compared to friends and romantic partners) because peer relationships are not stable enough to provide the level of emotional security that parents offer (see Kobak, Rosenthal, Zajac, & Madsen, 2007). Cui, Conger, Bryant, and Elder (2002) suggest that adolescents' choice of a parent as a primary attachment figure is developmentally appropriate and actually contributes to higher-quality friendships. Several studies have found support for this hypothesis. In one study, researchers found that in early and middle adolescence, those who selected peers (either romantic partners or friends) over parents as primary attachment figures were more likely to be involved in delinquent behavior (Nomaguchi, 2008), and those in middle to late adolescence who nominated peers over parents tended to show more anxiety (Freeman & Brown, 2001).

It makes theoretical sense that adolescents who have an ongoing secure attachment to a parent will transfer and generalize their sense of security, experience of trust, and supportive nature to their friendships. In a direct comparison of attachment to parents, peers, and a close friend, Wilkinson (2010) found that maternal attachment was the strongest predictor of positive adolescent adjustment. Nevertheless, security of attachment to friends was also important. High levels of anxious and avoidant attachment with a best friend predicted higher depression, lower self-competence, and lower positive attitudes toward school above and beyond attachment to parents and peers in general. In contrast, other studies have found that although adolescents who are securely attached to both parents and peers are the most well adjusted, security of attachment to peers alone is more closely related to positive adjustment than security of attachment to parents alone (e.g., Laible, Carlo, & Raffaelli, 2000; Laible & Thompson, 2000).

Perhaps the most compelling argument about the relative contributions of parent and peer attachments to adolescent functioning is that parent and peer relationships (including friendships) both serve important functions in adolescence—some overlapping and some distinct (Doyle, Lawford, & Markiewicz, 2009; Furman, Simon, Shaffer, & Bouchey, 2002). For instance, it may be that parents serve as important sources of security, and best friends and romantic partners meet other attachment needs such as comfort, support, and reassurance (Allen & Land, 1999; Hazan & Zeifman, 1994; Markiewicz, Lawford, Doyle, & Haggart, 2006). It is also likely that at different times in adolescence, these attachment relationships have different meanings; in other words, it may be that the most important and developmentally appropriate shift in attachment takes place in late adolescence when there is a tendency to turn to peers more due to increased and timely autonomy from parents (Steinberg, 1990).

Attachment in adolescence is clearly a changing system as the adolescent becomes more autonomous and emotionally mature. Additional research into attachment and friendship in adolescence will help guide researchers to a more in-depth understanding of which aspects of attachment can be best satisfied with friends and which are best satisfied by parents. Also, it is likely the case that as the intimacy in adolescent friendships matures, friends become better able to help each other as true attachment partners.

Adolescent Adjustment Based on Support from Parents and Friends

A third way to consider the significance of relationships with parents and peers in adolescence is to examine the social support adolescents receive from parents and friends and how that support contributes to adjustment. In general, there are several possibilities. First, support from parents and support from friends could both be related to adjustment. In fact, Laursen and Mooney (2008) found a high correlation between support in the two relationships; in other words, some individuals have "sets" of supportive or unsupportive relationships. So, parental support and friend support could be redundant and associated with the same outcomes, or parental support and friend support could be associated with different outcomes (e.g., parent support might relate to academic outcomes, and friend support could be most related to loneliness or internalizing distress). Second, support from one relationship might be more important across the board (e.g., parent support is always more strongly associated with well-being than is support from friends). Third, as long as one relationship is supportive, that support provides a buffer against the deleterious effects of low support in other relationships (threshold model of support) (Laursen & Mooney, 2008). Fourth, the support from various relationships might accumulate in an incremental way so that, for example, two highly supportive relationships are better than one, and one is better than none (additive model of support) (Laursen & Mooney, 2008).

The available evidence does not overwhelmingly favor any particular one of these models but together suggests that adjustment and well-being hinge on both support from parents and support from friends. Yet, these two types of relationships seem to be complementary, and the associations between relative levels of support and adjustment are complicated at best. Four recent studies illustrate the lack of a simple answer to the question about how support from parents and friends contributes to adolescent well-being.

First, in a sample of Dutch 12- to 20-year-olds, Scholte, van Lieshout, and van Aken (2001) found that nearly two-thirds of adolescents had average or better overall support from both best friends and parents and were well adjusted. For the other one-third of adolescents, however, compromised social support from important others was associated with various patterns of maladjustment. First, adjustment problems were evident in those who had no best friend coupled with low parent support—these adolescents were lonely and socially inept but highly focused on their academics. Interestingly, they did not compensate for the lack of a friend by seeking more support from their parents. Second, those with an unsupportive best friend and unsupportive parents showed both internalizing and externalizing difficulties, with low self-ratings of well-being and high bullying and delinquency. Third, adolescents with a highly supportive best friend but unsupportive parents were aggressive, had low self-esteem, and showed problem behavior at home and in the classroom. For this group, a highly supportive friendship did not buffer the negative effects of poor parental support, and perhaps exacerbated the problems. The most obvious conclusion is that support from both parents and friends is optimal, and not surprisingly, low support from both parents and friends is a risk factor for considerable maladjustment. The findings argue against the idea that a friend can make up for low parental support and may reflect important individual differences based on who the friend is (as discussed in Chapter 5). It may be that adolescents without supportive parents are those whose primary support comes from deviant peer groups, thus contributing to problem behavior.

Second, Rueger, Malecki, and Demaray (2008) asked adolescents how often they receive various types of support from different people (parent, teacher, classmate, friend). For example, they were asked how often their parents listen to them when they are mad and how often their close friend gives them advice. Girls reported receiving more support from friends than from parents, but boys did not differentiate between levels of support from parents and close friends. However, for girls, particular adjustment outcomes depended on whether support came from parents or friends. Specifically, greater parental support was associated with lower aggression and conduct problems, but greater support from a best friend was associated with more externalizing problems. For boys, there was not a clear link between support from parents or close friends and various aspects of adjustment.

Third, Laursen and Mooney (2008) compared a threshold model (one high-quality relationship with a parent or a friend is enough) with an additive model (each additional high-quality relationship will improve outcomes) by examining the number of supportive relationships an adolescent has, regardless of whether those relationships are with mothers, fathers, or friends. The findings were somewhat consistent with an additive model because adolescents with the most positive and fewest negative relationships had the best outcomes. Adolescents with few positive and many negative relationships had the worst outcomes. The threshold model was not supported—adolescents with one supportive relationship were no better off than those with none.

Fourth, Vaughan, Foshee, and Ennett (2010) considered maternal support and closeness with friends as predictors of depression symptoms from ages 12 to 16. Although closeness with friends predicted depression symptoms at age 12, this effect disappeared when controlling for maternal support. Thus, although support in the form of closeness with friends was important for warding off depression, it was not as important as support from Mom.

How do we make sense of these myriad findings to answer the question about the significance of support from close friends vis-à-vis support from parents in adolescence? The most obvious (and not surprising) conclusion is that support from both is optimal and they may be complementary. It will be important to determine whether there are particular domains in which support from a particular kind of relationship is more valuable than another. Person-centered approaches (vs. variable-centered approaches) allow us to consider individual differences in different patterns or configurations of support. Such patterns may include adolescents who do not have a close friend but have very supportive parental relationships or adolescents who have a high-quality friendship but unsupportive relationships with their mothers and fathers. It is clear that there is not one relation between parental support, friend support, and adolescent adjustment. That is too simple. Considering the (sometimes small) groups of adolescents with different patterns of support—high support from one relationship and low support in another, for example—provides ways to evaluate the various possibilities described above. These person-centered approaches were used by both Scholte and colleagues (2001) and Laursen and Mooney (2008). Indeed, what these two studies illustrate is that it is the "mixed" groups that are the most interesting and provide more nuanced information about the relative contributions of parents and friends to how adolescents feel about themselves, how well they are accomplishing important development tasks, and how well they are functioning with regard to behavioral and emotional problems. Most notably, additional research in this area could contribute to intervention efforts focused on building networks of support in the various environments in which adolescents live (Rueger et al., 2008).

Establishing an Identity

Consider the following self-description by an adolescent girl:

> " ... and then everybody, I mean *everybody* else is looking at me like they think I'm totally weird! Then I get self-conscious and embarrassed and become radically introverted, and I don't know who I really am! Am I just trying to impress them or what? But I don't really care what they think anyway. I don't *want* to care, that is. I just want to know what my close friends think. I can be my true self with my close friends." (Harter, 1990, pp. 352–353).

This excerpt from a prototypical adolescent's self-description highlights the social nature of the self and the critically important role that close friends may play in the process of self- and identity formation. According to Erikson (1959), it is adolescents' uncertainty about themselves that causes them to identify with "in-groups," become "clannish," stereotype themselves and others, and put themselves and others through a "loyalty test." Throughout these processes, friends necessarily serve as sources of social comparison, as sources of information about how the self is perceived, as providers of feedback and emotional support, and as role models and illustrations of possible selves.

Components of the Self and the Role of Friends

The idea of "self" includes multiple components, including self-understanding, self-esteem, and identity. Self-understanding incorporates our conceptions and knowledge of the "self-as-known" and the "self-as-knower" (Damon & Hart, 1982). It thus includes knowledge about attributes, material possessions, roles and relationships, thoughts, and other characteristics as well as self-reflections and feelings that the self is distinctive and unique. *Self-understanding* can be considered the cognitive component of self-concept. In contrast, *self-esteem* is the evaluative component of self-concept that defines how we feel about our worth and value. Adolescents have a general self-esteem that includes their overall sense of themselves as valuable and worthy individuals and more specific domains of self-esteem, including academic, social, physical appearance, friendship, romantic appeal, and job competence (Harter, 1998, 2006).

Identity development is considered a major developmental task in adolescence, and it is a multifaceted process that involves defining the self, identifying values, and determining life goals and directions. The environment offers varying levels of support and opportunities for exploration and commitment (Bosma & Kunnen, 2001; Grotevant, 1987). Peers and friends do so by providing role models and opportunities for exploring and "trying on" different identities. For example, in late adolescence, career development is an important identity-related task, and friends provide comfort and security that may encourage and help adolescents explore and take risks related to career decision making. Felsman and Blustein (1999) found that attachment and intimacy with friends were central in promoting confidence and competence related to the successful transition to work roles. In addition, identity development is fostered by interaction with diverse peers, such as in extracurricular activities that encourage exploration of values and roles (Barber, Stone, Hunt, & Eccles, 2005).

The content of one's self-concept changes from childhood to adolescence and from early to middle to late adolescence. Adolescents' self-concept contains more abstract ideas about the self that become possible with advancements in cognitive abilities and the emergence of what Piaget calls formal operational thought. In early adolescence, in particular, personal characteristics that are important for social status and friendships are salient features of self-representations (Damon & Hart, 1988; Harter, 2006)—for example, an early adolescent might emphasize that she is "good-looking, funny, and generally fun to be around." Compared to children, adolescents' more complicated and diverse social experiences can result in the emergence of *different selves* in different relationships. As is evident in the excerpt at the beginning of this section, adolescents may describe being different with parents, close friends, and other peers. Contradictions in descriptions of these different selves can lead adolescents to wonder about the "real me," and by middle adolescence, youth are capable of discerning these contradictions but are not yet able to integrate them effectively (Harter, 2006). This ability does not emerge fully until late adolescence. Nevertheless, adolescents' self-descriptions are more integrated than children's, and as adolescents include enduring attitudes, beliefs, and goals in their self-concept, they move toward a unified and coherent self that fosters identity development.

Social Influences on Self-Concept

Adolescents' self-concepts incorporate attitudes and beliefs that valued others hold about them, and they rely on social comparison and others' opinions about them as feedback in the process of developing a sense of self. By mid-adolescence, preoccupation with what important others think about them is at its height (Harter, 2006). Cooley (1902) described the "looking-glass self" to suggest the importance of the social world in the development of self. "Each to each a looking glass/Reflects the other that doth pass" (Cooley, 1902, p. 152), and Mead (1934) suggested that adolescents' self-perceptions are based on beliefs about how they are perceived by others. Through social experiences with peers and friends, adolescents come to understand that the self can be an object of others' perceptions. This understanding leads to the emergence of a "generalized other"—those norms and social behaviors that are appropriate to particular social groups and social settings. According to Mead, perspective-taking abilities and a self-concept develop hand in hand, and interactions with others, including peers and friends, are crucial to the development of self.

We could also conceptualize the role of friends in the development of self as an "arena of comfort" (Call & Mortimer, 2001; Simmons & Blyth, 1987). An arena of comfort is described as a "soothing and accepting context or relationship" that allows an adolescent to feel safe while managing challenging or stressful experiences in other domains of life. If friendship serves as an arena of comfort, it is viewed as a protective factor. This comfort allows an adolescent to manage normative developmental transitions (e.g., school transitions) and tasks (e.g., identity development) as well as non-normative stressors (e.g., parental divorce) more successfully. In addition, adolescents' selection of particular friends and the comfort and security they feel with friends help to determine the kind of feedback they receive about the self. Indeed, empirical findings show that comfort with friends is associated with high self-esteem (Call & Mortimer, 2001).

Empirical Research on Friendship and Self-Esteem

Although there is rather extensive theoretical discussion of the important role peers and friends play in the development of self for social comparison, for emotional support and comfort, and for specific feedback, it is surprising that very little recent empirical attention has investigated these functions of friends. As indicated earlier in this chapter, most often this research takes on the question of identifying which is more important—parental influence or peer influence—in determining identity development. One study showed that adolescents with close, supportive ties to peers more actively explored what they value in relationships and were more committed to a relational identity (i.e., commitment to a relationship and interest in exploring the other person in the relationship) than those with less attachment to peers and friends (Meeus, Oosterwegel, & Vollebergh, 2002). Attachment to parents, in contrast, had no association to adolescent relational identity but was associated with commitment to school. These findings support the hypothesis that peer versus parent influences differ and that future-oriented issues of identity (e.g., school) are more closely tied to parental influence whereas attachment to peers is most related to present-day situations (e.g., relational identity).

Self-esteem in adolescence may be both a determinant and an outcome of friendship experiences, meaning that having a friend or having a high-quality friendship may promote self-esteem and also that adolescents with high self-esteem may be more capable of establishing positive friendships than those with low self-esteem. Sullivan's (1953) conceptualization of friendship suggests that friendship and self-esteem are closely intertwined. He notes that friends are primarily concerned with "what should I do to contribute to the happiness or to support the prestige and feeling of worth-whileness of my chum" (p. 245) and suggests that intimacy between friends "permits validation of all components of personal worth" (p. 246). As such, supporting one another's self-esteem is a primary feature of friendships, and enhancing one another's sense of self-worth may be a crucial function of friendships. To be fair, Sullivan also suggested that children who emerge from what he called the juvenile era with various forms of maladjustment (i.e., "warps") may be able to form a close friendship in preadolescence. If so, the experience of "get[ting] a look at oneself through the chum's eyes" (p. 254) serves the function of "expanding" and in a sense correcting the self-system. These are exceptions to the rule, however, and from a normative perspective, Sullivan's view is that friendships foster the development of the self and contribute to self-worth (see also Berndt, 2004).

Empirical research allows for more modest conclusions about friendship as a determinant of self-esteem in adolescence than Sullivan (1953) suggested. There is some evidence that adolescents without a friend have lower self-concepts than adolescents with a friend (Mannarino, 1978) and that having a reciprocal friend (vs. being chumless) in adolescence is associated with higher self-worth in young adulthood, even after controlling for the adolescents' earlier levels of self-worth (Bagwell et al., 1998).

Among younger children, chronic friendlessness in elementary school is associated with low self-concept the next year (Ladd & Troop-Gordon, 2003). One study of preadolescents confirms that the association between having friends or not and self-esteem may also operate in the other direction with self-perceptions in part determining whether adolescents have a friend or not (Salmivalli & Isaacs, 2005). Specifically, among preadolescents, negative self-perceptions predicted friendlessness 4 months later, but being friendless did not lead to changes in self-perceptions the following year.

An often-cited hypothesis is that *high-quality* friendships contribute positively to self-esteem. This link has been found in numerous correlational studies (see Berndt & Murphy, 2002; Hartup, 1993; Hartup & Stevens, 1997; Klima & Repetti, 2008). In a recent qualitative analysis, Azmitia, Ittel, and Radmacher (2005) evaluated adolescents' narratives about their friendships and found that adolescents with high self-esteem included trust and loyalty as key characteristics of their friendships more than adolescents with low self-esteem did even though trust and loyalty were equally important expectations of friendships in general. Similarly, adolescents with high self-esteem named many experiences in which their friends were important sources of emotional support, but those with low self-esteem recounted experiences where their friendships did not provide the emotional support they needed. Consistent with the theoretical idea that friendships serve as important sources of social comparison, Azmitia and colleagues also found that boys with low self-esteem much more frequently recalled and described examples of public social comparisons with friends that were negative (e.g., being teased for coming in last in a race or doing poorly on an assignment) than did boys with high self-esteem. Girls in early adolescence with low self-esteem were more likely to describe experiences with friends that involved social exclusion (e.g., ignoring, excluding her from playing at recess) than girls with high self-esteem. In all of these examples, it may be that adolescents with low self-esteem are more attuned to or more adversely affected by these negative experiences with friends, or it may be that they actually occur more often for adolescents with low self-esteem. Importantly, these findings capture instances in which adolescents link friendships and the self on their own, without prompting. When adolescents with low self-esteem make these connections, they describe experiences that are negative.

In contrast, and as we discuss further in Chapter 6, longitudinal studies that can evaluate whether friendship quality predicts changes in self-esteem have not consistently supported the role of friendship in self-esteem enhancement (Berndt & Murphy, 2002; Klima & Repeetti, 2008), at least above and beyond the importance of support from family (Greene & Way, 2005; Way & Greene, 2006). In these studies, the question asked is whether friendship quality measured at one point in time predicts self-esteem at some later time, after controlling for self-esteem at the earlier time point. In other words, is friendship quality predictive of changes in self-esteem over time? This research question sets a high bar for friendship quality as a predictor because in order to show a statistically significant effect, having a high-quality friendship must predict *changes* in self-esteem even though self-esteem is relatively stable, particularly over a period of several months, such as from the beginning to the end of a school year (a typical length of longitudinal studies). Nevertheless, the available evidence suggests that it is having a friend versus being chumless that is most related to an adolescent's self-esteem. It is less clear that variations in the quality of that relationship result in differences in self-esteem. In fact, Berndt and Murphy (2002) concluded that the hypothesis that high-quality friendships promote self-esteem is a myth. At the very least, we need to avoid making the long-held and seemingly logical assumption that high friendship quality fosters positive self-esteem—an assumption easily found in theory (e.g., Sullivan, 1953) as well as in our everyday understanding of friendship in adolescence as reflected in anecdotal memories, novels, television shows, and other media.

Developing Romantic Relationships

As childhood blends into adolescence, a major change occurs in the central relationships in the lives of many youth. They develop a significant interest in establishing romantic relationships. Indeed, Sullivan (1953) describes the establishment of romantic relationships as the key developmental task in adolescence. Interactions with members of the other sex and thinking about romantic relationships occupy a significant amount of adolescents' time. Although fifth- and sixth-grade youth spend an hour or less each week with members of the opposite sex, high school seniors spend 5–8 hours each week thinking about members of the opposite sex on top of the 5–10 hours they spend in the company of other-sex peers (Richards et al., 1998). Being a part of a close romantic relationship may take time away from friends (Laursen & Williams, 1997), yet the effect of romantic relationships on peer and friendship relations varies greatly (Connolly, Craig, Goldberg, & Pepler, 2004; Furman & Shaffer, 2003). Most typically, the significance of friendship does not decrease as adolescents embark on these new relationships; instead, friendships influence the development of romantic relationships and may be an important precursor to healthy romantic relationships.

We discuss two ways that friendships contribute to the development of romantic relationships in adolescence. First, friendships and other peer relations provide a context within which romantic relationships can emerge. In this way, friendships provide a social structure conducive to the development of romantic relationships. Second, adolescents learn many of the skills necessary for successful romantic relationships within their same-sex friendships. This is because friendships and romantic relationships serve some of the same functions for adolescents. Unfortunately, the research on adolescent romantic relationships focuses almost exclusively on heterosexual relationships. Thus, we limit our discussion to romantic relationships between boys and girls, and it is not clear to what extent the conclusions generalize to the romantic relationships of gay, lesbian, or bisexual youth (see Diamond & Lucas, 2004; Diamond, Savin-Williams, & Dubé, 1999).

Friendships Provide a Context for Romantic Relationships to Emerge

First, friendships contribute to the emergence of romantic relationships by providing opportunities for adolescents to meet and interact with potential romantic partners. In other words, friendships are an important peer *structure* for promoting the initiation of romantic relationships in adolescence. Over four decades ago, Dunphy's (1963) ethnographic study of adolescents led him to propose a developmental progression of structural changes leading from same-sex friendships to romantic relationships. He suggested that adolescents are involved in two different types of peer groups—small groups of same-sex friends that he called cliques and larger groups of mixed-sex peers that he called crowds. In early adolescence, the cliques exist in relative isolation. Then they begin to be close with other small cliques of opposite-sex peers, and eventually, large mixed-sex crowds result from the joining together of many same-sex cliques.

According to Dunphy (1963), the function of cliques and crowds differs. Cliques provide friends opportunities for talking and disclosure, and crowds provide a setting for social activities. Importantly, crowds promote the development of romantic relationships because they provide access to potential partners and opportunities for social activities that foster initial dating experiences. In addition, these mixed-sex groups provide models of romantic relationships for adolescents who are not yet in a relationship (Connolly et al., 2004). Dunphy suggests that by late adolescence the crowd breaks up into small groups of heterosexual couples. In this model, same-sex friendships are essential for the participation in crowds that leads to the emergence of romantic relationships.

Surprisingly, Dunphy's theory has not been subjected to rigorous empirical study, yet as Brown (1990) says, "the validity of [his] stage model is rarely questioned" (p. 187). Connolly and colleagues provide evidence that much of Dunphy's (1963) model holds true for today's adolescents. The number of adolescents' same-sex friends predicted the size of their network of opposite-sex friends, which then predicted whether they were in a romantic relationship the next year (Connolly, Furman, & Konarski, 2000). Thus, involvement in a romantic relationship was indirectly associated with same-sex friendships through the association with other-sex friends. Adolescents involved in a romantic relationship had larger peer networks and more opposite-sex friends than those without a boyfriend or girlfriend (Connolly & Johnson, 1996). Another investigation of students in grades 5, 6, 7, and 8 showed that affiliations in mixed-sex groups and dating activities waxed and waned as would be predicted by Dunphy's model (Connolly et al., 2004). Over the course of the school year, neither type of activity increased for fifth graders. Activities in mixed-sex groups increased for sixth graders. Both mixed-sex affiliations and dating activities increased for seventh graders, and only dating increased for eighth graders. Overall, then, adolescents appear to move from same-sex friendships to mixed-sex group affiliations to dating to a romantic relationship. Nevertheless, these changes occur more fluidly than some strict stage theories suggest, and new romantic relationships do not replace old friendships but instead coexist (Connolly et al., 2004; Connolly & Johnson, 1996).

Competence in Friendships and Competence in Romantic Relationships

The second way in which friendships contribute to romantic relationships in adolescence is that many of the skills that are important for successful romantic relationships also indicate social competence in friendships and are first developed in friendships. Put simply, same-sex friendships and romantic relationships have many features in common (Fehr, 1993). Given that participation in friendships precedes the establishment of romantic relationships, the degree to which adolescents develop the social and emotional skills and competencies that promote high-quality friendships may forecast their success in romantic relationships. Furman (1999, p. 139) refers to this as the "carryover into romantic relationships." Specific skills that are important in both same-sex friendships and romantic relationships include companionship, conflict management, and providing intimacy and support.

Furman and colleagues have described four functions that romantic partners serve (Furman & Buhrmester, 2009; Furman & Wehner, 1994, 1997). Over time they become central to the four behavioral systems of attachment, caregiving, sexual, and affiliative. According to this view, competencies associated with affiliation, such as cooperation and collaboration, are developed with friends and are then important in romantic relationships (Furman, 1999). Thus, the similarity in features of friendships and romantic relationships emerge because both relationships serve an affiliative function. Likewise, Furman and colleagues suggest that adolescents' views or representations of romantic relationships and friendships are similar (Furman & Wehner, 1994). In this conceptualization, views of relationships include both relationship styles and working models of relationships that incorporate ideas about the self, the partner, and the relationship.

Several studies confirm that adolescents' perceptions of features of their friendships and features of their romantic relationships are indeed related. Perceptions of positive characteristics of friendships, including help and aid, nurturance, affection, and intimacy, are strongly related to those same characteristics in current romantic relationships (Connolly & Johnson, 1996), and perceptions of current romantic relationships in turn predict perceptions of romantic relationships 1 year later (Connolly et al., 2000). The same pattern holds for negative features such as conflict. Negative friendship features are highly related to negative features of romantic relationships (Connolly et al., 2000). Importantly, adolescents' perceptions of social support from their best friend do not differ for adolescents with and without a romantic partner or among adolescents with shorter versus longer enduring romantic relationships (Connolly & Johnson, 1996). These findings support the conclusion that support from best friends remains very important to adolescents even when they can turn to a romantic partner as well.

In a comparison of the features and provisions of tenth-graders' relationships with a best friend, a romantic partner, and their mothers and fathers, romantic relationships were much more similar to friends than to parents. Both friends and romantic partners provided intimacy and companionship, but parents were more likely to provide affection, help, and a sense that the relationship will endure (Furman, 1999). Similarly, relationships with parents and relationships with best friends both contributed to the quality of adolescents' romantic relationships. Overall support from friends is higher than from romantic partners in seventh and tenth grades but equal by college age. By this time, older adolescents and emerging adults have likely had a good bit of experience in various romantic relationships and learned what can be expected from romantic partners in general. Also, specific romantic relationships tend to last longer by this time so that there is an opportunity for developing a relationship that fulfills more diverse needs—not only affiliative and sexual but also attachment and caregiving (Furman & Wehner, 1994).

Although it could be expected that the similarities in features of friendships and romantic relationships may be strongest in early adolescence before romantic relationships take on additional attachment and caregiving functions (Furman, 1999), other evidence indicates significant overlap between friendships and romantic relationships beyond early adolescence. For example, when college students describe their actual romantic relationships (dating or marriage), friendship and companionship emerge as the primary types of love described by at least two-thirds of the partners (Hendrick & Hendrick, 1993). And even among married adults, women rate their relationship with their same-sex best friend similar to their relationship with their husbands in terms of the encouragement, support, and general positive feelings it provides. They even rated their friendship as providing more security and comfort than their relationship with their husbands (Voss, Markiewicz, & Doyle, 1999). There is also considerable similarity in the desirable traits in a friend and a romantic partner, in other words, in an ideal relationship. When given a large list of possible attributes and asked to choose the six they would most want in a best friend and the six they would most want in a spouse, college students chose many of the same qualities for the two partners—men chose four of the same and women chose five of the same. They want friends and romantic partners who are communicative, open and honest, and trusting (Laner & Russell, 1998).

In sum, the developmental significance of friendship in adolescence hinges in part on the contributions friendships make to developing romantic relationships. Activities and interactions with friends often lead to group activities with both boys and girls, which allow for dating and romantic relationships to flourish. Competence in friendships forecasts competence in romantic relationships. Once adolescents form romantic relationships, they seem to coexist rather than replace friendships. The children's song about friendship that urges "Make new friends / but keep the old / one is silver and the other gold" holds true as adolescents develop romantic relationships, too. Their friendships continue to prosper and retain considerable significance for them.

More research using a person-centered approach would allow for the consideration of different configurations of relationships and different quality relationships. As an illustration, using a person-centered approach, Laursen, Furman, and Mooney (2006) found that many adolescents have multiple relationships that are intertwined. Additional research could further inform us about whether adolescents who have both a high-quality friendship and a high-quality romantic relationship show the most optimal adjustment and what happens when an adolescent finds support in one friendship or romantic relationship but conflict and difficulty in the other.

CONCLUSIONS

There is no doubt that friendships are significant relationships to adolescents. They spend countless hours with their friends, talking to their friends, and thinking about their friends. Friends are the heroes of numerous novels, movies, and television shows aimed at an adolescent and young adult audience, reflecting the presumed importance of these relationships. The popularity of Facebook and MySpace and other social networking sites also attests to the importance adolescents place on their social world, and especially keeping up with their friends. The fact that adolescents consider their friends to be significant is a foregone conclusion.

The task for empirical research, then, is to consider the significance of friendships for adolescents' successful mastery of the developmental tasks before them. Does having friends, especially good friends, make contributions to developmental outcomes and to adjustment and well-being that cannot be accomplished any other way? Empirical research aimed at answering this question took off in the 1970s and particularly the 1980s. The research subsequently expanded to consider individual differences in adolescents' experiences with friends (e.g., the quality of the relationship, the characteristics of the friends) as predictors of various outcomes—school achievement, externalizing behavior problems, internalizing distress, self-esteem, and social competence, to name a few of the more commonly studied.

What conclusions can we draw about the developmental significance of friendships in adolescence? Adolescence is filled with developmental challenges—renegotiating relationships with parents as one seeks greater independence and autonomy; becoming keenly aware of how one fits in at school and preoccupied with social comparisons and others' perceptions of oneself on the way to developing a more nuanced sense of "Who am I?"; and thinking about and analyzing various interactions with same-sex and opposite-sex peers and figuring out what dating is all about. In sum, adolescents must determine how to accomplish the developmental tasks of balancing parents and peers, establishing an identity, and developing romantic relationships. Friendships play a role in all of these processes.

With regard to establishing autonomy and renegotiating relationships with parents, most adolescent–parent relationships remain close. They are likely to experience minor perturbations in the relationship, but parents are still expected to be primary attachment figures throughout adolescence. For most youth, friends do not "take over" from parents; instead, youth turn both to parents and peers for support. For the most well-adjusted children, parents and friends are complementary, and support from each may forecast different aspects of well-being.

Adolescents may seem preoccupied with self-exploration, with fitting in, with the opinions others hold of them, and with trying to reconcile what they view as apparent contradictions in who they are. Integrating these seemingly contradictory self-descriptions will come later in adolescence with more advanced cognitive abilities (Harter, 2006). An adolescent's best friend may provide an important sounding board while managing these challenges of self-representation and identity development. In their classic work on the roles of parents and friends, Youniss and Smollar (1985) note this valuable aspect of a good friendship:

> Friends will listen, take [adolescents] seriously, and work with them toward clarification. The result is that adolescents believe that they learn more about reality and about themselves from their friends than from anyone else. Indeed, it is within friendship that adolescents feel least as if they are living out a role and most like themselves—the personalities they believe themselves to be. (p. 143)

Surprisingly, there are few empirical studies that directly examine the processes through which friends contribute to identity development despite the strong theoretical arguments that they do. Empirical research is becoming clearer, however, that despite the often-cited hypothesis that having high-quality friendships promotes and enhances self-esteem, we have rarely been able to confirm this link in rigorous longitudinal studies. There is some evidence, in contrast, that being friendless—failing to establish a close friendship—is associated with low self-esteem (e.g., Bagwell et al., 1998).

Perhaps the strongest evidence for the significance of friendship in helping adolescents master developmental tasks is the contribution of friends to adolescents' development of romantic relationships. An adolescent's network of friends and the new inclusion of opposite-sex friends may provide an important context from which a romantic relationship can develop. In addition, the skills and competencies learned in friendships provide the building blocks for successful romantic relationships, especially cooperation, collaboration, and conflict resolution. Adolescent friendships have normative significance by providing a context for the expression of and receipt of intimacy, and this provides a foundation for the interpersonal intimacy in romantic relationships.

In order to really see how friendships matter and to uncover the role friendships play in development during early, middle, and late adolescence, we need longitudinal studies that can help us to tease apart the unique role of friends. Theoretically, it is during adolescence that friendships take on a singularly important role in promoting social and emotional adjustment and well-being (Sullivan, 1953). Surprisingly, despite frequent calls for such research (e.g., Hartup, 1996a), there are few longitudinal studies aimed at identifying links between adolescent friendship experience and later adjustment. In contrast, there are a number of investigations of peer acceptance or peer rejection or other global assessments of peer problems as predictors of later functioning (e.g., Coie, Lochman, Terry, & Hyman, 1992; Coie, Terry, Lenox, Lochman, & Hyman, 1995; DeRosier, Kupersmidt, & Patterson, 1994; Dodge et al., 2003; Laird, Jordan, Dodge, Pettit, & Bates, 2001; Ollendick, Weist, Borden, & Greene, 1992; Parker & Asher, 1987; Woodward & Fergusson, 1999).

Our own work examines whether having a friend in adolescence is associated with long-term adjustment by comparing the adjustment in young adulthood of adolescents with and without friends (Bagwell et al., 1998; Bagwell, Schmidt, Newcomb, & Bukowski, 2001). In 12- and 18-year follow-up studies of a sample of chumless and friended fifth graders, having a reciprocated friend in fifth grade was related in meaningful ways to adjustment in early adulthood. In the first follow-up study (at age 23), having a stable reciprocated friendship in fifth grade uniquely predicted more positive relations with family members, lower likelihood of depressive symptoms, and higher general self-worth (Bagwell et al., 1998). The second follow-up study (at age 28) revealed that having a close friend in preadolescence continued to be associated with a decreased likelihood of depressive symptoms. Not having a friend in preadolescence, combined with being rejected in preadolescence, predicted an increased risk for maladaptive adult adjustment (Bagwell et al., 2001). These long-term longitudinal studies provide evidence of the lasting effects of being without a close friend in adolescence.

As we discuss in Chapter 3, we do not know the direction of these effects. It is possible that missed socialization opportunities associated with failing to establish a stable mutual friendship in preadolescence lead to poor adjustment, including symptoms of depression and low self-worth. It is possible that failing to establish a friendship is simply a marker of other problems that cause maladaptation. And, it is possible that a combination of these models is the best explanation—underlying vulnerabilities contribute to difficulties establishing and maintaining a friendship in adolescence, and these vulnerabilities as well as missing out on the close, supportive, collaborative friendship in adolescence contribute to negative outcomes in early adulthood. Another possibility with this last model is that experiences in friendships attenuate the link between underlying vulnerabilities and later problems such that the negative outcomes are not as bad as they might otherwise be. Controlling for aspects of adjustment in adolescence and noting the unique contributions of friendship and peer rejection to particular dimensions of adult adjustment offer some measure of confidence in the findings described above (Bagwell et al., 1998, 2001).

Additionally, we know that simply the *presence* of a friend does not ensure positive social, emotional, psychological, and cognitive outcomes. Some children with friends have more success both within and outside their friendships than other children with friends do. As Pettit (1997) wrote in a review of Bukowski, Newcomb, and Hartup's (1996) edited volume on friendship over a decade ago:

> To be friendless is to be without an important source of social support, without a mirror with which to see oneself, and without a compan-ion with whom one can pursue pleasurable interests. However, being friended by no means guarantees that one's social development will be enhanced. (p. 808)

At the same time, Hartup (1996a) contended that the data consistently show that children with friends are never worse off than those with-out friends (cf. Bukowski et al., 1999). So, we remain, as in Chapter 3, with the questions, What individual characteristics of the adolescents in a friendship and what characteristics of the friendship dyad account for more or less positive adjustment of adolescents *with* friends? These questions require an idiographic or individual differences perspective on the experience of friendship, and we focus on each in turn in Chapters 5 and 6.

Future Research Directions

There are four other lines of research that seem particularly important for allowing us to make more clear conclusions about the unique devel-opmental contributions of friendships in adolescence. Here we provide brief descriptions.

1. Much of the friendship literature describes positive features of friendship and positive psychosocial adjustment. It could be argued that not enough attention has been paid to what can go wrong in friendships. Yet, it has been acknowledged that highly negative friendships can be damaging (Berndt, 2004). As examples, stability of friendship has been examined more closely than instability of friendship; the ways in which similarity between friends has fostered friendship has been investigated more than the ways in which dissimilarity either fosters friendship or interrupts friendship; the notion that girls are more intimate in their friendships than are boys has been widely accepted, but we have not closely examined the causes and consequences of low intimacy in some

girls' friendships or the nature of intimacy in boys' friendships. Future research efforts should focus on a more thorough examination of the "flip side" of some of our research findings. In addition to gaining a better understanding of adolescent friendships, we also might be better able to create interventions for children and adolescents who are less successful at making and keeping friends (see Chapter 8 for a discussion of friendship interventions).

2. Researchers have begun to address the developmental processes that underlie changes in friendship. We know that cognitive advances contribute to the more sophisticated nature of friendship in adolescence. We also know that social forces external to the child can influence friendship selection, maintenance, and termination. Finally, puberty drives the adolescent to seek new romantic relationships, which, in turn, have the potential to change the nature of friendships. Particularly given the amount of literature that describes friendships, the literature describing the "how" and "why" of adolescent friendships is scarce. Future research should more closely examine the underlying processes that drive changes in friendship with age—for example, advanced stages of reasoning can be linked to compromise and negotiation in relationships, both of which are fostered by and practiced with friends (Piaget 1932/1965; Selman, 1981; Youniss, 1980); complex reasoning can be related to friendship in that this more developed ability allows for better differentiation of levels of friendship in adolescence (Berndt & Perry, 1986; Furman & Bierman, 1984); and perspective taking—"being able to see things through the eyes of the other"—is an important component of intimacy, particularly as it relates to the more mature level of intimacy achieved in late adolescence (Paul & White, 1990, p. 377).

3. Much of the empirical research on adolescent friendship in the last decade focuses on large-scale studies surveying large groups of adolescents (e.g., all the students in one school or all eighth graders at multiple schools) with self-reports as the common methodology. These studies can be especially valuable for testing models of individual differences in friendship (e.g., friendship quality) as predictors of various outcomes. In addition, with large samples, person-centered analyses can allow for the identification of many different groups of adolescents, even small groups (e.g., adolescents with supportive friends but unsupportive parents [e.g., Scholte et al., 2001]; adolescents with a high-quality romantic relationship but no mutual same-sex friend). At the same time, smaller-scale studies, including lab-based studies and observational studies, may be particularly helpful in furthering our understanding of the normative significance of friendship. These kinds of studies provide a better avenue for exploring what happens in friends' interactions—How do friends talk

together? How do they solve problems together? How do they engage with one another? Understanding the processes that occur within friends' moment-to-moment interactions is necessary for a richer, more nuanced and complete understanding of the significance of friendships.

4. Arnett's (2000) theory proposes that there is a stage of development, "emerging adulthood," that occurs after adolescence and before full-blown adulthood (approximately ages 18–25). This increasingly accepted and influential theory is particularly relevant to our discussion of friendship in adolescence because historically, articles published on late high schoolers and college students have used the term *late adolescents* to describe these same youth. Therefore, there is an important intersection between research on friendship in late adolescence (often described as age 18 and older) and emerging adulthood (ages 18–25). According to Arnett (2007), although the literature on friendships of emerging adults is "sparse," friendships of those who are post-high school in industrialized cultures are different from those of adolescents in the following ways: (1) friends play a less prominent role due to a "less peer-centered context" (with the exception of the minority of emerging adults who enter a residential college setting), (2) friends are less influential due to emerging adults' increasing ability to make their own decisions, and (3) friendships are more emotionally deep and complex as the emerging adult is dealing with issues of great importance to him or her. Arnett (2007) concludes that friendships may become more important in emerging adulthood compared to adolescence for some components of socialization but also recognizes that "little research has addressed this question directly." It is important for researchers to reconcile differences in terminology. There is a reality that a 19-year-old is a 19-year-old, whether he or she is referred to as a "late adolescent" or an "emerging adult." So, although they may be conceptualized differently, in reality, we are studying the same people. As the theory of emerging adulthood continues to grow in its prominence in the developmental literature, friendship and peer relations researchers need to better understand the nature of the friendships as youth mature and exit the stage of adolescence.

PART III

INDIVIDUAL DIFFERENCES IN THE EXPERIENCE OF FRIENDSHIP

Chapter 5

The Individuals within a Friendship

Is friendship more important for some children than for others and which characteristics or conditions moderate its importance? Does well-being mediate (i.e., explain) the association between family environments and adequate functioning with peers? The association between friendship and well-being is likely to be complex and friendship is likely to interact with other variables. Brave researchers will happily and profitably pursue these important questions.

—William Bukowski (2004, p. 9)

How is your friendship with David different from your relationships with other kids you know?

I don't try to beat him up as much. And he doesn't bug me as much.

—Charlie, a fourth grader,
describing his relationship with his best friend

What's the best thing about your friendship with Lucas?

I like how much he sticks up for me and that it seems like he's a real friend if you stick up for someone else and I love that about our friendship. He's a really good friend.

When does he stick up for you?

Can I say an example? OK, I joined a kickball game late because my class decided to come out late because kids were cutting up in my class. And I was going to join the kickball game on Lucas's team and I was stepping to the line, and I

157

waited a while until it was my turn to kick and then they
said I couldn't play, and Lucas stood up for me, and said
I could kick a home run, and then I kicked a home run. It
made me feel good because Lucas kept telling everyone just
to give him a chance ... give him a chance at least, and I
kicked a home run. And they kept me on the team.
—JAMES, A FOURTH GRADER,
DESCRIBING HIS RELATIONSHIP WITH HIS BEST FRIEND

Characteristics that children bring to a relationship are key determinants
of individual differences in the friendship experience. Simply stated,
because children are not all alike and because children do not all choose
similar peers as friends, the context or shared environment that is created with any particular friendship is unique. These different contexts
are illustrated in the examples above. Charlie is a highly aggressive child
(based on teacher and peer reports), and his best friend David is special
because this particular relationship does not involve high levels of aggression. James's story, in contrast, suggests that the context provided by his
friendship with Lucas is one in which loyalty, support, and security are
central and highly valued. Considering individual differences in friendships highlights the necessity of examining how friendship is embedded
within multiple levels of social complexity—such as processes at the level
of the individual (e.g., aggression) and the larger peer group (e.g., peer
rejection) (Hinde, 1997; Rubin et al., 2006).

Chapter 5 examines characteristics of individual children and how
those characteristics might affect the formation and maintenance of
friendships and the effects of those relationships. Thus while Chapters
3 and 4 consider friendship as a normative experience in childhood and
adolescence, Chapter 5 considers individual differences in the experience
and effects of friendship based on the characteristics of individual friends.
There are numerous individual characteristics that might have an impact
on children's ability to form and maintain friendships, on the quality of
those relationships, or on the effect of those relationships on their own
adjustment and well-being. We have chosen three to consider in this chapter: (1) attachment history, (2) aggression and antisocial behavior, and (3)
peer victimization. These three characteristics were chosen because they
have been studied extensively so that we can draw conclusions about
their effects based on a substantial literature, they have both positive
and negative effects on friendship, and they represent both previous (e.g.,
attachment history) and ongoing (e.g., aggression) experiences that are
relevant for the friendship context. For example, considering attachment
history as a determinant of friendship assumes that each child brings to
a friendship expectations for the self and others, which affect the child's
behavior within friendships. Another example is the impulsive and often

hurtful behavior associated with aggression that makes aggressive children unpredictable play partners and interferes with their ability to form and then to maintain friendships. Likewise, peer victimization may be both a cause and consequence of friendship difficulties. Victims of peers' aggression have troublemaking and keeping friends, and lacking good friends may increase children's vulnerability to victimization.

ATTACHMENT AND FRIENDSHIP

Theoretical Background

John Bowlby set forth the basic tenets of attachment theory in the 1930s drawing from ethology, information processing, developmental psychology, and psychoanalysis (Bretherton, 1992). By 1950, Bowlby proposed that infants become attached to individuals who consistently and appropriately respond to proximity-promoting signals and behaviors. He later proposed that infants construct internal working models of their attachment figures that constitute representations of the adult's attributes (Bowlby, 1973). These internal working models continue to be formed through early childhood and are one mechanism for explaining continuity in relationships and in the child's developmental pathway.

In initial conceptualizations, the term *internal working model* described the individual's hypothetical, internal mental representation of the self, attachment figures, the environment, and the relations among these components (Bowlby, 1973). Main, Kaplan, and Cassidy (1985) subsequently defined the internal working model as "a set of conscious and/or unconscious rules for the organization of information relevant to attachment, and for obtaining and limiting access to that information, that is, to information regarding attachment related experiences, feelings, ideations" (pp. 66–67). Still more recently, Baldwin (1995) described internal working models from a social cognitive perspective as relational schemes, which function as memory structures to organize information.

According to these theorists, individuals behave differently due to variations in their internal working models of relationships. Early experiences contribute to the development of the internal working model by providing rules to direct and organize attention and memory, to guide behavior, and to appraise situations (Main, 1991). These rules govern the inclusion or exclusion of certain information about self, others, and relationships into the model, and affect the organization of thought. Internal working models are thus influential sources of information and play an active part in guiding behavior. Bowlby (1969) wrote, "The more adequate the model the more accurate its predictions; and the more comprehensive the model the greater the number of situations in which its predictions apply" (p. 81).

According to Bowlby, early interactions with the caregiver lead the child to develop models of self and other that will be complementary, as they both represent aspects of the same relationship (Bowlby, 1973). Infants whose attempts at proximity are appropriately and consistently responded to in a warm and nurturing way will develop qualitatively different internal working models than those infants whose attempts are ignored or are responded to unpredictably. The child who receives sensitive and responsive caregiving will develop an internal working model of others as loving and supportive, and of self as worthy of others' help and love. The child will be able to predict successfully what others will do in future situations. In contrast, the child who receives inconsistent and unpredictable responses from the caregiver, or who is ignored or rejected by the caregiver, will develop an internal working model of others as rejecting, and of self as unworthy of others' attention and nurturing (Bretherton, 1985). In sum, internal working models represent hypothetical models of the world and enable individuals to act in new situations without rethinking each situation (Main, 1991).

Empirical Evidence Linking Attachment with Friendship

Driven by the early work of Mary Ainsworth, attachment researchers have extensively studied the nature and consequences of early child–caregiver attachment relationships. Researchers who find support for the link between quality of attachment and peer relations are advancing the working model concept. From this perspective, children with a healthy internal working model are more likely to have relationships with peers and friends that are characterized by positive expectations, reciprocity, behavioral flexibility, self-confidence, and an ability to modulate negative arousal. Research over the past three decades has provided a great deal of empirical evidence in support of this proposition.

It is widely accepted that children who form secure attachment relationships with their caregivers tend to be more successful in forming and maintaining positive relationships with their peers (Cohn, 1990; LaFreniere & Sroufe, 1985; Park & Waters, 1989; Sroufe & Fleeson, 1986). Belsky and his colleagues (e.g., Belsky & Cassidy, 1994; Freitag, Belsky, Grossmann, Grossman, & Scheuerer-Englisch, 1996) proposed that relationships with peers, more generally, may be related to heritable factors such as sociability, but close friendships should be better predicted by specific characteristics of early attachment relationships. Intimacy characterizes both attachment relationships and friendships and is expected to be the common link between the two. Thus, although early attachments with parents are conceptually and empirically linked with later social competence, including popularity and acceptance in the peer group (which do not involve intimacy), the concept of internal working models suggests that the intimacy within early family relationships would be most important as a determinant of intimate friendships.

To synthesize studies of attachment and peer relations from 1970 to 1998, Schneider, Atkinson, and Tardif (2001) completed a meta-analysis of 63 studies that considered attachment as a predictor of children's peer relations. They reported a global effect size of .20 (a small but not negligible effect) and found that the effect size for predicting friendship was larger than the effect size for predicting aspects of social competence with peers more generally. More recent research adds to the body of work Schneider et al. summarized a decade ago and demonstrates that early attachment security predicts the number of nominations as a "best friend" children have 1 to 2 years later (Wood, Emmerson, & Cowan, 2004), that securely attached adolescents report higher levels of trust in others (Larose & Bernier, 2001), and that attachment security is associated with relying on a best friend for emotional support (Allen, Porter, McFarland, McElhaney, & Marsh, 2007).

Children who have insecure relationships with their caregivers are at risk for concurrent as well as later behavioral, emotional, and social problems. Insecurely attached children have heterogeneous internal working models in part based on the type of attachment insecurity they experience (Doyle & Markiewicz, 1996). Some children will avoid friendships, whereas other insecurely attached children may have friends but possess unrealistic expectations of those friends, which ultimately make them less likely to keep the friends (Selman & Schultz, 1990). For example, children with avoidant attachment histories at 15 months were in friendships characterized by more instrumental aggression at the age of 3 years than those with secure or resistant attachment histories, yet children with resistant attachment histories displayed less self-assertion when interacting with friends than those with avoidant histories (McElwain, Cox, Burchinal, & Macfie, 2003). Other studies have reported that avoidant attachment histories may place children at the highest risk for social isolation (Jacobsen & Hofmann, 1997; Larose & Bernier, 2001). These findings underscore the role that secure versus insecure attachment histories may play in friendship success and suggest that various categories of insecurity may be associated with specific expectations and beliefs about self, other, and relationships (McElwain et al., 2003).

Compared to early childhood, there has been relatively little research on attachment relationships in middle childhood and adolescence (Kerns, 1996; Kerns, Klepac, & Cole, 1996; Verschueren & Marcoen, 2005).

From a theoretical perspective, it is believed that the attachment system becomes a true negotiated partnership during these periods of development (Waters, Kondo-Ikemura, Posada, & Richters, 1991). Although both the intensity and frequency of child–parent interactions demonstrating attachment behaviors may decline in early adolescence, managing the availability of the attachment figure (when needed) is still a goal (Bowlby, 1973). Older children continue to need a secure base, but both the child and the parent now take on shared responsibility for maintaining contact with one another (Kerns, 1996).

Although not abundant, the existing empirical research on attachment and friendship in middle childhood and adolescence sheds light on the continued importance of internal working models in guiding individual behavior and relationships. Several studies have demonstrated that secure attachment histories are associated with more positive interactions with a close friend in fourth grade (Lucas-Thompson & Clarke-Stewart, 2007), a better ability to make friends and to choose friends who also have secure attachment histories (Elicker, Englund, & Sroufe, 1992), and higher friendship competence (Freitag et al., 1996) in middle childhood.

Friendship is also concurrently associated with parent–child attachment. Children and adolescents who rate their parents as more available and who rely on their parents more during stressful times and report feeling very secure with parents have higher-quality friendships and less conflict in their close friendships (Howes, 1996; Lieberman, Doyle, & Markiewicz, 1999) and have more reciprocated friendships in early adolescence (Kerns et al., 1996) than children with less secure attachments. Negative interactions with mothers is associated with adolescents' poorer communication and greater difficulty discussing problems with their best friend, and consistent with attachment theory, adolescents with relatively more dismissing versus secure working models have trouble talking with a best friend about concerns and problems (Shomaker & Furman, 2009).

Another possibility is that friendship quality may mediate or moderate the relationship between early attachment and psychosocial adjustment (Booth-LaForce, Rubin, Rose-Krasnor, & Burgess, 2005; Rubin et al., 2004). Bowlby (1973) suggested that adjustment and well-being at any point is determined by both past experiences and current relationships (Booth-LaForce et al., 2005). As a result, a high-quality friendship may compensate for poor relationships with parents and moderate the association between parent–adolescent attachment and adolescent adjustment. Several studies have investigated these hypothesized associations between attachment, friendship, and psychosocial functioning. One study found that, as expected, adolescents who were securely attached to both parents and friends (friends generally, not a specific close friend) fared best in terms of low externalizing and internalizing problems. Interestingly, adolescents who were securely attached to friends but insecurely attached to parents were better adjusted than those who were insecure with friends but secure with parents, highlighting the central importance of friends in adolescence (Laible et al., 2000). Although their earlier work did not find that a supportive best friend protected against the negative consequences of insecure attachment (Booth, Rubin, & Rose-Krasnor, 1998), Rubin and colleagues (2004) found that for boys, low maternal support was related to poor social competence only when the boys' friendship quality was also poor, and for girls, high-quality friendships buffered the negative effects of low maternal support on internalizing distress.

Together, these findings suggest the potential for a close friend to protect against the negative outcomes associated with poor-quality parent–child attachment relationships. Nevertheless, as we discuss in Chapter 4, adolescents with highly supportive relationships with both their parents and their best friends are the most well adjusted across a variety of important domains. Thus, the buffering hypothesis of friendship receives some support, but the existing evidence does not frame friendship as a solution for all ills, and the associations seem more complex than simply friendship making up for problems in other important relationships, such as poor-quality relationships with parents.

Summary

More than three decades of research has linked attachment with parents to children's experiences with friendship in early childhood, middle childhood, and adolescence. The last meta-analysis of this literature was completed in 2001 and showed a small but meaningful effect size for the association between attachment and friendship. These studies cannot demonstrate causality, yet they are grounded in developmental theory and suggest that attachment history is a critical individual difference variable that may help determine children's ability to make and keep close friends, the features and characteristics of those relationships, and the developmental significance of friendships.

There are a number of remaining questions about the role of attachment in predicting friendship success. First, if we conceptualize attachment history as an individual difference variable that children bring with them to their friendships, then we would want to know about the attachment history of both friends. This dyad approach recognizes that the features and quality of a friendship a securely attached child forms with a peer may depend in part on the partner's attachment history, whether secure or insecure (Kerns, 1996).

Second, greater specificity about what aspects of friendship are influenced by attachment experience is desirable. As we have discussed, friendship is multidimensional, and attachment may be differentially related to particular components of friendship. Children with secure attachment histories may have an easier time initiating and forming friendships, and they are also expected to have higher-quality friendships with greater intimacy and support. As described above, children with secure attachments are also likely to form friendships with children who also have secure attachment histories. By determining and specifying particular challenges that children with insecure attachments face when forming and maintaining close friendships, we would be better able to develop intervention strategies to help them overcome those challenges. For example, is a key problem forming friendships in the first place, or is maintaining high-quality friendships with positive features more of a concern?

Third, initial questions about attachment and friendship focused on uncovering direct effects of attachment on children's success in friendships. More recent research has considered a more complex association in which children's experience in friendships moderates the link between parent–child attachment security and later outcomes (e.g., Booth et al., 1998; Rubin et al., 2004). This view represents a compelling way of thinking about the significance of friendships—in particular, that friendships may compensate for early problems with parent–child relationships or may provide a buffer against insecure attachment by weakening the association between insecure attachment and later adjustment difficulties (e.g., internalizing distress). Conceptualizing friendship as a moderator variable has shown promise as well in explaining the significance of friendship in the experience of peer victimization.

Finally, research on attachment and friendship is typically grounded in the theoretical concept of internal working models, yet as Hinde (1988) and others have cautioned, we need to be careful about using the concept of internal working models "to explain anything" (p. 378) and instead specify more clearly the mechanisms and limitations of the internal working model. Although finding associations between attachment and friendship are entirely consistent with theoretical ideas of the role and influence of internal working models, they offer no "proof" for their existence. It is also likely that the experiences that lead to secure attachment also foster the development of particular social and relationship skills that are advantageous in friendships—the tendency to approach social relationships with a prosocial orientation, and the experience and expectation of reciprocity (Booth-LaForce et al., 2005; Elicker et al., 1992). Additional research that includes multiple measures of parent–child relationships, including attachment security, cognitive representations of relationships, parenting styles, and other features of parent–child interactions, would allow for testing multiple predictors of friendship success and for further specifying the observed link between attachment and friendship experiences.

THE DARK SIDE OF FRIENDSHIPS

For parents of young children entering school for the first time, typical concerns center on questions such as Will they be successful academically? How will they adjust to the demands of school? and Will they fit in with peers and make good friends? A few years later as their children transition to middle school, questions often reflect concerns about the dark side of friendship: Will they get caught up in the "wrong crowd"? and Will their friends lead them astray? Empirical evidence suggests that this concern may be valid for at least some parents.

Attention to how friends might contribute to one another's antisocial behavior (i.e., a class of behaviors including aggression, delinquency, substance abuse, property damage, and other behaviors that inflict harm or property damage on others) soared in the mid-1990s, especially following the publication of several seminal articles by Thomas Dishion and colleagues in the mid-1990s (e.g., Dishion, Andrews, et al., 1995; Dishion, Capaldi, et al., 1995; Dishion et al., 1994, 1996). These studies focused on the features of friendships between aggressive and antisocial boys and documented the powerful process of deviancy training. Research questions centered on the way that interactions between friends promote deviant behavior and predict later antisocial behavior. Surprisingly, this literature on the dark side of friendship has not been well integrated with research on the positive outcomes of friendship. This integration is a critical aspect of understanding individual differences within friendships because it speaks to the idea that their may be adjustment tradeoffs associated with friendships—ways in which particular friendships contribute in both positive and negative ways to well-being and adjustment.

Children who are aggressive and display antisocial behavior in childhood are often rejected by peers. Thus, they have limited opportunities to form friendships with others. Nevertheless, many rejected and/or aggressive children have a mutual friend (e.g., Grotpeter & Crick, 1996; Ladd & Burgess, 1999; Mrug, Hoza, & Bukowski, 2004). Their unfavorable characteristics do not automatically exclude them from involvement in friendship networks or keep them from forming mutual friendships. Although significantly fewer low-accepted children have a mutual friend than do average- or high-accepted children, roughly half of the low-accepted group studied by Parker and Asher (1993) had a mutual best friend. Relationally aggressive children are no less likely than non-aggressive children to have a friend (Grotpeter & Crick, 1996; Rys &

Bear, 1997). Often, the friends and frequent companions of rejected or low-accepted children are themselves not well liked (Ladd, 1983; Parker & Asher, 1993), and although pairs of low- and average-accepted friends are common, it is rare to find a friendship between low-accepted and high-accepted children.

The pairing of two children who are not well liked in their peer group and/or are aggressive is likely due to a combination of two factors. First, because rejected children have few peers who like them, they do not have many choices of peers with whom to form a friendship, and they associate with one another by default. Second, an active process of friendship selection also leads to friendships between two rejected and/or aggressive children. Children seek peers who are fun, who enjoy the same activities, and who provide reinforcement for them. Aggressive children often reinforce aggressive and deviant behavior in others; thus, aggressive children are attracted to peers with similar characteristics, and friendships form between two similar peers. Indeed, aggressive children are liked by peers who are also disruptive, likely to start fights, and less cooperative than other peers (Nangle, Erdley, & Gold, 1996). Friends are even similar in aspects of social information processing associated with aggression. Reciprocal friends' hostile attribution biases predicted adolescents' own hostile attribution biases even when accounting for friends' and adolescents' own aggressiveness (Halligan & Philips, 2010).

Patterson and colleagues refer to this process as a "shopping model"—children shop for peers who are reinforcing to them, and this attraction forms the basis of the friendship (Dishion et al., 1994; Patterson, Littman, & Bricker, 1967). These two processes—association by default and active selection—may differ in salience in childhood and adolescence with the latter occurring more in adolescence than in childhood (Vitaro, Pedersen, & Brendgen, 2007; cf. Werner & Crick, 2004). One test of these processes comes from comparing who aggressive children want to have as friends and who they actually have as friends. Comparisons of preferred friends (unilateral friendship nominations) and realized friends (reciprocated friendship nominations) showed that highly aggressive and nonaggressive boys preferred similar friendships, but their actual relationships differed—highly aggressive boys were more likely to have a friendship with other aggressive boys. Furthermore, their relationships provided low levels of emotional support even though they looked for emotional support in their friendships. These findings support the conclusion that aggressive boys form friendships with others by default—they are "stuck with" friends like themselves (Sijtsema, Lindenberg, & Veenstra, 2010).

As we discuss in Chapter 4, over time, friends may influence one another, and their aggression may increase (socialization effects). The relative importance of selection effects (friendships forming between similar youth) and socialization effects in explaining friends' similarity in aggression has been debated. A recent analysis suggests that the effects may operate differently for subtypes of aggression with selection effects for instrumental aggression but not reactive aggression and socialization effects for both (Sijtsema, Ojanen, et al., 2010).

The Friendships of Aggressive and Antisocial Youth

The features and quality of friendships between aggressive or antisocial children may differ from those of other children because of the individual characteristics that aggressive children bring to their friendships. Compared to nonaggressive children, aggressive children do not have the repertoire of social skills and social competence that are important for establishing and maintaining friendships. Thus, they may not provide the emotional support, skills in conflict management, and careful balancing of intimate exchange that are key elements of high-quality friendships. The context created by a friendship with an aggressive child has particular characteristics and norms that likely differ from other friendships.

There are mixed findings about the quality of the relationship between aggressive or antisocial friends, in part based on whether you ask the friends about their relationship or rely on outside observers' impressions. What do aggressive and antisocial youth say about the qualities of their friendships? The general conclusion is that they describe their relationships in quite similar terms as nonaggressive/nonantisocial youth. When differences do emerge, they indicate lower-quality relationships for antisocial youth and their friends. In one study, antisocial adolescent boys rated their friendship more negatively than nonantisocial boys but did not differ in their perceptions of the positive features of their friendship (Poulin et al., 1999). Notably, the antisocial boys and their friends did not agree about the features and quality of their relationship—the target boys' views and their friends' views of the same relationship were not correlated. In another sample of adolescents, antisocial and nonantisocial friends did not differ in their reports of positive and negative features of the relationship and the time they spent together (Piehler & Dishion, 2007). The friends differed, however, in their assessment of one another's positive personal characteristics, and as expected, antisocial youth reported that their friends had fewer positive characteristics than did nonantisocial adolescents. In our own study of preadolescent boys, we found no differences between aggressive and nonaggressive boys' reports of companionship, closeness, help, security, and conflict with their best friend (Bagwell & Coie, 2004). In addition, the friends of aggressive and nonaggressive boys also reported similar levels of these features in their relationship.

Some clarification of findings about whether and how the friendships of antisocial and nonantisocial youth differ in quality may come from examining different types of aggression—reactive versus proactive or relational versus overt. Proactive aggression (aggression that occurs to achieve a goal) and reactive aggression (hostile, emotionally intense aggression in response to provocation) are associated with friendship quality and satisfaction in opposite directions. Proactively aggressive boys have more supportive, less conflictual, and more satisfying friendships, yet reactively aggressive boys have less supportive, more conflictual, and less satisfying relationships with their best friend. Over time, however, proactive aggression predicts increases in conflict and thus predicts deteriorations in stable friendships (Poulin & Boivin, 1999).

The distinction between relational and overt aggression also illuminates links between aggression and friendship. Grotpeter and Crick (1996) examined 12 characteristics of friendships as a function of children's relational (i.e., aggression aimed at harming another's status and interpersonal relationships) and overt (i.e., including physical and verbal aggression) aggression. Only two characteristics differentiated relationally aggressive and nonaggressive children. Relationally aggressive children reported more exclusivity and intimacy in their friendships. Two characteristics also differed between overtly aggressive boys and girls and nonaggressive peers. Overtly aggressive children reported higher levels of aggression toward others and lower levels of intimacy in their friendships. Interestingly, overtly aggressive children reported that they and their friends engaged in high levels of aggression against others, regardless of whether the friend was aggressive. This finding speaks to the context that a friendship with an aggressive child provides—one in which the friend may be drawn into aggression even if he or she is not otherwise aggressive (Grotpeter & Crick, 1996).

The picture of friendship quality painted by children's and adolescents' own reports ("insider views") of their friendships described above is quite different than the one that emerges from outsider views. In Chapter 2 we discuss potential explanations for this discrepancy between friends' perceptions and outside observers' impressions of friendship quality, including a positive illusory bias for aggressive children or the fact that aggressive children may derive pleasure and satisfaction from interactions with friends that observers view as problematic. In contrast to preadolescent boys' self-reports about their friendships in our own work (described above), when interviewers rated the quality of the friendship based on the boys' open-ended descriptions of their friendship, these ratings showed dramatic differences—nonaggressive boys and their friends were rated as having higher-quality friendships than aggressive boys and their friends (Bagwell & Coie, 2004). When the friends' interactions were observed in a lab setting, nonaggressive boys and their friends displayed more positive social skills (such as cooperation and helpfulness, attentive communication, and warmth), reciprocity, and balance in their interactions. Conversely, aggressive dyads tended to demonstrate more negative styles of interaction that included aggressive and rude behaviors and statements, competitiveness, and an overall negative tone. Interestingly, the nonaggressive and aggressive friends did not differ in the degree to which they seemed to have fun and enjoy being together. This finding is consistent with self-reports that aggressive and nonaggressive boys do not differ in how much fun they have together (Crick & Grotpeter, 1996). Other observational studies conclude that antisocial adolescents have difficulty with the responsive, reciprocal, and positive behaviors that are generally considered important features of friendships (Panella & Henggeler, 1986). Mutuality has also been observed to be lower among antisocial adolescents (Piehler & Dishion, 2007). Teacher ratings provide another "outsider view." For example, among preschool children, teacher ratings of friendship quality show that physically and relationally aggressive children have more conflict in their friendships, and relationally aggressive children also have more exclusivity and intimacy in their friendships (Sebanc, 2003).

When relying on qualitative measures or observer ratings, the findings from these studies converge to suggest that the friendships of aggressive children and adolescents are compromised not only by negative styles of interaction with friends but by a lack of the sometimes subtle positive interplay and mutuality that reflects social competence in intimate peer relationships. Nevertheless, most friendships include a lot of laughter, positive affect, and discussion of common interests, and the friendships of antisocial or aggressive youth are not substantially different in this regard (Dishion et al., 1996).

Deviancy Training within Friendships

In addition to documenting similarities and differences in the features and quality of aggressive and nonaggressive friends, a critical question is what processes occur within the friendships of aggressive children and adolescents that might account for the "dark side" of these relationships. By far the most attention has been paid to the process of deviancy training (e.g., Dishion et al., 1996; Granic & Dishion, 2003). It is a dyadic process in which positive affect between the friends is contingent on deviant talk—talk about rule-breaking behavior and talk that violates social rules or is not appropriate to the setting. Thus, the concept of deviancy training is grounded in learning theory with a focus on identifying contingent patterns of behavior (Dishion et al., 1996).

Deviancy training has been investigated most thoroughly by Dishion and colleagues in a series of lab-based studies in which pairs of male adolescent friends engage in short videotaped conversations. A consistent finding is that antisocial adolescents engage in more deviant talk with friends than nonantisocial youth (Dishion et al., 1996). In addition, examinations of the moment-to-moment sequences in their interactions show that antisocial youth laugh in response to deviant talk, and laughter elicits more deviant talk. In nonantisocial dyads, there is no link between laughter and deviant talk. Thus, the sequential patterns within the friends' conversations are qualitatively different for antisocial and nonantisocial youth, and deviant talk emerges as an important organizing feature within the friendships of antisocial youth (Granic & Dishion, 2003; Piehler & Dishion, 2007). It is clear that conversations with friends provide a context for the transmission of values, beliefs, and attitudes. As such, antisocial friends communicate tolerance for deviant behavior.

The power of deviancy training is quite remarkable. Assessments of deviancy training within merely 25 minutes of conversation between friends predict increases in delinquent behavior (Dishion et al., 1996), escalations in substance use (Dishion, Capaldi, et al., 1995; Dishion & Owen, 2002), participation in violence (Dishion et al., 1997), and amount of aggression toward female romantic partners in late adolescence (Capaldi, Dishion, Stoolmiller, & Yoerger, 2001). Particularly when friends' interactions are well organized (as opposed to chaotic and unpredictable), high levels of deviancy training in adolescence predict high levels of antisocial behavior in adulthood (Dishion et al., 2004), highlighting the powerful nature of deviant talk as an organizing principle for at least some high-risk friendships. In addition, recent work identifies deviancy training in younger and older samples. It occurs between peers as early as kindergarten (Snyder et al., 2005) and is associated with antisocial talk with romantic partners in early adulthood (Shortt, Capaldi, Dishion, Bank, & Owen, 2003).

In our own work, we examined friends' rule-breaking talk as well as rule-breaking behavior (Bagwell & Coie, 2004). Aggressive and nonaggressive preadolescent boys and their best friends were observed interacting in a lab setting where there were opportunities to engage in rule-breaking behavior by cheating on a word scramble task using an answer key, taking candy and other snacks off of a shelf they were told not to bother, and committing other minor rule violations. Pairs of aggressive boys and their friends committed more rule violations than nonaggressive boys and their friends. In addition, they engaged in more rule-breaking talk.

We also assessed talk that represented explorations of potential rule violations but did not involve actual rule-breaking talk, and we labeled this "temptation talk" (Bagwell & Coie, 1999)—for example, talking about the candy on the shelf or wondering aloud about the answers on the answer key without actually taking the candy or using the answer key. We suggest that this kind of talk is an important process in middle childhood because it enables children to get feedback on their ideas and helps them mutually negotiate and figure out the norms of the friendship. Interestingly, the aggressive and nonaggressive friends did not differ in the amount of time they spent in this kind of talk. What appeared to distinguish the two groups is that nonaggressive friends tended to engage in temptation talk and then return to normative topics. For the aggressive friends, in contrast, this exploration was more likely to lead them to action, and they actually then engaged in rule-breaking behavior.

Two examples serve to illustrate. In the first exchange between Nate and Josh (a nonaggressive boy and his friend, respectively), the two boys discuss cheating on the word puzzle with the answer key but eventually go back to work without cheating.

NATE: Let's look on the answer sheet.

JOSH: No.

NATE: (*Laughs.*)

JOSH: I won't, but you can.

NATE: And I'll give you the answers, right?

JOSH: No, not right.

NATE: This is hard. I was kidding. I don't want to look on the answer sheet.

In the second example, Steve and Mark (an aggressive boy and his friend, respectively) are sitting at the table and discuss taking candy off of the shelf. By the end of the interaction, both boys are eating food from the shelf.

STEVE: Let's just get a cookie.

MARK: No, get a tongue twister (*referring to a particular kind of candy on the shelf*). They ain't gonna come in here. Remember, they talking (*referring to the experimenters*).

STEVE: Oh yeah.

MARK: Go get it! A tongue twister.

STEVE: (*Runs to the shelf and picks up a small candy bar*).

MARK: No, not those. A tongue twister.

STEVE: It gonna be too long (*referring to the size of the candy*).

MARK: No, we can just stuff them in our mouth. Just get it. Get it.

STEVE: I'll get you one, and I'll get me a cookie.

MARK: All right.

STEVE: (*Brings Mark the candy he wants.*)

It is not clear what causes these different responses to the initial discussion and exploration of potential rule breaking. Taken together with the research on deviancy training, these findings indicate that there are distinct and predictable ways of interacting between aggressive and nonaggressive children and their friends. The characteristics of a child's friends, such as having an aggressive or antisocial friend, are critical factors in determining the characteristics and outcomes of the friendship experience. Interestingly, Dishion and colleagues' longitudinal studies show that even as specific friends come and go, children and adolescents seem to form other friendships with similar peers. Thus, they argue for "the importance of the specific qualities or characteristics of adolescent friendships and their impact on a youth, rather than the specific people involved in the friendship per se" (Dishion et al., 1997, p. 220).

Models Explaining the Link between Deviant Friendships and Maladjustment

To what extent does deviancy training, or any other process within friendships, cause problematic outcomes such as increased antisocial behavior? There are several models that potentially explain the links between friendships and delinquency. The *causal* and *incidental* models were described by Parker and Asher (1987) in their review of research on links between peer relations and adjustment more generally. We describe them here with a specific focus on friendships and delinquency. Variations of the third model have been described more recently and have been called by a variety of names.

In the causal model (also called the *peer influences model*), there is a direct link between peer relations, such as a friendship between aggressive or antisocial youth, and a particular negative outcome. In this model, associations with deviant friends is a *necessary* component of the pathway that leads to delinquent and other problem behavior (e.g., Elliott, Huizinga, & Ageton, 1985; Simons, Wu, Conger, & Lorenz, 1994). There is some evidence for a sequential model proposed by Patterson and colleagues in the late 1980s and early 1990s (e.g., Patterson, Capaldi, & Bank, 1991; Patterson & Yoerger, 2002) in which early disruptive behavior leads to peer rejection in childhood, which in turn leads to associations with deviant friends in early adolescence. These associations then lead to adolescent delinquency (Vitaro et al., 2007). With regard to deviancy training, the causal model suggests that the process of deviancy training causes increases in problem behavior—friends encourage and promote this behavior during their interactions, and friends even model and engage in that behavior together (Bagwell & Coie, 2004).

In support of a causal model, Dishion and Andrews (1995) report that high-risk youth who were randomly assigned to an intervention to reduce problem behavior that involved group sessions with other high-risk youth showed increases in tobacco use and behavior problems at school 1 year later compared to youth assigned to an intervention that did not involve group sessions. These iatrogenic effects persisted even 3 years later (Dishion, McCord, & Poulin, 1999). The authors hypothesize that the deviancy training that took place even in these highly structured and supervised sessions and the introduction to other high-risk youth that was provided by the intervention group were responsible for the escalations in deviant behavior (Dishion & Andrews, 1995; Dishion et al., 1997).

An *incidental* model suggests that underlying risk factors cause both the problem behavior and poor peer relations. In this model, poor peer relations are a marker for (and are correlated with) negative outcomes, like delinquency, but do not contribute independently to the problem behavior. For example, early disruptive and aggressive behavior, coercive parent–child interactions, difficult temperament, and other factors are responsible for deviant behavior in adolescence. In other words, there is continuity in aggressive and antisocial behavior from childhood through adolescence. Children with these risk factors also form friendships with other antisocial or aggressive youth, and deviancy training within these relationships is thus correlated with later problem behavior but does not contribute in a causal way (cf. Gottfredson & Hirschi, 1990). There is some empirical support for this model (also known as the *individual characteristics* model) with some researchers finding that characteristics of friends do not add to or explain the link between early disruptive behavior and later problem behavior, including substance use and delinquency (Dobkin, Tremblay, Masse, & Vitaro, 1995; Laird et al., 2001; Tremblay, Masse, Vitaro, & Dobkin, 1995). In addition, there is some empirical support for a combination of the causal and incidental models—individual characteristics *and* peer relations both play a role in the trajectories leading to delinquency (Vitaro et al., 2007).

A more middle-ground position that combines elements of the causal and incidental models—called the *enhancement model* (Vitaro, Brendgen, & Wanner, 2005)—suggests that friendships with other aggressive or antisocial youth moderate the association between early problem behavior and later antisocial behavior. In other words, association with deviant friends strengthens the path from early behavior to later delinquency, and may be especially influential for some youth. Tremblay and colleagues (Dobkin et al., 1995; Tremblay et al., 1995) provide evidence to support this model. In a very large sample of boys, there was a link between target boys' aggressiveness and their best friends' aggressiveness between the ages of 10 and 12, but once the target boys' early problem behavior was taken into account, the aggressiveness of the best friends did not predict the boys' delinquent behavior the following year. These findings support the selection aspect of friendship—birds of an antisocial feather flock together. The story does not end here, however. For certain subgroups of boys, friends' aggressiveness *was* associated with later problem behavior. For the two extreme groups—the most disruptive boys and the most nondisruptive, conforming boys—later delinquency was not associated with friends' delinquency (Vitaro, Tremblay, Kerr, Pagani, & Bukowski, 1997). For the moderately disruptive boys, however, the influence of their friends was more profound. If they had aggressive, disruptive friends, the moderately disruptive boys had levels of delinquency in adolescence that were similar to the highly disruptive boys.

In addition, aspects of the causal, incidental, and enhancement models may fit subgroups of children and adolescents differently. Vitaro and colleagues (2005) identified subgroups of children who fit different trajectories of affiliations with deviant friends. Early affiliates appeared to be delinquent before they began to associate with deviant friends and then became more delinquent as their association with deviant friends continued (enhancement model). Late affiliates did not associate with delinquent peers in preadolescence, but by adolescence their friends were very delinquent. Their own level of delinquency increased similarly—it was negligible before they had delinquent friends and considerable once they had these friends (causal model). Also supporting the causal model, the friendless children, who by definition did not have delinquent friends, did not become delinquent (Vitaro et al., 1997, 2005). In another study, there was no association between aggressiveness and teacher-reported externalizing problem behavior for friendless children (Hoza et al., 1995). For children with a mutual friendship, though, the more aggressive they were, the more teachers reported behavior problems at school, suggesting again the potential negative influences of friends for aggressive children.

Two related and influential models explaining the development of antisocial behavior in general suggest two pathways to delinquency in adolescence. On the life-course-persistent (Moffitt, 1993) or early-starters (Patterson et al., 1991) pathway, children engage in antisocial behavior beginning in early childhood, and their problem behavior continues into adulthood. In contrast, on the adolescence-limited (Moffitt, 1993) or late-starters (Patterson & Yoerger, 2002) pathway, youth begin offending in adolescence, and their behavior tends to desist by adulthood. Both theories propose a different set of causes and influences on these two groups. In terms of peer relations, it may be that association with deviant friends amplifies the delinquent behavior of the early starters, but consistent with the incidental or individual characteristics model, other factors, including personal characteristics and dispositions and family factors, cause delinquent behavior. For late starters, however, deviant peers may play a more influential role in the initiation and escalation of problem behavior in adolescence (see Vitaro, Tremblay, & Bukowski, 2001, for a review).

Summary

There are a number of predictable ways in which the friendships of aggressive and nonaggressive children and adolescents differ. But because these findings have not been well integrated with research on the normative developmental significance of friendships, there are a number of critical questions left to answer. Most important is the question of what aggressive and antisocial children "get out of" their friendships. Despite the problematic aspects of the relationships, do they also afford emotional support, validation of self-worth, and many of the other positive functions that Sullivan (1953) and others describe as critical functions of friendship? In other words, are there benefits of friendship—any friendship—that outweigh the deviancy training and other negative outcomes of friendships between two aggressive or antisocial youth? And to be even more concrete, should we encourage those relationships, despite the problems, or would aggressive children be better off friendless? For example, at least according to the aggressive or antisocial children and adolescents themselves, they enjoy and have fun with their friends. In a comparison of early adolescents with deviant friends, nondeviant friends, and no mutual friends, those with friends, regardless of whether the friends were deviant, were not as lonely as their peers without friends, suggesting that even deviant friends protect against feelings of loneliness and social isolation (Brendgen, Vitaro, & Bukowski, 2000).

A related point is that friendships are not expected to transform a well-adjusted, socially competent, prosocial child into a troubled and troublemaking youth. In part, it would be relatively rare to find a close relationship between two friends with such opposite competencies and characteristics. Nevertheless, friendships clearly have the potential to promote the maintenance and escalation of existing antisocial tendencies and even to foster the development of more severe antisocial responding to the external world.

In evaluating this research on friendships of aggressive and antisocial children, there are at least three important caveats to consider. First, much of the research, especially on the process of deviancy training, has been limited to boys with only a few studies including girls (Dishion, 2000; Piehler & Dishion, 2007; Snyder et al., 2005). These studies indicate that boys may engage in higher levels of deviancy training than girls (Dishion, 2000; Piehler & Dishion, 2007). Additional research is needed to examine whether deviancy training serves a different function in boys' and girls' friendships and whether the predictive power of deviancy training is similar for both.

With regard to friendship quality, there are overall differences between boys and girls (see Chapter 6), and these seem to hold for aggressive and nonaggressive children (Grotpeter & Crick, 1996). In addition, there is not strong evidence that more general peer problems contribute differently to aggressive and antisocial behavior or to other behavior problems for boys and girls (Coie et al., 1992; Kupersmidt, Burchinal, & Patterson, 1995; Laird et al., 2001). However, there is at least some evidence that the link between association with delinquent friends and antisocial behavior might differ for girls and boys (van Lier, Vitaro, Wanner, Vuijk, & Crijnen, 2005). Girls who are delinquent appear to be more affected by poor relationships with normative peers (peer rejection) and less affected by association with deviant friends as compared to boys. Nevertheless, the fact remains that the friendships of aggressive and antisocial girls have not been studied with the same intensity as boys, and this is a significant limitation to our understanding of individual differences in friendship experiences.

Second, the research we have reviewed in this section focuses on specific dyadic relationships—relationships with a child's best or good friend rather than relationships with his or her friends in general. This is in keeping with our interest in the contexts that specific relationships provide and individual differences in those relationships. Nevertheless, as discussed in detail in Chapter 2, most children and adolescents have multiple friends and also participate in broader friendship and peer networks. Recognition that peers serve an important function (or even necessary, in some cases) in the developmental trajectories leading to aggression and antisocial behavior predates the empirical studies of friendship discussed here. Sociologists and criminologists have long argued that association with deviant peers is strongly correlated with, if not a cause of, delinquency (e.g., Elliott et al., 1985; Sutherland, 1947; Thornberry & Krohn, 1997). Indeed, association with deviant peers is one of the strongest proximal predictors of antisocial and delinquent behavior in adolescence and predicts the maintenance, escalation, and even the onset of deviant behavior (Elliott et al., 1985; Keenan, Loeber, Zhang, Stouthamer-Loeber, & Van Kammen, 1995; Patterson et al., 1991). Examination of individual friendships complements this focus on broader peer networks in several ways. It allows for the study of specific processes in friends' ongoing interactions that might explain the strong associations between deviant peers and delinquency, and it allows for integration with our substantial knowledge about the features, quality, and function of friendships in general.

Third, because of convenience and because it is easy to assess reciprocity of friendship nominations in school settings, most studies of children's friendships only include school-based relationships. For aggressive children, in particular, including friends outside of school may be especially important (cf. Vitaro, Brendgen, & Tremblay, 2000). Many aggressive and antisocial children and adolescents have difficulty making and maintaining friendships with peers in school, and they do not have strong ties to school. As a result, their closest relationships may be with children in their neighborhood and with children who are different ages—friendships that would not be identified if the typical classroom- or grade-based reciprocal friend nominations are used to identify friendships. In both childhood (Bagwell & Coie, 2004) and adolescence (Dishion, Andrews, & Crosby, 1995), aggressive boys seem to form relationships of convenience with others who live close to them. In our study, over one-third of the aggressive boys had best friends who did not attend school with them, and over half had friends who lived within walking distance. More than friendships based on interactions at school, it is likely that these neighborhood relationships are based on spending unsupervised time together when there are limited constraints on the children's activities and behavior. This unsupervised time may yield increased opportunities for troublemaking. Indeed, preadolescent aggressive boys indicated that adults were less likely to supervise their activities with friends when compared to nonaggressive boys (Bagwell & Coie, 2004). Furthermore, associations between substance use with a friend (i.e., "co-use") and individual levels of substance use were strongest when parental monitoring was low and when the time spent with the friend was out-of-school time (Kiesner, Poulin, & Dishion, 2010).

Future Research Directions for the Dark Side of Friendships

There are at least three critical future directions for better understanding the dark side of friendships. First, the field is ripe for the exploration of other processes within the friendships of aggressive and antisocial youth that might promote increased problem behavior and that might function differently within this kind of friendship context compared to a more normative relationship. Reinforcement (deviancy training) is the only process explored extensively to date, yet others include imitation or direct modeling of deviant behavior. As we discuss in Chapters 3 and 4, the normative friendship literature has considered conflict as an important feature of friendships and has examined both the negative and positive functions of conflict (e.g., Laursen, 1993). For example, conflict may lead to friendship dissolution, disrupting other positive functions of the relationship, yet it may also promote skills in negotiation, compromise, and cooperation. Clearly, conflict management may be a particularly important process within the friendships of aggressive children. On the one hand, aggressive behavior between friends requires some kind of conflict management. On the other hand, aggressive and antisocial children might have particular difficulty managing conflicts with friends because they lack skills in emotion regulation and self-control, because they may be more likely to engage in coercion rather than cooperation and conflict instigation rather than conflict resolution, and because their relationship may provide a context for the development of norms supporting impulsive and aggressive displays of emotion and escalation rather than deescalation of affective arousal.

Second, now that we know a good bit about the effects of associating with deviant friends on problem behavior, we are ready to ask what factors might moderate this association—might strengthen the relationship between friends' bad behavior and the child's behavior or might protect a child from the influence of deviant friends. The search for moderator variables should consider at least three different kinds of variables. First are individual characteristics of the youth. The question we then ask is what might make *this child* more susceptible to the negative influences of aggressive friends. Van Lier and colleagues (2007) found that for young children having aggressive friends was a risk factor for aggression, but this was strongest for children who were also genetically vulnerable for aggression. Pubertal status is another biologically based variable that has been shown to moderate the link between friends' delinquency and adolescent's delinquency—early puberty strengthened that association, and late puberty appeared to serve as a protective factor for adolescents with delinquent friends (Fergusson, Vitaro, Wanner, & Brendgen, 2007). Other potential moderator variables include having other friends who are or are not deviant (Vitaro et al., 2000) and family factors such as parental monitoring and attachment to parents (McElhaney, Immele, Smith, & Allen, 2006; Vitaro et al., 2000).

A second group of possible moderator variables are those that describe aspects of the friendship. The question here is whether there are characteristics of *this specific relationship* that might weaken or strengthen the impact it has on a child's behavior and adjustment. For example, Piehler and Dishion (2007) considered mutuality within antisocial youths' friendships with the hypothesis that deviancy training would be stronger in higher-quality friendships. As expected, for friends who engaged in relatively low levels of deviant talk, greater mutuality was associated with low antisocial behavior. In contrast, friends whose interactions were characterized by a lot of deviant talk had higher levels of antisocial behavior when their interactions were observed to be more mutual and reciprocal, an indicator of generally higher-quality friendships. The relationships characterized by high levels of mutuality in their interactions and high levels of deviant talk in their conversational content may be most problematic as these friendships may reflect greater investment by the friends and a stronger allegiance to the antisocial norms in the relationship (Piehler & Dishion, 2007). Whether or not the friendship is reciprocated may also have implications for the promotion of aggression. Adams, Bukowski, and Bagwell (2005) found that for youth initially high on aggression, aggression was most stable over the course of the school year when the child's friend was also aggressive, and this was particularly true for unreciprocated friendships. Adams and colleagues suggest that in these unreciprocated relationships, the adolescents' need for intimacy (Sullivan, 1953) is not being met even though they are seeking common ground with this peer, likely around aggression.

A third type of potential moderator variable is characteristics of the friend, and these variables have received limited attention to date. They answer the question of whether individual characteristics of *this specific friend* make this friend's influence stronger or weaker. For example, do friendships with antisocial children who are better accepted by peers or who have personal characteristics such as leadership skills or who are aggressive yet also socially competent exert a greater influence and strengthen the association between deviant friends and deviant behavior than friendships with antisocial peers who are rejected or less socially competent? These kinds of variables hold promise but have not been addressed in any systematic way.

The third future direction for studying and understanding the dark side of friendships is to move beyond thinking only of externalizing behaviors and broaden our view of potential negative outcomes of some friendships. For example, several research teams have considered the role of friends and friendships in adolescent depression. Here are four illustrative studies. Brendgen, Lamarche, Wanner, and Vitaro (2010) found three trajectories of depressed mood between the ages of 11 and 13 years— low stable, increasing, and high stable. Compared to friendless youth, having nondepressed friends predicted less of an increase in depressed mood, but those with depressed friends experienced steeper increases in depressed mood. The authors conclude that not having friends is indeed a risk factor for increasing depression in adolescence but that having friends who are depressed themselves may be just as significant a risk factor for depression. Chan and Poulin (2009) used an interesting method to explore associations between friendships and depression symptoms. On a monthly basis, they traced the stability of adolescents' friendships and changes in depression. Findings suggested that high depression symptoms at one point predicted instability in friendships the next month, again demonstrating a complex link between depressed mood and friendship experiences. Rose (2002) identified the process of corumination that involves rehashing problems and dwelling on negative affect with a friend. Although corumination is associated with high friendship quality, it is also linked with depression and anxiety symptoms. Finally, Prinstein and colleagues (2010) found that friends influence girls' nonsuicidal self-injurious behavior (NSSI) in both community and clinic samples. Even after controlling for depression symptoms, friends' NSSI predicted increases in girls' NSSI a year later. Together, these converging findings suggest that friendships with certain others and particular processes that occur within some friendships serve as risk factors in the development of internalizing symptoms, such as depression and anxiety. Further exploration of these dark sides of friendship is needed.

FRIENDSHIP AND PEER VICTIMIZATION

Peer victimization can take many different forms, including victimization by physical aggression, verbal aggression, social exclusion, and various social manipulations by others (e.g., spreading rumors). The term *victimization* implies a power differential between the aggressor and the victim, and for many children peer victimization is a chronic experience. Approximately 10–15% of students report regularly experiencing peer victimization and harassment at school (Boulton & Smith, 1994; Kochenderfer-Ladd & Wardrop, 2001). One of our most fundamental expectations for friends is that they stick up for us and help us. Friends protect us and provide support. Thus, having friends and having good friends should provide protection against peer victimization. But if children do not have a friend, or have a poor-quality relationship, or have a friend who is also victimized, this function of friendship may be compromised.

There are at least three important questions about associations between friendship and peer victimization. First, the most basic question is whether victimized children have fewer friends than nonvictimized children. Second, what are the characteristics of those friends and the nature of those friendships? For example, are they lower in quality? Third, can friendship serve as a buffer to victimization or protect against the potential negative consequences of victimization?

Do Victimized Children Have Few Friends?

The answer to the first question is a clear "yes." Children without a mutual friend are more likely to be victimized than children with a mutual friend (Hodges et al., 1999). Moreover, correlations between the *number* of friends children have and victimization suggest that highly victimized children have fewer friends than nonvictimized children and that children with more friends are less likely to be victimized (Bukowski, Sippola, & Boivin, 1995; Fox & Boulton, 2006; Hodges, Malone, & Perry, 1997; Hodges & Perry, 1999; Scholte et al., 2009). This relationship appears to hold true for children as young as kindergarten age (Hanish, Ryan, Martin, & Fabes, 2005) and to be particularly strong for relational forms of victimization (e.g., social exclusion, spreading rumors; Malcolm, Jensen-Campbell, Rex-Lear, & Waldrip, 2006). There is also longitudinal evidence that changes in friendship covary with changes in victimization. In one study, children who lost a friend over the course of the year experienced increases in victimization, and children who gained a friend showed decreases in victimization (Bowker, Rubin, Burgess, Booth-LaForce, & Rose-Krasnor, 2006).

There are many reasons why we would expect this link between few friends and high levels of peer victimization. Some possibilities are these: If bullies are to maintain their status, they would not be likely to target peers who have strong social affiliations (Pellegrini & Long, 2002). Children with friends are less likely to be alone. As a result, there are fewer opportunities for them to be victimized. Children with friends may successfully turn to those friends for advice on how to deal with a bully and thus may be less likely to be targets of continued victimization (Hodges et al., 1997).

What Is the Nature of Victimized Children's Friendships?

The second question asks about the nature of the friendships that victimized children have. Although they tend to have fewer friends than nonvictimized children, many victimized children establish a reciprocal friendship with at least one peer. It is here that we see most clearly the importance of an individual differences perspective when evaluating the developmental significance of friendship—How does the context of a friendship formed with at least one child who is victimized by peers differ from that of other relationships, and in turn, How does this friendship context affect the children involved? There is increasing evidence that victimized children have friendships that are lower in quality than nonvictimized children. They report lower support, companionship, and intimacy from friends and more conflict in their relationships (e.g., Bollmer, Milich, Harris, & Maras, 2005; Champion, Vernberg, & Shipman, 2003; Erath, Flanagan, & Bierman, 2008; Malcolm et al., 2006; Rubin et al., 2004). Youth who are victimized are also less satisfied with their friends (Gini, 2008). In addition, the characteristics of victimized children's friends are expected to change the context of the relationship. Victimized children tend to have friends who are weak (Hodges et al., 1999; Malone & Perry, 1995), who experience internalizing symptoms (Hodges et al., 1997, 1999), who are poorly adjusted socially (Scholte et al., 2009), and who are themselves victimized by their peers (Browning, Cohen, & Warman, 2003; Hodges et al., 1997).

A primary shortcoming in the existing literature is that it does not clearly establish whether friendship difficulties make children vulnerable to victimization or victimization makes children vulnerable to friendship difficulties or both. One possibility is that poor friendship quality is a precursor to victimization. In this view, only high-quality friendships are expected to contribute to children's positive adjustment, and low-quality friendships might place children at risk for negative outcomes, including victimization. Social support theories suggest that children and adolescents who do not have close, high-quality friendships do not receive the emotional support they need in times of stress and might be more vulnerable to adjustment difficulties and psychological problems (e.g., Garmezy, 1983; Sandler, Miller, Short, & Wolchik, 1989).

Moreover, children who lack good friends may be at risk for victimization because they do not have someone to stand up for them or to retaliate against aggressors (Bollmer et al., 2005; Hodges & Perry, 1999). Aggressive children may seek out children who appear more vulnerable because they lack good friends. In addition, experience in high-quality friendships is expected to promote the development of prosocial skills and competencies, and high-quality friendships may also provide children links to other classmates and thus to other positive relationships with peers (Berndt, 2002). In contrast, low-quality relationships that are high in negative features may contribute to an overall conflictual and negative style of interaction that promotes disruptive behavior and poor adjustment (e.g., Berndt & Keefe, 1995) and that may increase risks for peer victimization.

Findings that changes in friendship quality correspond to changes in victimization provide strong support for this hypothesis. For example, one study found that children who experience a decrease in positive friendship qualities over time are more likely to experience corresponding increases in levels of victimization (Goldbaum, Craig, Pepler, & Connolly, 2003). Another found that young victimized children who report that they respond to peer aggression by "having a friend help" were less victimized by the end of the school year (Kochenderfer & Ladd, 1997), suggesting that even very young children successfully seek assistance from their friends to cope with victimization by other peers. Indeed, having friendships characterized by high levels of companionship, intimacy, and support is associated with low levels of overt and relational victimization (Malcolm et al., 2006).

A second possibility to explain the association between friendship and peer victimization is that victimization is a precursor to friendship difficulties. Children who are victimized often have trouble forming new friendships (Ellis & Zarbatany, 2007) as well as maintaining high-quality friendships. Ellis and Zarbatany (2007) suggest that victimized children may not be able to create a friendly and welcoming context for a friendship to develop. Personal characteristics, such as social anxiety and withdrawal, may make victimized children less desirable as friends because they are not fun to be around. In addition, victimized children may have trouble providing the kinds of companionship and support to friends that would allow a relationship to flourish. Potential friends may also be wary of associating with disliked children, and victimized children are at risk for increases in peer rejection over time (Hodges & Perry, 1999).

Several studies have examined this possible direction of effect. Goldbaum and colleagues (2003) found that as victimization experiences increased, youth reported decreasing trust and affection with friends. They suggest that victimized youth lose trust in friendships over time because of their friends' inability to help them overcome the peer abuse. Ellis and Zarbatany (2007) found that higher levels of victimization interfered with children's ability to form new friendships later in the school year. In addition, friendships between a victimized and a nonvictimized girl were highly unstable relationships. The authors suggest that the nonvictimized friends may face significant social sanctions from peers for befriending victimized girls, and these negative social consequences (e.g., threats to their own peer status) may make the relationships short-lived. In addition, Hodges and Perry (1999) found that victimization predicts increases in *friends'* victimization and internalizing problems. Although they did not investigate it directly, these changes may also be associated with changes in friendship quality. In other words, victimized children's friendships change for the worse over time, regardless of whether they form new friendships with more victimized peers or lose the good friendships they have. These studies collectively suggest that being victimized may be a precursor to friendship difficulties.

The evidence tells a likely story of a vulnerable child who is victimized by peers and could benefit from the help and support of a good friend. This child, though, has difficulty establishing and holding on to such a relationship. Potential friends are wary of associating with this child, and the child struggles to be a fun, supportive companion. The child manages to form a friendship but it may be short-lived, the friend may also be victimized, and the possible benefits of having a high-quality friend to protect against victimization and the internalizing stress that may come from being a victim of peer aggression are never realized. In time, the child suffers repeated victimization experiences at the hands of peers. Friendship difficulties are thus expected to be cause and consequence of peer victimization.

The Protective Function of Friends

Do Friendships Protect against Peer Victimization?

Consistent findings that children with friends are less likely to be victimized establishes some support for the "friendship protection hypothesis," suggesting that the presence of friends may ward off potential victimization (e.g., Bukowski et al., 1995; Hodges et al., 1997, 1999; Hodges & Perry, 1999; Pellegrini, Bartini, & Brooks, 1999). The buffering effect of having friends may even become stronger over time. In one study following children from kindergarten through fifth grade, having a friend in kindergarten was not associated with peer victimization in kindergarten. However, children with kindergarten friends showed much steeper declines in victimization over the course of elementary school compared to children without friends in kindergarten (Reavis, Keane, & Calkins, 2010). The authors suggest that friendships provide important contexts for developing and honing skills and competencies that, over time, make children less vulnerable to victimization.

Even more compelling evidence for the protective function of friendship comes from longitudinal studies showing that friendship attenuates the risk for peer victimization from other known risk factors. For example, we know that internalizing problems increase children's risk for peer victimization. However, having a friend who offers high levels of protection (i.e., a high-quality friendship) completely mitigated the risk such that internalizing problems were not associated with victimization for children lucky enough to establish this kind of friendship. In contrast, for children with a friend unable to serve this protective function, the link between internalizing problems and victimization was strengthened (Hodges et al., 1999). In addition, who the friend is, or the characteristics of the friend, matters in terms of whether the association between individual risk factors and peer victimization is buffered. For example, the link between internalizing problems and victimization was significantly reduced for children with friends who were themselves not victimized or who were physically strong, but the link was strengthened when friends were also highly victimized or were physically weak (Hodges et al., 1997). The quality of the friendships is also important in determining whether friendships buffer against victimization. For example, a link between relational aggression and increases in relational victimization was only found for children with low-quality friendships but not those with high-quality friendships (Kawabata, Crick, & Hamaguchi, 2010).

In two studies, Schwartz and his colleagues have demonstrated the powerful protective effects of friendships. In one study, externalizing behavior problems in kindergarten and first grade were associated with peer victimization in third and fourth grade for children with few friends but not for children with many friends (Schwartz, McFadyen-Ketchum, Dodge, Pettit, & Bates, 1999). In another study, there was a clear link between early harsh treatment at home and peer victimization in later elementary school for children with few friends, but this association did not exist for children with many friends (Schwartz et al., 2000). These studies suggest that children who are able to establish friendship, despite individual and social risk factors (Hodges et al., 1999), may receive significant protective benefits from those relationships. Importantly, the studies also demonstrate that these protective benefits of friendships during the early transition to elementary school extend over the period of several years. Friendship thus appears to serve a particularly important function in helping children (especially vulnerable children) integrate successfully into the peer world of elementary school during the early years (Schwartz et al., 1999). Furthermore, the buffering effects of friendship are found across multiple dimensions of friendship—having a friend, having many friends, having a high-quality friendship, and having friends with particular characteristics (e.g., physical strength, nonvictims) all serve to reduce the impact of various risk factors on peer victimization.

Schwartz and colleagues (2000) considered friendship as a buffer for distal risk factors that lead to peer victimization, yet there are also more proximal experiences in children's social worlds that also increase the likelihood of being a victim of peers' aggression. Being highly disliked by the peer group increases children's risk for victimization, yet having a close friend, especially a high-quality friendship, may serve a protective function for children who are rejected. For children with low peer acceptance, those with high-quality friends (Malcolm et al., 2006) and those with at least average or high numbers of friends (Lansford et al., 2007) were less likely to be victimized. Similarly, the link between poor social skills and peer victimization was weaker for children with many friends compared to those with few friends (Fox & Boulton, 2006).

An important next question, then, is *"How* does friendship serve a protective function?" The central idea here is that there are a number of risk factors for peer victimization, including behavioral vulnerabilities (e.g., shy and withdrawn behavior, externalizing problems), stressful home environments, rejection by peers, and social-cognitive deficits. However, these risk factors are more likely to result in victimization when the child also experiences social vulnerabilities that encourage others to act aggressively toward the child and/or that fail to ward off potential aggressors (Hodges et al., 1997). Being friendless and having low-quality friendships are some of the most consequential of these social vulnerabilities.

Unfortunately, we are left to speculate about the particular processes through which friends exert their positive influences on reducing victimization. One set of mechanisms highlights the significance of friendship in protecting against the establishment of bully–victim relationships. In a very tangible way, friends can offer protection. They can stand up for the child in the face of a potential bully just as James described at the beginning of this chapter and even threaten retaliation. To the extent that a victimized child's friends are socially skilled, they may be able to help negotiate a challenging social situation (e.g., Lamarche et al., 2006). The mere presence of friends may discourage potential aggressors who might prefer to bully a peer who is often alone (Hodges & Perry, 1997). Friends may provide advice and good ideas about how to handle aggression from peers, or they may provide emotional support and validation for a child after a bullying episode.

An alternative set of mechanisms focuses on the skills and competencies children learn within friendships. Skills in conflict management, in help seeking (and help giving), in effective coping strategies, and in emotion regulation that might be practiced and honed in interactions with friends may minimize risk for victimization. For some children, the development of these social and emotional competencies may even compensate for early risk factors and help vulnerable children progress on a more adaptive developmental pathway that does not lead to victimization. Over the long term, supportive experiences with friends and the development of social skills may promote the child's development of a positive social reputation that is inconsistent with vulnerability for victimization (Schwartz et al., 1999, 2000).

Do Friendships Protect against the Negative Effects of Victimization?

As discussed above, friendships provide an important protective function in buffering children against peer victimization. In this way, friendship alters the link between risk factors and peer victimization. Friendship may also serve a protective function in buffering children against the negative consequences associated with peer victimization—altering the link between victimization and distress. Internalizing problems, including depression, anxiety, and loneliness, are common outcomes of peer victimization (Hawker & Boulton, 2000), and there is some evidence that friendship can mitigate these effects. For example, Hodges and colleagues (1999) found that physical and verbal victimization predicted increases in internalizing problems only for children who did not have a mutual friend.

Friendship quality and the characteristics of a child's friends may be even more important than simply having a friend or not when considering whether friendships provide a buffer against the negative effects of victimization. It is anticipated that only high-quality friendships would serve this protective function. Similarly, having friends who are aggressive, who are themselves victimized, or who have other risk factors may interfere with their ability to protect against the consequences of victimization. In our own work, we found that a friendship characterized by a high degree of help buffered children from social concerns when faced with overt and relational aggression. Likewise, friendships with a high level of security protected against depression associated with victimization (Schmidt & Bagwell, 2007). Hodges and colleagues (1999) also found that the link between victimization and internalizing problems varied according to the quality of the friendship. Surprisingly, for children with high levels of companionship in their friendship, victimization predicted increases in internalizing problems. The authors suggest that these very high levels of companionship may indicate an exclusive relationship where friends employ preoccupied coping strategies (which are associated with internalizing distress) to handle stress from victimization.

In terms of the characteristics of children's friends, there is evidence that the aggressiveness of a child's friends influences the degree to which friendships mitigate or exacerbate the association between peer victimization and academic difficulties (Schwartz, Gorman, Dodge, Pettit, & Bates, 2008). In one recent study, Schwartz and colleagues (2008) considered the number of highly aggressive friends children had and the number of nonaggressive friends children had. Peer victimization predicted declines in grade point average (GPA) over the course of a school year for children who had few nonaggressive friends and for children who had many aggressive friends. However, both having many nonaggressive friends, especially for boys, and having few highly aggressive friends buffered against the academic declines associated with peer victimization. Establishing close friendships with prosocial, nonaggressive peers may help victimized children engage more positively at school, may facilitate their liking of school, and may offer effective social support that allows them to maintain their academic functioning despite the experience of negative interactions with other peers.

Summary

In sum, the associations between peer victimization and friendship are strong. Victimized children tend to have fewer friends and lower-quality relationships. The direction of this effect is not completely clear, but current understandings point to a mutually reinforcing cycle in which peer victimization leads to challenges in forming and maintaining close friendships, and difficulty in friendships makes children vulnerable to increases in peer victimization over time. Despite this cycle, one of the most compelling arguments for the developmental significance of friendship is that friendships have the potential to serve valuable protective functions related to peer victimization. Peer victimization takes place in a social context, and having friends, especially having friendships of high quality, protects vulnerable children against victimization by other peers. Similarly, friendship moderates the link between peer victimization and negative consequences, such as internalizing distress and academic declines. In other words, having good friends provides some measure of protection and may promote resilience so that even in the face of peer victimization, substantial negative outcomes are less likely to be realized. These conclusions are particularly important given evidence that bullying often occurs within friendship networks and that within these groups, bullying is a group norm (Duffy & Nesdale, 2009).

At the beginning of this chapter, James recounts a compelling story in which his friend Lucas encourages others to give James a chance and wards off the social exclusion other peers are about to level at James. This is a very specific example of a direct intervention by a friend to stand up for a child. There are many other less direct mechanisms as well: Friends provide positive socialization experiences that might help children compensate for early risk factors. In their experiences with friends, children learn conflict management and emotion regulation skills that keep them from becoming a victim. Friends offer emotional support, encouragement, and validation so that even if a child is victimized, those experiences do not precipitate internalizing distress.

Just as we discussed with the effect of friendship on the development of antisocial behavior, the links between friendship and peer victimization may be explained by the *incidental* model. As Schwartz has articulated, this model assumes that friendship may simply be a marker variable that correlates with coping skills, social skills, and other individual characteristics and protective factors (Schwartz et al., 2000, 2008). It is these child attributes that protect against victimization or that mitigate the negative effects of victimization, and these same characteristics foster the formation of good friendships. However, friendship may not have a direct influence on adjustment and well-being.

Directions for future research on victimization and friendship are clear. The role of friendship as a moderator variable has been clearly established, yet we could learn more about other outcomes associated with victimization that might be moderated by friendship, including externalizing behavior, loneliness, and other aspects of school adjustment in addition to GPA. Similarly, we have only begun to consider ways in which friendship quality and characteristics of children's friends serve a protective function. In all future research, we need to carefully keep in mind the relational context of victimization (see Card, Isaacs, & Hodges, 2009). The interactions that occur between bullies and victims can be conceptualized as dyadic relationships. For example, most peer-directed aggression occurs within particular dyads rather than being doled out indiscriminately across a number of peers. In an intensive observational study of boys' interactions in small play groups, Dodge, Price, Coie, and Christopoulis (1990) observed that 50% of aggressive behaviors took place in only 20% of the dyads, and in another play group study with mutually aggressive dyads, relational factors accounted for as much of the variability in aggressive episodes as characteristics of either the actor or the partner (Coie et al., 1999).

In terms of peer victimization, specifically, it is most common in dyads characterized by mutual dislike (i.e., mutual antipathies; Card & Hodges, 2007; see Card, 2010, for a meta-analysis of antipathetic relationships). Nevertheless, some children are victimized by their friends. Relational victimization, which by definition involves harm to social relationships, occurs within friendships (e.g., Grotpeter & Crick, 1996). Far from offering protection from victimization, these particular friendships may contribute to adjustment problems, such as social anxiety, social avoidance, and externalizing difficulties (Crick & Nelson, 2002). Victimization by a friend involves a violation of generally held expectations of friendship—betrayal instead of loyalty, harm instead of protection and validation, criticism instead of support. As a result, victimization within a friendship may be associated with considerable confusion (Mishna, Wiener, & Pepler, 2008) and even more damaging effects than victimization from others in the peer group (Crick & Nelson, 2002). An alternative view is offered by Card and Hodges (2007), who find that victimization within mutually antipathetic relationships is more strongly linked with internalizing distress and low self-concept than is victimization within other dyadic relationships, including friendships. As the authors note, however, these correlational findings may be explained by the fact that victimization from mutually disliked peers is especially harmful or that victimization from a particular peer is more likely to lead to the formation of a mutual antipathetic relationship than a friendship. Nevertheless, the bottom line here is that our understanding of the role of friendship in peer victimization will be greatly enhanced by further consideration of the dyadic context of victimization.

CONCLUSIONS

The purpose of this chapter was to focus on the idea that children's experiences in friendships and outcomes of those experiences are in part determined by characteristics they bring to the relationship. This idiographic perspective complements the normative perspective presented in the previous two chapters and is necessary for capturing a more complete picture of the significance of friendships. We have examined three specific individual characteristics—attachment history, aggression and antisocial behavior, and peer victimization—but there are countless others that may be important. We selected these three in part because although we have called them "individual characteristics," they represent links between friendship and other levels of social complexity (Hinde, 1997). Attachment history is another dyadic-level, relationship variable; aggression and antisocial behavior could be considered individual-level variables; and peer victimization is a process that occurs at the level of the larger peer group.

The discussion necessarily considers as well the characteristics of children's friends. After all, there are two individuals in the relationship, each bringing with them a history of experiences in other relationships and individual characteristics including behaviors, skills and competencies, emotions, cognitions, and personality characteristics, to name a few. These characteristics that friends bring to their relationship affect the relationship itself, and in turn, that relationship has the potential to influence and change the individuals in a transactional way. Although this transactional influence over time is relatively easy to describe theoretically, it is much more difficult to evaluate empirically, and as described in this chapter, such empirical work is in its infancy. Nevertheless, the overall conclusion from the theoretical and empirical research examined in this chapter is that what children and their friends bring to their relationship has a significant influence on the characteristics and course of the relationship as well as the potential outcomes for the children involved. By far, the most attention has been paid to aggression and antisocial behavior as individual characteristics that affect friendships. Lest we not get carried away, however, in assuming that the influence of friends and the impact of friends' characteristics is unidimensional, we must remember that friends' influence is certainly not always, and not even usually, negative (Berndt & Murphy, 2002).

As this chapter describes, characteristics of individual children, such as their attachment history, their level of aggression and antisocial behavior, and their experience of peer victimization, are associated with friendship in multiple ways. All three of these factors have been studied as outcomes of friendship with the idea that attachment history, aggression, and peer victimization influence children's participation in friendships and the quality of their relationships with friends. Nevertheless, the developmental significance of friendship is highlighted more clearly by evidence of reciprocal influences that occur between friendship on the one hand and aggression or peer victimization on the other. Finally, consideration of friendship as a moderator variable holds considerable promise. Children's experience with friends has been shown to moderate the link between early aggression and later delinquency and antisocial behavior. Likewise, having friends and friendship quality can provide a buffer against the negative outcomes associated with peer victimization and perhaps with insecure attachment, though this latter association has not been studied extensively. Continued work identifying the role of friendship as a moderator and specifying transactional models involving friendship and these and other characteristics and experiences should prove fruitful for further explicating the developmental significance of friendship.

Chapter 6

Friendship Quality

A close friend is someone who sticks by you through the good
and bad and they always have your back so you never have to
worry.
> —AN ADOLESCENT DESCRIBING WHAT'S IMPORTANT ABOUT A FRIEND

Wilbur never forgot Charlotte. Although he loved her children
and grandchildren dearly, none of the new spiders ever quite
took her place in his heart. She was in a class by herself. It is not
often that someone comes along who is a true friend and a good
writer. Charlotte was both.
> —E. B. WHITE, FROM *CHARLOTTE'S WEB*

I found out that one of my friends was talking badly about me
behind my back. It made me feel badly because someone I put
my trust in would go behind my back and deliberately hurt me.
> —AN ADOLESCENT DESCRIBING A RECENT BETRAYAL BY A FRIEND

Friendships are developmentally significant across the life span.
The meaning assigned to these relationships changes relatively
little with age, although the behavioral exchanges between
friends reflect the ages of the individuals involved. Whether
friendships are developmental assets or liabilities depends on
several conditions, especially the characteristics of one's friends
and the quality of one's relationships with them.
> —HARTUP AND STEVENS (1999, p. 79)

We often idealize friendship and focus on the security and support that
friends provide and the dependability, loyalty, and faithfulness of friends.
These are some of the features that we appreciate and value most in

relationships with friends. Yet friendships vary considerably. Some are defined by intimacy and self-disclosure; others by social and emotional support; others by closeness, coupled with intense disagreements. There are some friends children turn to for support on a bad day, and others they call just when they want to have fun. Some friendships are fleeting, yet others are "go to" friends who can be counted on for years. Children spend lots of time with some friends, and they may interact with others only in specific settings, such as on a sports team. The quality of a friendship is determined by the relative amounts of positive (e.g., companionship, closeness) and negative (e.g., conflict) features, and thus varies significantly from friendship to friendship. From this perspective, quality is viewed as one index of the developmental context that particular friendships provide and the outcomes associated with those relationships. This chapter is devoted to understanding friendship quality as one of the most important determinants of individual differences in the friendship experience for children and adolescents.

The idea that the quality of a relationship may have important developmental implications is not surprising. For example, the extensive theoretical and empirical literature on parent–child attachment has at its core the assumption that relationships differ along qualitative dimensions, and that relationship quality has implications for the relationship itself and for the individuals involved in the relationship. It is somewhat surprising, then, that the quality of children's friendships has not been addressed more extensively. Studies comparing friends and nonfriends rest on the assumption that there is something qualitatively different about a friendship compared to other associations with agemates, yet these comparisons often neglect the fact that friendships vary substantially. Furthermore, having a friend is assumed to be synonymous with having a *high-quality* relationship. Having friends versus not having friends clearly tells us something important about a child and his or her developmental trajectory, yet we contend in this chapter that the quality of the friendship also has important implications for determining the developmental significance of friendship.

WHY IS FRIENDSHIP QUALITY IMPORTANT?

There are several reasons to expect that the quality of a friendship affects children's adjustment and well-being. High-quality relationships are likely to be more stable and long lasting than poor-quality friendships, and this might translate to more enduring influence (Berndt, 2004). High-quality friendships are more likely to serve the functions that would contribute to children's positive adjustment than are low-quality relationships

(Hartup, 1992b). Compared to poor-quality relationships, high-quality friendships are more likely to serve as emotional and cognitive resources that help children adapt to stress and that provide a sense of security and protection. Lacking a high-quality friendship may make children more vulnerable to adjustment difficulties in times of stress because they do not receive the social support they need (e.g., Garmezy, 1983; Sandler et al., 1989). Experience in high-quality friendships is expected to promote the development of prosocial skills and competencies. To the extent that friendships provide models for future relationships (Hartup, 1992b; Sullivan, 1953), high-quality relationships are those that would provide experience with intimacy, collaboration, and mutual negotiation and thus serve as positive relationship templates. Similarly, high-quality friendships may also provide children links to other classmates and thus to other positive relationships with peers (Berndt, 2002). On the flip side, low-quality relationships that are high in negative features may contribute to an overall conflictual and negative style of interaction that promotes disruptive behavior and poor adjustment (e.g., Berndt & Keefe, 1995).

Much goes into determining the quality of a friendship. The characteristics of the individual children—whether they are aggressive or cooperative or fun—play a role. Nevertheless, the features that the two children bring to a relationship do not completely determine its quality. The quality of a friendship also emerges over time as friends develop norms for their interactions, gain a history of shared experiences together, and learn what can be expected from this particular friendship. The goal of this chapter is to evaluate what effects friendship quality has on the developmental significance of friendships. We organize the chapter around three questions:

1. What determines the quality of a friendship?
2. What are the correlates of friendship quality?
3. How does friendship quality affect developmental outcomes?

WHAT DETERMINES
THE QUALITY OF A FRIENDSHIP?

Why is it that some children and adolescents have a relatively easy time establishing high-quality friendships, yet others struggle to establish good friendships or have friendships with low levels of support and intimacy or high levels of conflict and rivalry? In this section, we examine associations between friendship quality and other aspects of children's personal or social relationships that might suggest answers to these questions. In most cases, the study designs do not permit conclusions about causal or determining factors but rather indicate associations among variables. We consider three types of variables shown to be associated with individual differences in friendship quality—family relationships, gender, and peer rejection.

Family Relationships as Determinants of Friendship Quality

Early research on the family's contributions to children's success in peer relationships centered on the parent–child relationship, including the security of the attachment relationship and the parents' childrearing style. As we discuss in Chapter 5, there are strong theoretical and empirical links between secure parent–child attachment and children's success in friendships, including establishing high-quality friendships. The quality of parent–child relationships and interactions is one component of a tripartite model explaining the role of parents in promoting children's social competence, including friendships (McDowell & Parke, 2009; Parke, Burks, Carson, Neville, & Boyum, 1994). Parents who are overly controlling (e.g., Putallaz, 1987) or who engage with children in coercive interactions (e.g., Patterson, 1995, 2002) tend to have children with poor social competence. Overall, authoritative parenting styles—warm and supportive yet appropriately demanding—are most closely associated with peer competence (see Ladd & Pettit, 2002, for a review). Recently, authoritative parenting has been linked specifically with high levels of intimacy in adolescents' friendships (Sharabany, Eshel, & Hakim, 2008).

Specific parenting practices and behaviors also contribute to children's high-quality friendships. For example, adolescents with parents who were more involved in consulting and helping them mediate peer relationships reported higher levels of positive friendship features. Likewise, higher autonomy granting by parents was associated with adolescents' reports of lower conflict in their friendships (Mounts, 2004). In a sample of preadolescents, those whose parents engaged in more monitoring of their behavior reported low levels of conflict with friends. For girls, high levels of parental monitoring were also related to positive friendship features (disclosure, help, support; Simpkins & Parke, 2002b).

Traditional socialization theories suggest that parenting influences children's peer relations and friendships. However, new research examining genetic and environmental influences on peer relations calls into question this direction of causal influence. For example, Pike and Eley (2009) found moderate genetic influences for the prosocial and antisocial characteristics of adolescents' peer groups, indicating perhaps that adolescents are attracted to peers similar to themselves in heritable traits. More specific to dyadic friendships, significant genetic influences on friendship satisfaction highlight the fact that each member of the dyad contributes to the quality of the relationship, and many of the characteristics the two friends bring to their relationship are heritable. In addition, the fact that there are large nonshared environmental effects indicates that children's friendships are important and powerful influences on their adjustment and development beyond the influence of the family.

Parents' Relationships and Children's Friendship Quality

More recently, broader conceptualizations of the family's influence have led to a consideration of how family relationships other than parent–child relationships, including those in which children are not directly involved (such as the marital relationship), can have a significant influence on the quality of the relationships children form with their peers and friends. There are multiple theoretical explanations for why and how parents' relationships affect children's friendship quality. From the perspective of attachment theory, the quality of parents' marital relationship is expected to affect children's and adolescents' attachment security, and in turn (as discussed more thoroughly in Chapter 5), security of children's attachment with parents influences children's friendship quality (see Markiewicz, Doyle, & Brendgen, 2001). From a social learning perspective, parents' marital relationships and friendships serve as models for children's friendships. Children learn important social skills and friendship skills through direct instruction and by observing their parents interact, and parental relationships provide children with cognitive models for conflict resolution (see Kitzmann & Cohen, 2003; Lucas-Thompson & Clarke-Stewart, 2007). From the perspective of family systems theory (Lindsey, Colwell, Frabutt, & MacKinnon-Lewis, 2006; Minuchin, 1974, 1988), the family context and interactions between multiple family members (marital interactions, sibling interactions, parent–child interactions, etc.) are expected to influence children's adjustment, including children's relationships with peers and friends.

Markiewicz and colleagues (2001) found support for both attachment theory and social learning theory explanations of the link between parents' relationships and adolescents' friendship quality. In support of attachment theory, marital quality was linked to the security of adolescents' attachment to their mothers, which in turn predicted attachment to friends and friendship quality. In support of social learning theory, adolescents' perceptions of their mother's marital quality and their mother's friendship quality was associated with their own prosocial behavior and in turn their own friendship quality, suggesting that adolescents model the parental relationships they observe.

The associations between parents' marital quality and children's friendship quality have emerged in several studies. In one, marital quality predicted children's friendship quality, yet similar to the model proposed by Markiewicz and colleagues (2001), attachment security partially mediated this association (Lucas-Thompson & Clarke-Stewart, 2007). In other words, parents with positive marital quality tended to have children with high-quality friendships, in part because marital quality led to more secure parent–child attachment, which in turn led to good friendships. Another study demonstrated that conflict between parents was associated with children's friendship quality (Kitzmann & Cohen, 2003). In particular, when parents did a poor job of resolving conflicts, their children had lower-quality friendships, characterized by high levels of conflict, poor conflict resolution, and low intimacy and companionship. Triangulation in marital conflict (i.e., when the adolescent is pulled into parents' marital conflict) puts adolescents at risk for low friendship quality (Buehler, Franck, & Cook, 2009). The link between marital conflict and children's friendship quality may also depend on family structure. The findings from another study suggest that high levels of marital conflict were associated with high levels of conflict and animosity in boys' best friendships, but only for boys from divorced families (Lindsey et al., 2006).

Children may model parents' poor resolution strategies, attributions about their parents' conflict may affect children's expectations for intimate relationships with friends, and exposure to poorly resolved conflicts between parents may promote poor coping strategies for handling stressful situations with friends (Kitzmann & Cohen, 2003). In addition, Lindsey and colleagues (2006) suggest that children's friendships may be affected as marital conflict "spills over" into other family relationships involving the child. Along with attachment theory explanations, these are all possible mechanisms for explaining links between marital quality, especially conflict between parents, and children's friendship quality.

In addition to the marital relationship, the quality of parents' friendships and their participation in social networks is also predictive of children's friendship quality. For example, mothers who rated their own friends as supportive had children who reported more closeness and intimacy in their best friendships (Doyle & Markiewicz, 1996; Doyle, Markiewicz, & Hardy, 1994). In studies that have examined both mothers' and fathers' relationships, the links between parent friendships and child friendships have varied between the two parents. In one study, various dimensions of mothers' and fathers' friendships were linked to dimensions of children's friendships when both parents and children rated the quality of their best friendships (Simpkins & Parke, 2001). For example, high levels of help and validation in mothers' relationships with their best friends were associated with low levels of conflict in daughters' best friendships, and positive characteristics of fathers' best friendships predicted high-quality friendships for their daughters. Oliveri and Reiss (1987) reported that positive aspects of fathers' friendship networks (but not mothers') were associated with positive aspects of their children's friendships (help, feelings of need, positive feelings), especially for daughters. Further specification of the particular contributions of mothers' and fathers' relationships will be important.

Sibling Relationships and Children's Friendship Quality

Parents often comment that having a sibling is "good" for their child because it teaches cooperation, sharing, empathy, conflict management, and other prosocial skills that are important for friendships, too. To what extent do children's relationships with siblings influence their relationships with their friends? On the one hand, skills that develop and exist in sibling relationships might transfer to peer relationships, and especially to friendships given that they are both close dyadic relationships (e.g., Brody, 1998; Kramer & Gottman, 1992; Parke & Buriel, 1998). Similarly, internal working models of relationships could guide children's experiences and expectations of both sibling and friendships in the same way (Bowlby, 1973). On the other hand, there are fundamental differences between siblings and friends that suggest these relationships are distinct and may not be related. Choice, for example, is a critical element of friendships that does not exist between siblings. Tom can end his friendship with David at any time, but he can't get rid of his brother Joe! The voluntary nature of friendship may create expectations for friendship (e.g., reciprocity, conflict management) that simply do not exist between siblings. Most siblings differ in age as well, creating an imbalance that often does not exist between friends.

To the extent that sibling relationships provide a valuable training ground for skills and competencies that generalize to peer relationships, children without siblings may be missing out on important opportunities. Nevertheless, Kitzmann, Cohen, and Lockwood (2002) found no difference in the number of friends or the quality of friendships as a function of whether the child had siblings. The authors suggest that the quality or specific features of the sibling relationship may better predict friendship quality than the mere presence or absence of siblings.

Yet there is mixed evidence for similarity in the quality of children's relationships with their siblings and friends, suggesting that the associations are complex and there is no simple "carryover" from one relationship to the other (Stocker & Dunn, 1990). Correlations between the quality of best friendships and sibling relationships among twins were moderate for positive features (e.g., affection, caring, intimacy) and negative features (e.g., conflict and hostility) (Pike & Atzaba-Poria, 2003). Lindsey and colleagues (2006) report that boys who use high levels of reasoning to manage conflicts with their siblings have warm friendships with little animosity. In contrast, Mendelson, Aboud, and Lanthier (1994) found that features of kindergartners' same-sex sibling relationships were related to the features of their same-sex friendships in opposite directions—children who reported positive feelings and little conflict with siblings had low-quality friendships. Likewise, Stocker and Dunn (1990) found that children who were reported by their mothers to have very positive friendships were competitive and controlling when observed in interactions with their sibling. And children who reported high levels of closeness in their friendships were reported by their mothers to have negative sibling relationships, characterized by competition, jealousy, and aggression.

There are several reasons why these associations are complicated and why high-quality sibling relationships may not lead simply to high-quality friendships. Mendelson and colleagues (1994) suggest that when children's time must be split between siblings and friends, one will inevitably detract from the other, or one relationship may simply reduce the need for the other relationship, contributing to distinct sibling and friend relationships. Alternatively, high-quality friendships may compensate for difficult relationships with brothers and sisters, or challenging relationships with siblings may encourage the development of social-cognitive skills that allow for especially close friendships (Stocker & Dunn, 1990).

Twin studies provide a very interesting research methodology for investigating similarities between sibling and friend relationships. In one study of adolescent twins, Pike and Atzaba-Poria (2003) evaluated the features and quality of sibling relationships and best friendships. Although genetic, shared environmental, and nonshared environmental influences contributed to variations in sibling relationship quality, nonshared environmental influences were the most important component of variations in friendship quality. Shared environmental influences accounted for a moderate portion of variance for only the friendship feature of conflict and betrayal. Nevertheless, even for this friendship feature, the contributions of the nonshared environment were stronger. Thus, even adolescent twins have very different experiences in their friendships.

Gender as a Determinant of Friendship Quality

By far, the variable that has been studied most frequently and linked most consistently with friendship quality is gender. Gender is included as a "control" variable in nearly all studies of friendship quality even if it is not a primary focus of the particular study. As such, we have much evidence about gender and friendship quality. Gender is hypothesized to be a source of variability in friendship quality in part because of the gender segregation in children's peer groups. Maccoby (1998) theorizes that hormonal differences between boys and girls lead them to prefer different play styles—calmer play styles for girls and rougher, noisier play for boys. Because of these differences in preferred play styles, children are drawn to same-sex peers as playmates. Gender segregation in playmates begins in preschool and continues throughout the elementary school years. Coupled with other forces (gender stereotypes and sex role socialization, for example), gender-segregated play means that boys and girls have different social experiences with peers that might in turn lead to differences in the features of their friendships and expectations for what makes a good friend.

Do boys' and girls' friendships differ in quality? This is actually a more complicated question than it seems because there are multiple ways boys' and girls' relationships may differ. Almost exclusively, the question has been asked regarding differences in the mean levels of various friendship features for girls versus boys—are girls' friendships closer than boys', for example? A second consideration is whether there are differences in the structure of friendship quality for girls and boys. Structural differences would suggest, for example, that the indicators of positive friendship quality are different for boys and girls—different behaviors or different provisions define positive friendship quality for girls compared to boys. A third consideration is whether the outcomes of friendship quality are different for boys versus girls. In other words, does having a high- versus low-quality friendship predict adjustment in different ways for boys or girls, suggesting that friendship quality has different meanings or different implications for boys compared to girls? These three ways of conceptualizing sex differences in friendship quality may be operating simultaneously.

Structural Differences in Friendship Quality between Boys and Girls

In one of the few studies that has specifically examined both mean-level and structural differences in friendship quality between boys and girls, Hussong (2000a) found support for both. In terms of structural differences, intimacy and peer control were defined by different behaviors for adolescent boys and adolescent girls. Companionship was a stronger component of intimacy for boys than for girls. In terms of mean-level differences, girls reported higher levels of intimacy than boys, and boys reported higher levels of peer control in their friendships than girls. Likewise, Camarena and colleagues (1990) found different pathways to emotional closeness for boys (through shared experiences and self-disclosure) and girls (only through self-disclosure). In contrast, Brendgen and colleagues (2001) suggest that high friendship quality is not achieved differently for adolescent boys versus girls. They found that correlations between children's perceptions of friendship quality and observations of their behaviors with friends were similar for boys and girls and concluded that the same behaviors are related to high versus low friendship quality for both girls and boys.

A different way of considering this question is to examine whether boys and girls differ in the activities they do with their friends and whether the association between particular activities and the quality of the relationship is different for boys and girls. Mathur and Berndt (2006) found that boys spent more time playing sports and engaging in media activities with their friends than did girls, and even though girls rated socializing with their friends as more important than did boys, they did not actually engage in more social activities with their friends. Most notably, however, youth who participated in socializing and school activities with friends perceived their relationships as more intimate, validating, and overall more positive, yet these correlations were not different for boys and girls. Thus, it was not the case that boys and girls achieved high-quality friendships through different activities.

Inconsistencies in definitions of friendship quality make it difficult to draw conclusions about gender differences. As we discuss in Chapter 2, some researchers include a separate dimension of positive features and negative features. Others consider only positive features. Still others combine positive and negative features into one dimension. To complicate matters further, the specific features used to index either positive or negative features also differ substantially. To choose one example that is especially relevant for discussions of gender, the construct of intimacy is particularly problematic. Sometimes intimacy is defined specifically as self-disclosure (Berndt, 1982; Buhrmester & Furman, 1987; Furman & Buhrmester, 1985). Other times definitions of intimacy focus on the affective feeling of emotional closeness with a friend (Camarena et al., 1990). Broader definitions of intimacy also incorporate behavioral aspects of spending time together, affective feelings of caring, and cognitive-affective experiences of loyalty (Buhrmester, 1990; Hussong, 2000a; Sharabany et al., 2008). Sullivan's (1953) definition of intimacy reflects a broader perspective incorporating validation of self-worth through mutual collaboration. Self-disclosure may be a more salient process for girls than boys, and overall emotional expressiveness may be more tolerated and encouraged for girls than boys due to a number of influences, including gender-role socialization and early sex segregation in play groups and resulting differences in social experiences. In contrast, boys may be more likely to express intimacy through shared activities and companionship (Camarena et al., 1990). As a result, gender differences in overall positive friendship quality and in the specific friendship feature of intimacy may be inflated when definitions of intimacy focus on self-disclosure or emotional expressiveness.

Mean-Level Differences in Friendship Quality between Boys and Girls

Turning to mean-level differences in friendship quality, findings are not entirely consistent—many studies show significant differences in friendship quality between boys and girls, but others do not. When gender differences are found, they tend to be in the direction of girls reporting higher friendship quality than boys. If specific friendship features are examined separately, girls consistently report higher levels of affection, closeness, validation and enhancement of self-worth, conflict resolution, intimacy, and empathic understanding (Bowker, 2004; Bukowski et al., 1994; Clark & Ayers, 1993; Furman & Buhrmester, 1985; Hoza et al., 2000; Parker & Asher, 1993; Pike & Atzaba-Poria, 2003; Prinstein, Boergers, Spirito, Little, & Grapentine, 2000; Sharabany et al., 1981). In contrast, no gender differences are typically reported for companionship and sharing mutual activities (Bukowski et al., 1994; Clark & Ayers, 1993; Furman & Buhrmester, 1985; Parker & Asher, 1993; Sharabany et al., 1981).

Some friendship features have shown inconsistent gender differences. The friendship feature that is labeled as security or reliable alliance or loyalty is sometimes found to be higher in girls (Bowker, 2004; Bukowski et al., 1994; Sharabany et al., 1981), but other times, no differences between boys and girls are reported (Clark & Ayers, 1993; Furman & Buhrmester, 1985). In part, these inconsistencies are due to differences in the kinds of behaviors and provisions tapped by the different measures of this friendship feature—confidence that the relationship will endure (e.g., Furman & Buhrmester, 1985) or a broader sense that the relationship will transcend problems and that the friend can be trusted (e.g., Bukowski et al., 1994). Likewise, several studies indicate that girls report more help and guidance from friends than do boys (Bukowski et al., 1994; Bowker, 2004; Parker & Asher, 1993). However, when the measure of help focuses more specifically on instrumental types of help—helping with homework or helping get something done—gender differences do not emerge (Furman & Buhrmester, 1985).

Researchers who have relied on composite measures of friendship quality that incorporate a number of friendship features—sometimes only positive features and sometimes both positive and negative features—also report overall higher friendship quality for girls than boys (Aikins et al., 2005; Berndt & Keefe, 1995; Brendgen et al., 2001; Buhrmester, 1990; De Goede, Branje, & Meeus, 2009; Furman & Buhrmester, 1992; Hussong, 2000a; Kingery & Erdley, 2007; La Greca & Harrison, 2005; Malcolm et al., 2006; McElhaney et al., 2006; Mounts, 2004; Ojanen et al., 2010; Phillipsen, 1999; Rose & Asher, 2004; Rubin et al., 2004; Sharabany et al., 2008; Way & Chen, 2000). In contrast, two studies showing no gender differences in positive friendship features were conducted with younger children, in kindergarten and second grade (Ladd et al., 1996; Stocker, 1994). These findings fit with the suggestion that gender differences may increase with age (e.g., Jones & Costin, 1995; Phillipsen, 1999). Aspects of intimacy are especially likely to show these enhanced gender differences in adolescence (Buhrmester & Furman, 1987; Sharabany et al., 2008).

As we discuss in Chapter 2, friendship quality is examined almost exclusively by self-report measures. In one study that used both an observational assessment of friends' interactions and self-report measures of friendship quality, gender differences were not apparent in the friends' play interactions even though early adolescent girls reported higher levels of positive friendship features than early adolescent boys (Phillipsen, 1999). In contrast, in adolescence, observations of friends' behavior during conversation tasks showed gender differences in a number of areas. Girls were rated as more responsive and showed more positive affect and self-disclosure and less negative affect, criticism, and conflict compared to boys (Brendgen et al., 2001). Notably, these observed behavioral differences paralleled the adolescents' perceptions of friendship quality as girls reported more positive features in their friendships than did boys.

In contrast to the mean gender differences in positive friendship features, conflict between friends does not show the same pattern. Most studies that have considered conflict independently of positive friendship features report no gender differences (Bowker, 2004; Bukowski et al., 1994; Furman & Buhrmester, 1985, 1992; Ladd et al., 1996; Parker & Asher, 1993; Phillipsen, 1999; Rose & Asher, 2004; Stocker, 1994). There is some suggestion that other negative features may be more frequent among boys than girls, such as peer control (Hussong, 2000a) and negative interaction patterns (La Greca & Harrison, 2005), and occasionally conflict is shown to be higher among boys (Brendgen et al., 2001). These findings support two recommendations. First, if gender differences are of interest, then measures of positive and negative friendship features should be considered separately rather than combined into one composite score. Second, indexing negative features other than conflict is likely to result in measures that highlight gender differences.

Gender Differences in Associations between Friendship Quality and Adjustment

Although boys and girls tend to report mean differences in levels of various friendship features, the association between friendship quality and adjustment is often similar for boys and girls. Typically this association is addressed statistically by examining whether the size of the correlations between friendship quality and adjustment differ for boys and girls or whether there is a statistical interaction between gender and friendship quality in the prediction of adjustment. There is considerable evidence that associations between friendship quality and various outcomes do not depend on gender. This conclusion holds for self-esteem and self-competence (Gauze et al., 1996; Keefe & Berndt, 1996), loneliness (Nangle et al., 2003; Parker & Asher, 1993), and other types of internalizing distress, such as anxiety and depression (Hussong, 2000b; La Greca & Harrison, 2005; Vernberg, Abwender, Ewell, & Beery, 1992). As we discuss in Chapter 5, the role of friendship quality in the link between early disruptive behavior and later delinquency also appears to be similar for boys and girls. Thus, although levels of friendship quality are often found to differ between boys and girls, and there is also evidence that the experiences that reflect a high-quality friendship may differ for boys and girls, the effects of friendship quality are generally consistent for boys and girls.

There are some exceptions to that general finding. Although the association between friendship quality and school involvement among adolescents did not differ for girls and boys (Berndt & Keefe, 1995), adjustment to kindergarten was particularly difficult for boys with high levels of conflict in their friendships (Ladd et al., 1996). In addition, two studies show that the link between friendship quality and emotional adjustment, particularly depression, is stronger for boys than girls (Demir & Urberg, 2004; Erdley et al., 2001). The measure of emotional adjustment used by Demir and Urberg (2004) included an assessment of happiness (in addition to depression). Interestingly, Hussong (2000b) found that positive friendship quality predicted positive affect for adolescent boys but not girls.

Together, these findings provide preliminary evidence to suggest that expressions of positive affect and positive friendship quality are strongly linked for boys. Nevertheless, it is not clear why these inconsistent gender differences emerge, and clearly, additional study of gender differences in friendship quality, particularly examinations of differences in predictors and outcomes of friendship quality for girls and boys, is warranted. Likewise, greater attention to potential structural gender differences in positive and negative friendship quality will provide further evidence to examine whether boys and girls achieve close, high-quality relationships in different ways, or whether the mean gender differences in friendship quality simply reflect an overall more harmonious and positive style of interaction for girls and their friends than for boys and their friends (e.g., Brendgen et al., 2001).

Peer Rejection as a Determinant of Friendship Quality

Despite the fact that low-accepted children are not well liked by class-mates, many are able to establish a close friendship. However, given the lower social skills and social information processing deficits of rejected children, we might expect that children who are not well accepted by peers have friendships of lower quality. There is a small literature investigating the associations between children's experience in other peer relations and the quality of their dyadic friendships. Rejected children's friends are younger, less accepted, and more likely to originate outside of school as compared to friends of high-accepted children. The friendships of low-accepted children are also less stable than the relationships of high-accepted children (George & Hartmann, 1996).

Observations of friends' interactions in play settings indicate that pairs of low-accepted friends show less positive social behavior, coordinated play, and sensitivity with one another and more disagreements than pairs of high-accepted friends. The two groups did not differ in their level of self-disclosure (Phillipsen, 1999). Observations of girls who are rejected by peers and their best friend showed that they have poorer conflict resolution skills and are more immature than better-accepted girls and their friends. Nevertheless, observers rated the overall quality of the friendships to be similarly rich and supportive for girls of varying levels of peer acceptance (Lansford et al., 2006).

When children of differing social status are asked about the quality of their friendships, differences are less consistent with some studies showing no differences between perceptions of friendship quality for low- versus high-accepted children (Lansford et al., 2006; Phillipsen, 1999). Other studies, however, indicate fairly robust differences—low-accepted children report less validation, help, and intimate disclosure than high-accepted children (Parker & Asher, 1993). In addition, conflict resolution is more problematic than for high-accepted children, and conflict overall is greater than for average-accepted (but not high-accepted) children. Children of all peer status levels report similar levels of companionship and shared activities with their friends. Interestingly, the low-accepted children showed a great deal of variability in their ratings of friendship quality as compared to other children (Parker & Asher, 1993), indicating that there are some low-accepted children whose friendships may be indistinguishable from the relationships of their better-accepted peers.

Clearly, the answer to the seemingly simple and intuitive question of whether children who are not liked by peers have lower-quality friendships is complicated. On the one hand, the well-known maladaptive behaviors, deficits in social skills and competencies, and problems in social information processing that characterize children who are not well liked would be expected to transfer to interactions with a specific friend and result in lower-quality friendships. Some research supports this conclusion. On the other hand, however, the competencies needed for success in the peer group at large may be quite different from those required to establish and maintain a high-quality friendship, and there is evidence that even rejected children experience close, supportive, and fun relationships with a friend.

Summary

Friendship quality is clearly determined by a number of factors, including family relationships, gender, and other experiences in the social world, such as peer acceptance versus rejection. There are numerous theoretical explanations for why we would see links between parent–child relationships, parents' marital relationships, parents' friendships, and children's friendships. Existing empirical research generally supports these links. Given that research suggests that different dynamics exist between fathers, mothers, daughters, and sons, future research should examine the different roles and influences of mothers and fathers on sons and daughters.

Although a good deal of research considers sibling relationships, very little compares the quality of those relationships to the quality of children's friendships. The few studies that do examine the links between siblings and friends usually examine only one of the sibling's friendships. Future studies should look more closely at both sibling's friendships, and should also consider the age of the siblings, the age difference between the siblings, the gender of the siblings, and other variables that contribute to the uniqueness of sibling relationships. In addition, in comparing sibling and friend relationships, we need to be aware that we are not examining culturally universal differences. In some cultures, the Yucatec Maya of Mexico, for example, children spend most of their time with siblings and other children who are family members (Gaskins, 2006). There is much overlap between the characteristics of friendships as we define them for European American children and the sibling relationships of the Yucatec Mayan children who rarely spend time with same-age peers outside of the family—companionship, intimacy, affection, closeness, and similarity of interests, for example.

We know the most about gender differences in friendship quality, and as discussed, it is important to think about the role of gender in several ways—structural differences, mean-level differences, and differences in associations between friendship quality and adjustment. Intimacy is the friendship feature that seems to show the most significant gender differences, including potential structural-level and mean-level differences. Specifically, depending on how intimacy is defined, different aspects of intimacy seem to contribute to high-quality friendships for boys versus girls, and consistently, girls report higher levels of intimacy in their friendships than do boys. Overall, continued exploration of differences in predictors and outcomes of friendship quality for boys and girls should help us better understand individual differences in friendship experiences and the developmental significance of high- versus low-quality friendships. Likewise, peer rejection is one component of children's experience in the broader peer world that is associated with friendship quality. Nevertheless, the substantial variability in the friendships of low-accepted children renders it difficult to make firm conclusions about peer rejection as a determinant of friendship quality.

WHAT ARE THE CORRELATES OF FRIENDSHIP QUALITY?

Assumptions about the developmental significance of friendship are captured in the theoretically based hypothesis that good, supportive, high-quality friendships lead to positive outcomes. In fact, this was accepted as a truism until recent empirical tests. The most straightforward way of addressing the question of whether the quality of a friendship affects children and adolescents is to correlate measures of friendship quality with measures of individual adjustment. Indeed, there are a number of studies that do precisely that. Many of these studies include assessments of other aspects of peer relations as well with the goal of figuring out whether friendship quality is uniquely associated with adjustment. In part because of the influence of Sullivan's (1953) theory, self-esteem, loneliness, and aspects of internalizing distress are the most frequently examined correlates of friendship quality. High-quality friendships have been hypothesized to stave off feelings of loneliness, to bolster self-esteem, and thus to protect against feelings of anxiety and depression.

Correlates of Friendship Quality in Childhood and Preadolescence

In preadolescence, friendship quality is associated with high self-worth and social competence and with low levels of anxiety, loneliness, and depression (e.g., Erdley et al., 2001; Gauze et al., 1996; Rubin et al., 2004; Stocker, 1994). However, the particular associations among various positive and negative features of friendships and these outcomes differ across studies. For example, 10-year-olds with friendships characterized by positive features had higher levels of self-worth and lower levels of anxiety (Fordham & Stevenson-Hinde, 1999). Conflict in the friendship was associated with lower self-worth, but overall, positive friendship features were more strongly associated with various outcomes than conflict. For younger children, however, these associations did not hold (Fordham & Stevenson-Hinde, 1999). In another study, positive friendship features were related to lower loneliness and depressed mood and higher self-worth and perceptions of appropriate behavioral conduct, but friendship conflict was unrelated to these aspects of adjustment (Stocker, 1994).

There is also evidence that friendship quality and popularity are both implicated in loneliness and depression. Some studies find that both friendship quality and popularity independently predict depression (Oldenburg & Kerns, 1997) and loneliness (Parker & Asher, 1993). Others find that friendship quality mediates the association between popularity and internalizing outcomes in preadolescence (Bukowski, Hoza, et al., 1993; Nangle et al., 2003). Specifically, popular children have more and higher-quality friendships, and in turn, children with high-quality friendships experience less loneliness and/or depression. One reason that both popularity and friendship quality are associated with loneliness is that there are different types of loneliness. Hoza and colleagues (2000) distinguish between peer network and dyadic loneliness. Dyadic loneliness reflects not experiencing support and companionship from a close friendship, and children who report high levels of positive features in their best friendship report low levels of this type of loneliness. Social preference among peers, in contrast, was associated with peer network loneliness.

It is not clear whether there are certain features of friendship that are most associated with specific aspects of individual adjustment. Parker and Asher (1993) found that validation, companionship, help, intimacy, conflict resolution, and conflict are roughly equally associated with loneliness, yet Oldenberg and Kerns (1997) found that validation and conflict were most consistently associated with depression. A number of methodological and measurement factors make this question about the independence of particular friendship features and particular domains of adjustment difficult to answer. Some studies rely on summary indices of friendship quality that incorporate both negative and positive features. Others separate positive and negative features into two dimensions. Still others focus on multiple indicators of positive or negative features separately (e.g., validation vs. intimacy vs. support vs. companionship). When studies include a separate positive and negative dimension, the positive dimension often includes different features, and there is no agreement on which specific positive features to include.

Friendship Quality as a Moderator Variable

Overall, though, some associations between good friendship quality and adjustment (high self-esteem, low loneliness, and internalizing distress) are consistently found in childhood and preadolescence. Friendship quality may also affect adjustment by acting as a moderator variable that either strengthens or weakens the association between another aspect of functioning and adjustment. One version of this general hypothesis is that friendship quality provides a buffer against the negative outcomes associated with other problematic experiences. In other words, having a high-quality friendship protects children from threats to their well-being that come from other relationships and other aspects of their lives, such as peer rejection and victimization or poor family relationships. In Chapter 5, we discuss ways in which high-quality friendships for children who are victimized by peers protect against anxiety, depression, and other negative outcomes of peer victimization.

Friendship quality has been investigated as a moderator of the association between a number of other factors, such as family relationships and adjustment. Gauze and colleagues (1996) find support for the hypothesis that among children with poorer family environments (low cohesion and adaptability), having a high-quality friend is important for promoting social competence and self-worth. When the family environment is positive, self-concept is adequate regardless of the quality of the friendship. Similarly, in adolescence, the link between perceptions of parental conflict and poor adjustment is exacerbated for adolescents with low friendship quality (Larsen, Branje, van der Valk, & Meeus, 2007).

A compensatory model between family relationships and friendships is also suggested by findings that children who have high-quality, warm relationships with their close friends, their mothers, or both have lower loneliness and depressed mood and more positive assessments of their behavioral competence than those with low levels of warmth with their mothers and their friends (Stocker, 1994). Children who have poor relationships with their mothers may turn to friends for support and overcome the vulnerabilities associated with lack of warmth with their mothers. It is also possible that children who are poorly adjusted may not be able to develop high-quality relationships with their friends or their mothers and in fact alienate both (Stocker, 1994). As we discuss in Chapters 4 and 5, adolescents with supportive and secure relationships with both parents and friends fare the best, but these findings are also suggestive of a buffering role for friendship quality.

Correlates of Friendship Quality in Adolescence

With young children, most investigations focus on internalizing symptoms and aspects of the self as correlates of friendship quality; however, with adolescents, there is a fairly equal focus on both internalizing and externalizing behavior problems as indicators of adjustment and well-being. With regard to internalizing symptoms in adolescence, friendship quality is often associated with anxiety and depression; however, the findings are somewhat mixed about whether it is the absence of positive features or the presence of negative features that is most significant. Three illustrative studies provide support for these different links.

La Greca and Harrison (2005) reported that adolescents with high levels of negative features in their best friendships reported greater social anxiety and depression. Having a best friendship with a high level of positive features seemed to protect against social anxiety but not depression (La Greca & Harrison, 2005). Burk and Laursen (2005) also found correlations between negative friendship features (but not positive features) and adolescents' and their mothers' reports of internalizing problems. Higher levels of positive features, however, according to the friends' reports, were associated with the adolescents' reports of lower internalizing problems. Demir and Urberg (2004), in contrast, found that *both* positive and negative friendship features were related to depressed mood and to happiness (in the expected directions). In this study, it was positive friendship features that were most strongly associated with adjustment when the quantity of friends and the degree of conflict in the relationship were taken into account. Also qualifying conclusions from this study was the finding that the effect of positive friendship features on adjustment held only for boys. Similar gender differences were also reported with younger children—friendship quality was associated with loneliness and depression for boys but not for girls (Erdley et al., 2001).

The link between friendship quality and depression does not always emerge, however. Hussong (2000b) found that the number of friends as well as positive and negative friendship features were not associated with depression, yet positive friendship features predicted greater expressions of positive affect. Among a group of clinically referred adolescents, low friendship support was not associated with depression symptoms but was directly associated with suicidal ideation (Prinstein et al., 2000).

As we discuss in Chapter 5, the associations between friendship quality and externalizing symptoms and behavior problems are complex. Across correlational studies, inconsistent findings emerge—conflict with friends was positively associated with adolescent delinquency and drug use (Mounts, 2004) and with externalizing problems (Burk & Laursen, 2005); having more friends and friendships with more positive features predicted adolescent substance use (Hussong, 2000b); and among Italian children (Menesini, 1997) and American adolescents (Burk & Laursen, 2005), positive friendship features were not related to aggression or externalizing problems. These findings parallel the inconsistent findings discussed in Chapter 5 about whether friendship quality is compromised for aggressive and antisocial youth.

In sum, more often than not, friendship quality in adolescence is correlated with adjustment indicators, yet the patterns of association vary considerably. There is some evidence to support each of these different conclusions: (1) highly conflictual and negative friendships are associated with internalizing distress, including depression; (2) high levels of positive features protect against internalizing distress, including depression; (3) associations between friendship quality and internalizing distress are strong for boys but not girls; (4) poor-quality friendships are not associated with depression; (5) highly conflictual and negative friendships are associated with externalizing problems; (6) high levels of positive features are associated with externalizing problems; and (7) positive friendship features are not associated with externalizing problems. Different measures of friendship quality, different ages of children and adolescents studied, and different indicators of internalizing distress and externalizing problems may help explain these inconsistent findings. Nevertheless, the bottom line seems to be a link between friendship quality and adjustment, and additional research, holding some of these variables constant, we hope will reveal more specificity about the particulars of those links.

Correlates of Friendship Quality Using Typological Approaches

All of the studies reviewed above consider one or more dimensions of friendship quality and assume that relationships can be differentiated by the amount of particular features—the degree to which positive or negative features are present. Another approach involves identifying meaningful patterns of friendship quality that might be important. Identification of these patterns fits with ideas from systems theory that particular relationships and relationship characteristics must be considered in the context in which they are expressed, for example, what other relationships or other features of relationships are present (Hartup, 1996a; Hussong,

2000b; Shulman, 1993). Does a high level of intimacy have different effects in the context of high versus low levels of conflict? What are the effects of a balance between cooperation and individual needs versus an emphasis on cooperation, cohesion, and mutual regulation at the expense of individual goals? What are the effects of perceptions of high levels of negativity in the context of a relationship where the friend also perceives a high level of negative features versus one in which the friend perceives a low or moderate level of negativity? These are questions that a systems perspective and a typological assessment of friendship quality can address. Below we discuss several examples of typological approaches.

Kerns (2000) used a categorical approach to assess friendship quality among preschoolers and compared three groups based on the combination of positive affect and interactive play—friends who displayed high levels of both, friends who displayed low levels of both, and friends who displayed much positive affect but little interactive play. To assess adolescent friends, Shulman (1993) applied systems theory and examined whether different types of friendships parallel a typology of family relationships (an area in which systems theory has been extensively applied). Two types of friendships were identified—interdependent friends in which the adolescents worked together in a coordinated and engaged way and disengaged friends in which the adolescents worked individually and did not coordinate their activities. In middle adolescence, there were more interdependent dyads, but in early adolescence there were more disengaged dyads. These two types of dyads reported similar activities together, suggesting that common ground and companionship do not distinguish them. However, they reasoned differently about friendship: Disengaged friends participated in friendship to stave off loneliness and interdependent dyads turned to friends for help and support.

Hussong (2000b) grouped adolescents into four categories based on their pattern of positive and negative friendship features—disengaged (low positive and low negative), positively engaged (high positive and low negative), negatively engaged (low positive and high negative), and mixed engagement (high positive and high negative). These categories were more strongly associated with adolescents' depression, positive affect, and substance use than were the dimensional measures of positive and negative friendship features. And, interestingly, this typological assessment of friendship quality revealed gender differences that were not apparent in analyses using dimensional assessments of positive and negative friendship features. Specifically, adolescent boys in the negatively engaged and mixed-engagement groups had higher levels of depression than those in the positive engagement group. For substance use, adolescents who were heavily involved in both positive and negative ways with their friends had higher levels of substance use than adolescents in the negatively engaged and disengaged groups. For positive affect, disengaged girls showed lower positive affect than the positively engaged or mixed-engaged groups, and for boys, positive engagement with their friend was associated with higher positive affect than all other patterns of engagement.

Selfhout, Branje, and Meeus (2009) identified two types of adolescent friendships based on trajectories of intimacy. Interdependent friendships were high in commitment with increasing balance across adolescence. These adolescents were able to balance commitment and individuality, but those in disengaged friendships had trouble accepting one another's views and needs and maintained lower levels of commitment. These typologies were associated with adjustment as well. Girls in disengaged friendships showed higher levels of depression across adolescence than boys and girls in interdependent friendships.

Finally, another typological assessment focused on both friends' perspectives on the relationship and compared six groups of dyads—three groups agreed in the level of positive or negative features (i.e., low, medium, and high), and three groups disagreed (i.e., one reported low and one reported medium, one reported medium and one reported high, and one reported low and one reported high). The most externalizing problems were found in pairs of friends who both reported high levels of negative features or who disagreed in their assessments of negativity (Burk & Laursen, 2005).

Such typological assessments are uncommon, yet they are promising alternatives to the dimensional approach because they assert the importance of examining multiple features together and recognizing patterns of features (e.g., Hussong, 2000b; Kerns, 2000; Selfhout, Branje, & Meeus, 2009; Shulman, 1993) and of incorporating both friends' perspectives on the relationship (e.g., Burk & Laursen, 2005). To date, however, there have been only limited attempts to identify what the key types of friendships might be. These typological approaches vary greatly by examining combinations of affect and activity (Kerns, 2000), coordination of activity (Shulman, 1993), and positive and negative features (Hussong, 2000b; Selfhout, Branje, & Meeus, 2009).

Furman and colleagues (Furman, 2001; Furman et al., 2002; Furman & Wehner, 1994) distinguish between adolescents' experiences with friends, their styles or perceptions of friendships based on self-report measures of friendship quality, and their working models of friendships that are internalized rules and expectations for friendships that affect thoughts, feelings, and actions and about which the individual may not be aware. The assessment of working models comes directly from working models of attachment based on parent–child relationships. Indeed, Furman and colleagues identify three types of working models of friendship—secure, dismissing, and preoccupied—based on representations of attachment, caregiving, and affiliation in friendships. Unlike the typological approaches described above, a focus on working models does not tap specific friendships but rather a more general view and representation of friendship as a kind of relationship. To date, we do not yet know whether or how these working models of friendship are associated with individual adjustment and functioning.

Summary

Friendship quality is clearly correlated with various aspects of adjustment. Having high-quality friendships is associated with low levels of loneliness and internalizing distress and high levels of self-esteem. Nevertheless, it is not clear what particular aspects of friendship quality are responsible for the links with positive adjustment. Typological approaches and consideration of friendship quality as a moderator of the link between risk factors and adjustment hold promise for further understanding why and how high-quality friendships correspond to positive adjustment.

HOW DOES FRIENDSHIP QUALITY AFFECT DEVELOPMENTAL OUTCOMES?

Finding a correlation between friendship quality and some aspect of adjustment could indeed mean that having higher-quality friendships leads to better adaptation. As described above, this conclusion is theoretically sound in that there are many reasons to expect that experiences with more intimate, close, supportive friends in relationships not disrupted by unmanageable conflict provide a developmental context for the acquisition of skills and competencies, for support during times of stress, and for protection against loneliness and depression. However, there is also good reason to anticipate that children and adolescents who are better adjusted are able to form higher-quality relationships with their friends. For example, depressive symptoms may elicit social rejection (Coyne, 1976), and peers may avoid depressed children (Peterson, Mullins, & Ridley-Johnson, 1985). Although longitudinal designs are still correlational in nature and thus suffer from the same critique, they do enable us to examine whether friendship quality can predict changes in adjustment over time and in that way strengthen support for the conclusion that friendship quality affects developmental outcomes.

Does Friendship Quality Affect Adjustment to Transitions?

If high-quality friendships do indeed help children and adolescents cope with stressful situations, we might expect these effects to be particularly noticeable during periods of transition. As we discuss in Chapter 3, school transitions represent a normative transition that encompasses significant change and therefore a potential period of stress. For most children, the transition from elementary to middle or junior high schools involves a shift in school context—from small schools with self-contained classrooms to much larger schools in which children must move from class to class with different teachers and students throughout the day. In addition, academic demands increase, and there are many changes in the peer context as well with much larger and more diverse peer groups and less adult supervision of peer group activities.

The stability and the quality of friendships are important factors in children's and adolescents' adjustment over a school transition. Higher-quality friendships before the school transition predict the stability of the relationship and in turn higher friendship quality and better school adjustment after the transition (Aikins et al., 2005). When high-quality friendships are stable across the transition, adolescents' sociability and leadership increase (Berndt et al., 1999). High-quality, stable relationships also seemed to protect adolescents from the potential negative effects of having a withdrawn friend—for these adolescents, their own isolation did not increase, but a low-quality friendship with a withdrawn friend elicited more isolation from the adolescent (Berndt et al., 1999). These effects have not always emerged so strongly. In one study, pretransition friendship quality predicted lower loneliness and greater school involvement after the transition, yet when adolescents' acceptance by peers was taken into account, friendship quality was no longer related to adjustment across the school transition (Kingery & Erdley, 2007).

The transition to elementary school among young children also presents significant challenges to children and provides a critical time for considering how friendships may help children negotiate these challenges and demands. Ladd and colleagues (Ladd, 1990; Ladd & Kochenderfer, 1996; Ladd et al., 1996) assert that stable friendships facilitate this early school transition by providing support and validation and by functioning as a critical attachment for young children. Among kindergarten children, more validating and less conflictual friendships were more stable. Over the course of the school year, boys with conflictual friendships felt more lonely, liked school less, avoided school more, and were less engaged in the classroom. When friends provided high levels of help and aid, children liked school more over the course of the year (Ladd et al., 1996).

Taken together, these findings support the notion that high-quality friendships promote adjustment across potentially stressful school transitions. Furthermore, they bolster the conclusions presented in Chapter 3 by suggesting that it is not only having a friend but having a high-quality, supportive friend that smoothes the rough patches of stressful school transitions. Nevertheless, many aspects of adjustment examined in these studies were not related to friendship quality, and we need to be careful not to overemphasize the importance of friendship quality as having comprehensive, overwhelming effects on individual adjustment and well-being.

Does Friendship Quality Affect Emotional Adjustment and Self-Concept?

Friendship quality is clearly correlated with emotional adjustment and self-esteem, yet the findings from longitudinal investigations are not as consistent. Concurrently, closeness with a best friend and other positive friendship features are associated with lower depression symptoms and higher self-concept in the areas of perceived social acceptance, scholastic competence, and global self-worth (Keefe & Berndt, 1996; Vernberg, 1990). Negative friendship features were associated with lower global self-worth and perceptions of behavioral competence (Keefe & Berndt, 1996).

Predictions over time, however, are less strong. For example, closeness with a best friend and other peer experiences (e.g., rejection experiences) predicted changes in depression over time, but greater closeness with a best friend was not uniquely associated with decreases in depression (Vernberg, 1990). In two studies, Berndt and colleagues (1999; Keefe & Berndt, 1996) found that positive friendship features did not predict changes in self-concept and self-esteem over the course of the school year or over the course of a school transition. Adolescents with conflict-ridden friendships in the fall perceived their behavioral competence to worsen over the school year (Keefe & Berndt, 1996), but hypothesized links between high-quality friendships and self-esteem were simply not found.

A recent study with Italian adolescents suggests stronger links over time between friendship quality and emotional adjustment and self-concept among older adolescents (Ciairano, Rabaglietti, Roggero, Bonino, & Beyers, 2007). Support from friends predicted decreases in depression and alienation and increases in positive self-perceptions. Improvements in friendship quality also forecast better adjustment. Adolescents with high-quality relationships across the year and those whose friendships improved from low to high quality had greater positive self-perceptions and lower alienation. If the friendship quality weakened over the course of the year, positive perceptions of the self decreased (Ciairano et al., 2007).

Changes in behavioral indicators of adjustment may also be predicted by friendship quality. For example, adolescents with close, supportive, intimate friendships became more involved in school over the course of the year. Those with conflict-ridden friendships showed increases in disruptive behavior from fall to spring if those relationships also had high levels of positive features (Berndt & Keefe, 1995).

Overall, then, there is some evidence that friendship quality affects adjustment over time. The empirical findings, however, are not as strong as theoretical ideas or common sense might suggest. Furthermore, the long-held belief that high-quality friendships promote self-esteem has received only mixed support in longitudinal studies. Rather, friendship quality seems to have more specific effects on adjustment. As noted above, having friendships high on positive features seems to help children cope with school transitions. Berndt (2002; Berndt & Murphy, 2002) suggests that supportive friends help children adjust to new school environments by promoting positive relationships with other peers and helping them connect with others after school transitions. This is demonstrated in part by students' increased school involvement.

There is increasing evidence, however, that having friendships with many negative features promotes disruptive behavior (Dishion et al., 1996; Keefe & Berndt, 1996). The long-term implications of high levels of negative features, such as conflict and rivalry, and the effects of having friendships high on both positive and negative features are important directions for future research. The negative effects of having a contentious friendship and of frequent negative exchanges and interactions with a friends appears to be strongest when that relationship is also characterized by many positive features—high levels of closeness and companionship, for example (Berndt & Keefe, 1995; Piehler & Dishion, 2007). In the context of a fun, rewarding, and intimate friendship, high levels of conflict, antagonism, and coercion may be particularly pernicious because children become increasingly skilled in those kinds of interactions, have many opportunities to practice and perfect negative behaviors, and generalize them to other social interactions with other peers, with parents, and with teachers. These more recent ideas about the effects of negative friendship quality have not yet been sufficiently studied, in part because Sullivan (1953) and others focused exclusively on the positive effects of good friendships. They come from observations in clinical settings, such as Dishion and colleagues' (1999) careful investigation of iatrogenic effects from peer reinforcement in group treatment sessions, and from empirical studies that include measures of both positive and negative friendship features over time.

Summary

Overall, then, the assumption that having high-quality friendships causes positive outcomes like high self-esteem and good socioemotional adjustment has not found overwhelming empirical support. It does seem that good friendships assist children with successful transitions in school—the transition to kindergarten and the transition to middle school or junior high. In addition, recent work on the effects of poor-quality friendships—including relationships high in conflict and other negative features—suggests that this is an important area to look for possible long-term associations between friendship quality and adjustment, in this case maladjustment.

CONCLUSIONS

The primary conclusion we draw is that friendship quality is a key indicator of how friendships differ from one another, and in turn, of the effects a particular relationship has on the children involved. Low-quality versus high-quality friendships differ in the developmental context they provide, in the experiences the friends have in the relationship, and in the effects they have on individual children. Interestingly, we do not know a whole lot about what determines the quality of a particular relationship, or in other words, what factors predict friendship quality. Much of the emphasis is placed on the characteristics of the individual children—for example, to what degree does a child's aggressiveness determine the quality of his or her friendships? As discussed above, however, parents' behaviors and children's relationships with their parents have implications for the quality of the friendships children develop. This research is valuable for demonstrating how friendships exist within and are affected by the broader social context around them.

Boys and girls clearly differ in the degree to which certain features tend to be present in their friendships. In fact, we know more about gender differences in friendship quality than about any other aspect of friendship quality. The conclusion is that in terms of mean levels of positive friendship features, girls report more—more intimacy, closeness, and validation. It is now time to ask whether there are other ways that the quality of boys' and girls' friendships differs. Specifically, do boys and girls achieve high-quality friendships in different ways, and do variations in friendship quality affect boys and girls in different ways? These kinds of questions about gender and friendship quality fit with gender socialization theories and other theories about the importance of dyadic relationships for boys and girls. Yet, simply knowing whether boys and girls report different levels of positive and negative features does not answer these questions, and it is quite possible that girls may report greater intimacy or closeness than boys *and* that the way high-quality friendships are realized is not the same for boys and girls *and* that a high-quality friendship buffers boys and girls differently from other experiences.

The importance of friendship quality as an individual differences variable associated with the developmental significance of friendship shines through in studies evaluating the correlates of friendship quality. Here we see that friendship quality is associated with self-worth, anxiety, loneliness, depression, and social competence in the directions one would expect—higher friendship quality is associated with better adjustment. It is perhaps surprising, then, that the findings about friendship quality as a predictor of adjustment over time are more limited. In many ways, drawing conclusions from these longitudinal studies requires choosing between a glass-half-empty and a glass-half-full approach. On the one hand, high-quality friendships predict school adjustment and sociability across school transitions. Friendships with much conflict predict worsening behavioral competence and disruptive behavior (Berndt & Keefe, 1995; Keefe & Berndt, 1996). Thus, having positive relationships with friends may help children cope with the demands of normative developmental transitions. There is good evidence, too, that high levels of negative features (especially in the context of otherwise warm, close relationships) forecast increases in disruptive and problem behavior. On the other hand, friendship quality is not as strongly associated with changes in adjustment over time than with aspects of current functioning. This is particularly true for the oft-cited claim, stemming from Sullivan's (1953) theory, that high-quality friendships promote self-esteem (Berndt & Murphy, 2002).

Most of the longitudinal studies examining the effects of friendship quality over time proceed as follows: assessments of children's adjustment and friendship quality are made at Time 1, and after some period of time, assessments of adjustment are made again at Time 2. In regression models, the effect of friendship quality on adjustment at Time 2 is evaluated, controlling for the stability of adjustment from Time 1 to Time 2. In these models, the question is whether friendship quality accounts for changes in adjustment over time. Typically, the domain of adjustment examined is fairly stable over the time span covered by the study; thus, there is not much change in adjustment left for friendship quality to predict. When friendship quality does not predict adjustment at Time 2 with adjustment at Time 1 in the model, it does not necessarily mean that friendship quality is unrelated to adjustment, only that friendship quality does not uniquely explain the often relatively small changes in adjustment over the course of a school year or two. Are there better ways to examine how friendship quality predicts adjustment and well-being over time?

The quality of the friendship accounts for some variability in outcomes associated with participation in this particular relationship with this particular friend. Friendship quality is thus developmentally significant and an important variable for considering individual differences in the experience of friendship. Yet, we need to avoid the tendency to idealize friendships, as novels, films, songs, and our own memories are wont to do. Instead, we need a more nuanced appreciation for ways in which our intuitive sense that a high-quality relationship must contribute to positive adjustment in every way depends on the outcome domain being considered and the way in which friendship quality is assessed.

Future Research Directions

Many of the most needed directions for future research involve questions of how we measure friendship quality. Chapter 2 discusses a number of issues related to the measurement of friendship quality that have implications for how we understand its effects. Here we discuss four important directions for future research.

1. First, the correlates and effects of various friendship features differ—most notably for positive versus negative features. Yet, many studies include a composite assessment of friendship quality that includes only positive features or that includes a combination of positive and negative features. It is clear that the correlates and outcomes associated with a friendship low on positive features are not necessarily the same as those associated with a friendship high on negative features. In other words, a lack of emotional closeness may not have the same effects as the presence of a high degree of conflict. Furthermore, a lot of conflict in the friendship is likely to have different effects if that conflict is in the context of closeness, support, and intimacy as opposed to a lack of emotional closeness. Thus, researchers studying friendship quality should, whenever possible, include separate dimensions of positive and negative features. These kinds of investigations also address the issue of whether negative features are more important than positive features. The argument here is that friendships are supposed to be supportive, positive, fun relationships. Thus, the presence of a high level of negative features is unexpected and particularly salient and may be more predictive of adjustment than variations in positive features (Keefe & Berndt, 1996; Rook, 1984). In other words, "bad is stronger than good" (Baumeister, Bratslavsky, Finkenauer, & Vohs, 2001, p. 323).

2. A related point is that we usually conceptualize friendship quality as a continuum. Any particular friendship exists at a particular location on this continuum (or on two continua if positive and negative features are considered separately). As such, our conclusions rest on the assumption that incremental changes—more positive features or fewer negative features are better. Alternatively, a categorical or typological approach would suggest that there are types of friendships that differ in important ways and these friendship types are associated with positive (or negative) outcomes. For example, perhaps there is a certain level of positive friendship features that define a good friendship, and variations in positive friendship features beyond this amount do not forecast even better adjustment. Likewise, perhaps whether friendships contain a low to moderate amount of conflict, rivalry, and other negative features has no substantial impact on adjustment, but beyond this level, negative features are associated with maladjustment. As noted above, high levels of conflict in the presence of many positive features as well may not be problematic, but conflict coupled with low support may lead to problems. With notable exceptions (Burk & Laursen, 2005; Furman et al., 2002; Hussong, 2000b; Shulman, 1993), this kind of typological approach has not been adequately considered. In part, this may be because we do not have clear agreement on what the important typologies might be (Hartup, 1996a)—presence or absence of some critical level of positive and negative features? Formulations akin to family systems theory such as interdependent versus disengaged friends? Agreement versus disagreement between friends on their relationship quality? Activation of specific relationship provisions and behavioral systems—attachment versus affiliation versus caregiving? All of these various typological approaches hold promise.

3. Another promising approach is the conceptualization of friendship quality as a buffer or moderator of the association between individual characteristics and experiences or characteristics of other relationships and outcomes. As discussed above and in Chapter 5, friendship quality has been found to buffer against negative outcomes associated with peer victimization, having a withdrawn friend, and difficult family relationships. Thinking of friendship in this way fits well with Sullivan's (1953) ideas of friendship compensating for or making up for problematic experiences in other domains. The existing evidence is not overwhelming, and having a high-quality friendship is certainly not a panacea. Nevertheless, thinking of friendship quality in relation to other experiences and relationships—as conceptualizing friendship quality as a buffer or protective factor necessarily does—is an important direction for future research. Similarly, examining complex associations between

friendship quality, the characteristics of children's friends (as we discuss primarily in Chapter 5), and other aspects of peer relations, such as peer status and children's place in the social network, is necessary for teasing apart the intersections among multiple dimensions of friendship and other peer relations.

4. Finally, readers may be struck by the lack of research examining processes through which friendship quality exerts its effects. Speculation about how and why friendship quality contributes to adjustment independent of the presence of friends or the characteristics of friends comes primarily from Sullivan's (1953) ideas about the importance of friendship. There are a number of possibilities. From Sullivan's perspective, poor-quality friendships are likely to fail in meeting the need for interpersonal intimacy and providing the collaborative experience that promotes adaptation and well-being. Alternatively, from a stress and coping perspective, poor-quality friendships may represent a significant stressor for children and require substantial coping mechanisms, especially if a low-quality friendship translates into daily experiences of conflict, victimization, or rejection experiences (Sandstrom & Zakriski, 2004). Identifying the processes that explain why and how friendships of varying quality contribute differently to adjustment is a key direction for future research.

PART IV

IMPLICATIONS AND LOOKING FORWARD

Chapter 7

Friendship and Culture

with Emily C. Jenchura

According to the contextual-developmental perspective ...
cultural influence on children's social competence is a dynamic
process, which is reflected at three levels: the changing cultural
context, the developing child, and the mediating role of social
interaction between the child and peers, parents, and others.
To understand the nature of children's social competence, it
is important to examine how the child's characteristics and
socialization practices contribute to the social interaction
processes, which in turn shape developmental outcomes in
cultural context.
—XINYIN CHEN AND DORAN FRENCH (2008, p. 607)

Researchers will discover and explore friendship as perhaps the
most human of relationships, because friends try to construct
their relationship in relative independence of, but not necessarily
against, the most respectable institutions of their society. For
that purpose they are a culturally based shared meaning system
because it enables them to negotiate their relationship in a
way that offers the best balance of personal desires and others'
demands in a given context. Relative to the respective context,
no relationship is less standardized than friendship. Because of
the diversity of cultural contexts, no relationship can be realized
in richer variations than friendship can be.
—LOTHAR KRAPPMAN (1996, p. 37)

Emily C. Jenchura, BS, received her degree in cross-cultural psychology from the University
of Richmond in 2008. She then spent one year in Trinidad and Tobago as a Fulbright Fellow investigating cross-ethnic friendships. Her research interests include close relationships
and cross-cultural studies.

The idea of studying similarities and differences in friendships across cultures and how cultural context influences children's experiences with friends seems obvious given several of the assumptions we make about friendships. After all, we assume that friendships are multidimensional, that there are individual differences in the effects of friendship on adjustment, that various aspects of friendship are affected by outside influences in systematic ways, and that friendships are situated within networks of other peer contexts and broader social contexts, such as schools and communities. Thus, culture is expected to play an important role in friendships as well. Nevertheless, the study of friendships cross culturally is still relatively limited even though it has expanded dramatically in recent years.

There are two primary questions at the heart of research on friendships and culture. First, what are the important similarities and differences in the presence of friendship, in the characteristics of children's and adolescents' interactions with friends, and in the quality of relationships with their friends across cultural contexts? Second, inasmuch as these differences exist, do they lead to different developmental outcomes? In the sections that follow, we discuss theoretical perspectives on understanding the cultural context of friendship and then review the empirical evidence on the cross-cultural study of children's friendships with particular attention to these two questions. The aspects of friendship that have been examined most extensively include the role of friendships vis-à-vis family and other relationships, the characteristics and quality of friendships, and the similarities between friends.

THEORETICAL PERSPECTIVES
ON CULTURE AND FRIENDSHIP

There are a number of ways to conceptualize the effect of cultural context on children's experience in friendships. One view defines culture as a set of values, norms, and practices that affects individuals' behavior and development. This perspective owes much to Bronfenbrenner's (1979) ecological model in which culture is a context that may directly shape peer relationships. In analytical terms, culture is seen as the independent variable that influences friendship, the dependent variable. A second view focuses on the dynamic nature of cultural processes and the role that children themselves play in becoming active participants in adult culture. In this latter perspective, friendship is a critical relationship that reflects the culture in which it is situated and that also provides a context for children's reproduction of their culture in an active, interpretive way (see Corsaro, 2003, for further discussion of the interpretive approach). Thus, friendship itself is a cultural practice (Way, 2006). In recent research, these two perspectives are becoming more closely related as researchers recognize the role of the child in the process of socialization and study reciprocal influences among culture, peer relationships, and the development of the individual child (e.g., Chen, French, & Schneider, 2006; Krappman, 1996). In much the same way, current views of friendship recognize that it both contributes to and is an outcome of developmental processes. Edwards, de Guzman, Brown, and Kumru (2006) describe this more recent view of friendship and culture stating: "Culture must be identified inside developmental contexts, for example, inside peer relationships ... rather than being modeled as a source of influence on human development with its own independent pathways" (p. 26).

Study of close relationships cross culturally is based on the assumption that similarities across cultures are evidence for universal processes (perhaps of an evolutionary origin), but differences highlight the unique practices specific to a particular culture (Reis, Collins, & Berscheid, 2000). The most convenient and often-used dimension to characterize cultures and explain differences in social relationships and social behaviors is the collectivism versus individualism dimension. Interest in individualism and collectivism within cross-cultural psychology stems from Hofstede's 1980 book *Culture's Consequences,* even though the roots of this distinction predate Hofstede considerably (e.g., Adam Smith and Jean-Jacques Rousseau in the late 1700s and Emile Durkheim in the late 1800s). Hofstede (1980) described four dimensions along which national cultures differ—power distance, uncertainty avoidance, collectivism/individualism, and masculinity/femininity.

According to Hofstede's definition, individualistic societies emphasize loose ties between individuals and a focus on the needs of the individual and his or her immediate family. In contrast, in collectivistic societies, individuals are a part of cohesive in-groups in which they are integrated throughout the lifespan. Behavior is based on concern and care for others. Individualism versus collectivism thus reflects ways in which people live together as well as societal norms and values (Hofstede, 2001). Triandis (1990) further identifies specific factors that characterize individualism versus collectivism. Family integrity and interdependence reflect collectivism, whereas self-reliance and separation from in-groups are associated with individualism. More recent reviews and meta-analyses emphasize that the key components of individualism are independence and uniqueness, and of collectivism are duty and obligation to and maintaining harmony with the in-group (Oyserman, Coon, & Kemmelmeier, 2002).

The definition of the in-group varies across cultures and may have important implications for considering how friendships differ across collectivistic versus individualistic societies. Collectivistic societies tend to have a stable in-group consisting of family and/or tribe with everyone else forming the out-group. In individualistic cultures, however, people tend to have more in-groups. One in-group may consist of the family, another of coworkers, another of members of a particular club or civic organization. If the demands that an in-group makes on a person in an individualistic culture are too high, the person may simply leave that in-group and form another. Thus, Triandis, Bontempo, Villareal, Asai, and Lucca (1988) characterize the demands of in-groups as "highly segmented" in individualistic cultures and as "diffuse" in collectivistic cultures (p. 324). Behavior toward in-group versus out-group members differs much more significantly in collectivistic than in individualistic cultures.

The collectivism/individualism dimension is sociological in nature in that it distinguishes societies and is not meant to be used at the level of the individual as a personality dimension. Triandis and colleagues (Triandis, 1995; Triandis et al., 1988) have described allocentrism versus idiocentrism as an individual-level variable that corresponds to collectivism versus individualism at the cultural level. At the sociological level, individualism and collectivism are viewed as opposite extremes of one dimension, but at the individual level, allocentrism and idiocentrism are separate dimensions, and a person can show both allocentric and idiocentric traits simultaneously (Hofstede, 2001). A similar individual-level variable focuses on how the self is perceived in relation to others. The independence view characterizes the self as an autonomous individual, whereas the interdependence view assumes that the self is tightly embedded in relationships (Markus & Kitayama, 1991).

Interestingly, hypotheses about how friendships might differ in collectivistic versus individualistic societies are implicit in some of the definitions and measures used to distinguish societies and individuals along this dimension. For example, Triandis and colleagues (1988) developed a measure to assess the idiocentrism–allocentrism dimension, and items include "I like to live close to my friends," "I am not to blame when one of my close friends fails," and "When a close friend of mine is successful, it does not really make me look better." These items assess concern for the in-group and distance from the in-group. The focus on friends suggests that friendship is an important in-group relationship and that individuals in collectivistic versus individualistic societies may have very different expectations and beliefs about and experiences with this relationship. In particular, one commonly discussed hypothesis is that people in individualistic cultures find it easier to make friends and are better skilled at entering and leaving social relationships and groups, but the term *friends* includes a wide circle of acquaintances and nonintimate relationships (French, Pidada, & Victor, 2005; Hofstede, 2001; Triandis et al., 1988). The contrasting hypothesis is that people in collectivistic cultures include among their friends only those with whom they have life-long, intimate relationships that are filled with mutual obligations. They are not as skilled in entering new relationships. These and other hypotheses about collectivism versus individualism as a determinant of cultural variations in children's and adolescents' friendships have received moderate support in the literature to date.

In this chapter, we refer to individualism and collectivism as a source for hypothesized differences between children and adolescents in different cultures and as a potential explanation for the differences that emerge because this is the primary dimension used in the existing literature. In doing so, friendship researchers are not unique. Estimates indicate that over one-third of studies on all types of cross-cultural comparisons invoke the individualism–collectivism distinction to explain observed differences (Hui & Yee, 1994, in Brewer & Chen, 2007). Nevertheless, there are limitations to this approach. First, the studies we describe do not actually assess individualism and collectivism directly. Instead, they rely on what Oyserman and colleagues (2002) call "applying Hofstede" (p. 7). In this approach, countries are deemed to be individualist or collectivist based on Hofstede's analysis rather than based on any current assessment of the constructs at the level of the individual. Second, although individualism and collectivism are often viewed as opposite ends of one continuum, more recent research suggests that they are orthogonal constructs and that all societies and cultures have at least some degree of both values. Third, although individualism seems to be a coherent and meaningful construct describing a particular worldview, collectivism is a much broader construct that includes many different values and attitudes (Oyserman et al., 2002).

Brewer and Chen (2007) propose a new theoretical model that distinguishes between *relational collectivism* and *group collectivism* and draws on distinctions between three levels of the social self—the individual, relational, and collective self. In this model, relational collectivism involves a focus on interpersonal relationships, including close dyadic relationships with strong attachment bonds, and the networks that build from those dyadic ties. The in-groups involved in group collectivism do not have close interpersonal bonds but are linked by shared (yet depersonalized) social categories. This model has not yet been applied in cross-cultural research on children's friendships.

SOCIAL NETWORKS AND THE ROLE OF FRIENDS

The research question that has been asked most consistently and extensively across cultures concerns the support, intimacy, and other social provisions received from various members of a child's social network. How does support from friends compare with support from parents, siblings, teachers, and others? This question relates directly to the functional characteristics of an individual's social relationships and stems from several sources. Sullivan's (1953) interpersonal theory contends that different needs arise throughout development, and specific social relationships emerge that are best suited for meeting that particular social need. Weiss (1974) carried this idea further and provides a framework for understanding the social provisions that different relationships offer. In his conceptualization, individuals seek different types of social support or provisions in their various relationships, and each relationship may provide a different kind of support.

The Role of Social Support Networks across Cultures

In developing the Network of Relationships Inventory (NRI; see Chapter 2), Furman and Buhrmester (1985) applied Weiss's theory to children's relationships with others in their social network. Indeed, children in U.S. samples consistently report that specific social provisions are gained in their relationships with different members of their network (e.g., mothers, fathers, siblings, friends, teachers, other relatives). Researchers investigating children's peer relationships and other social relationships cross culturally have seized on this type of question and measures like the NRI to examine whether cultural differences emerge in the provisions offered by specific network members. This work is promising for understanding children's perceptions of the role and function of their close friendships in very different cultural contexts in part because it does not treat friendships in isolation but considers them as one component of a potentially rich network of social relationships. Asking children about the perceived social support they receive from various others in their lives taps their cognitive appraisal of social support (as opposed to the support they actually receive). It is this element of support that best predicts mental health and other outcomes among adults (Sarason & Sarason, 1985).

Why might we expect the social provisions of specific relationships within a child's social network to differ across various cultural contexts? Tietjen (1989) proposed that the role of social support systems is to promote children's competence, and what connotes competence is culturally relative. Thus, network members foster the competencies that are important for successful adaptation to the norms and values of that particular culture. Using the individualistic versus collectivistic distinction to classify cultural systems offers several hypotheses for qualitative and quantitative differences in perceptions of the social provisions satisfied by various social network members. Put simply, in cultures that value and promote individual autonomy, the social network is organized to promote individual skills and achievement. In contrast, collectivistic cultures are more likely to promote competence within a social group. Thus, cooperation rather than conflict and strong bonds with family members may be emphasized. In collectivistic cultures, youth may rely on a larger network for their support needs, whereas individualistic cultures may promote reliance on a more limited range of others for social support. For best friends, in particular, this distinction might mean that they are more critical sources of support for youth in individualistic cultures.

Specific Findings from Empirical Studies

Empirical studies of children's and adolescents' social support networks have been conducted in a number of countries. Here we consider exemplar studies with youth from Indonesia, Costa Rica, Brazil, Turkey, Zimbabwe, Italy, Belgium, Canada, Australia, and the United States. The findings of these studies are summarized in Table 7.1, which includes a listing of cross-cultural similarities and differences. Only the findings from these studies that are directly relevant to friendship are included in the table. Canada, Australia, and the United States represent the extreme individualistic end of the individualism versus collectivism continuum (Hofstede, 1980, 2001). Indonesia and Costa Rica have both been considered highly collectivistic societies. According to French, Pidada, and Victor (2005), the agricultural-based economic history of many parts of Indonesia required a high degree of community organization, and the collectivistic values and behaviors there likely reflect this tightly coordinated community-based system. The nature of the Costa Rican society places special emphasis on strong ties with family members. There are strong ties between generations within a family, relatively large nuclear families, and significantly greater contact with relatives than with others outside the family (see DeRosier & Kupersmidt, 1991, for a review). Like other Latin American countries, Brazil is viewed as collectivistic, and Brazilian culture has a strong orientation toward family. Nevertheless, the industrialized nature of southern Brazil gives many southern Brazilians an individualistic orientation in terms of self-reliance (Van Horn & Marques, 2000). Similarly, although Turkey is rapidly adopting traditionally Western values, a focus on family is still the norm (Hortacsu, 1997), and Turkey (like Brazil) sits in the middle range of Hofstede's (2001) ranking of 53 countries and regions on individualism versus collectivism. The culture in Zimbabwe is clearly collectivistic and emphasizes the family. Historically, growing up in large extended families was typical (Harrison, Stewart, Myambo, & Teveraishe, 1995, 1997). In rural areas of Zimbabwe, extended families continue to live together and share

TABLE 7.1. Cross-Cultural Comparisons on Support from Social Networks

Study	Cross-cultural comparison (age)	Cross-cultural similarities	Cross-cultural differences
Claes (1998)	Italy, Belgium, Canada (11–18 years)	In all three countries, adolescents reported having the most intimate conversations with friends, followed by mothers, siblings, and fathers.	• Contact with social network: Italian youth have most contact with family, Canadian youth have most contact with friends, Belgian youth report equal contact with family and friends. • Shared activities with social network: Canadians report more shared activities with friends than Belgians and Italians. • Closeness with social network: Canadians closest to best friends, Italians closest to parents, Belgians equally close to parents and friends.
DeRosier and Kupersmidt (1991)	Costa Rica, U.S. (4th and 6th grades)	Costa Rican and U.S. children rated friends similarly on companionship, satisfaction, intimacy, and conflict.	• *Direct comparison:* Costa Rican children rated friends higher on instrumental aid and affection than U.S. children. • *Relative importance:* Costa Rican children view parents as primary source of support; U.S. children report best friends as primary source of support.
French, Rianasari, Pidada, Nelwan, and Buhrmester (2001)	Indonesia (5th and 8th grades), U.S. (6th and 8th grades)	Indonesian and U.S. children rated friends as their primary source of intimacy.	• *Direct comparison:* U.S. youth report higher companionship, satisfaction, and conflict in friendships than Indonesian youth. • *Relative importance:* Indonesian youth rate mothers and friends equally on companionship, U.S. youth rate friends highest. Indonesian youth rate parents and friends equally on conflict, U.S. youth rate friends lower on conflict than parents. Indonesian youth rate more satisfaction with mothers than friends, U.S. youth rate more satisfaction with friends than parents.

Reference	Countries (ages)	Findings
Harrison, Stewart, Myambo, Teveraishe (1995)	Zimbabwe, U.S. (13–15 years)	Rural Zimbabwean adolescents, urban Zimbabwean adolescents, and U.S. adolescents rated best friends similarly on instrumental help and intimacy. • *Direct comparison:* U.S. youth rated best friends higher on reliable alliance, enhancement of worth, affection, companionship, and satisfaction and lower on conflict than Zimbabwean adolescents. • *Relative importance:* Zimbabwean adolescents (urban): best friends highest on conflict, instrumental help, intimacy; mothers and teachers higher than best friends on reliable alliance and affection; fathers higher than best friends on enhancement of worth, companionship, and satisfaction. Zimbabwean adolescents (rural): best friends highest on intimacy and conflict; mothers and best friends highest on reliable alliance; fathers higher than best friends on enhancement of worth; teachers and mothers higher than best friends on instrumental help; teachers and best friends highest on companionship; parents higher than best friends on satisfaction. U.S. adolescents: best friends higher than anyone on enhancement of worth, companionship, intimacy, and satisfaction.
Hortacsu (1997)	Turkey, U.S. (12–17 years)	In Turkey and U.S., best friends rated equally important for overall satisfaction of needs. • Adolescents in Turkey perceived mothers as more able to meet needs than friends; U.S. adolescents made no distinction.
Keats et al. (1983)	Australia, France, Norway, U.S. (12, 15, 18 years)	Adolescents in all four countries reported that parents' opinions mattered most and friends' opinions were second in importance.

(continued)

TABLE 7.1. (*continued*)

Study	Cross-cultural comparison (age)	Cross-cultural similarities	Cross-cultural differences
Laursen, Wilder, Noack, and Williams (2000)	Germany, U.S. (11–18 years)	Equal numbers of adolescents in Germany and U.S. reported high and low closeness with friends.	• German youth rated mothers and friends as equal in reciprocity, U.S. youth rated friends as more reciprocal than parents. • More links between closeness, authority, and reciprocity across friend and parent relationships for German youth than for U.S. youth.
Li, Connolly, Jiang, Pepler, and Craig (2010)	China, Canada (mean = 16.6 years)	Friendship quality and mixed-sex group affiliation were positively correlated for both Chinese and Canadian youth. Friendship quality was directly linked to romantic experiences in both societies.	• Companionship (negative correlation) and intimacy (positive correlation) in friendships were associated with serious dating only in Canada. The link between friendship quality and romantic experiences was stronger for Canadian than for Chinese adolescents.
Shute, De Blasio, and Williamson (2002; Australia) and Reid, Landesman, Treder, and Jaccard (1989; U.S.)	Australia (9–11 years), U.S. (6–12 years)	Australian and U.S. children rated friends equally on companionship support; pattern of type of support provided by friends similar—companionship highest, then emotional support, then informational and instrumental support.	• U.S. children rated best friends higher on emotional, instrumental, and informational support than did Australian children.

Note. Only studies with direct comparisons between at least two countries are included. The similarities and differences reported are limited to findings about friends.

an economy in an interdependent way. Modifications to this traditional structure have occurred in urban areas where families continue to share close bonds but do not typically share living spaces or economic links. According to Hofstede's (2001) analysis, Belgium and Italy are both individualistic societies (in the top 15% of those he studied). Nevertheless, Italian culture provides an interesting comparison to these other cultural contexts because it generally espouses goals and values consistent with an individualistic orientation, yet involvement in the family remains a critical determinant of identity and source of support (Schneider, Fonzi, Tani, & Tomada, 1997). Figure 7.1 plots these various countries according to Hofstede's analysis of individualism and collectivism.

One way of assessing the importance of various members of a child's social network is simply by asking who are the important people in children's lives; these findings also show similarities across cultures. Adolescents in Australia, France, Norway, and the United States all ranked parents as the people whose opinions matter most to them, and friends were a close second (Keats et al., 1983), showing the primacy of both parents and friends in adolescents' lives across a variety of cultures.

More typically, cross-cultural studies of social support networks have used the NRI or similar measures and have assessed social provisions such as companionship, intimacy, closeness, enhancement of self-worth, affection, and help or instrumental aid. In addition, the level of conflict in the relationship is often assessed as one indicator of negative features of close relationships. One of the earliest cross-cultural comparisons using this methodology was conducted by DeRosier and Kupersmidt (1991) with children in Costa Rica and the United States. Children from both countries reported similar levels of companionship, satisfaction, intimacy, and conflict in their best friendships, but Costa Rican children report higher levels of instrumental aid and affection in their friendships. Nevertheless, comparisons across various relationships in children's social networks revealed that Costa Rican children overall rated their networks as more supportive than children in the United States. One of the most notable differences was that children in Costa Rica viewed their parents as the most important providers of support, but among children in the United States, these positive functions were frequently attributed to best friends (DeRosier & Kupersmidt, 1991).

Two very different comparisons of cultural contexts also show the reliance on parents in collectivistic cultures. First, adolescents in Turkey perceived their parents, particularly mothers, as more able to satisfy their needs than their friends, but adolescents in the United States made no distinction between parents and friends in terms of meeting their needs for companionship, disclosure, affection, help and support, and other interpersonal needs (Hortacsu, 1997). Second, younger and older Brazil-

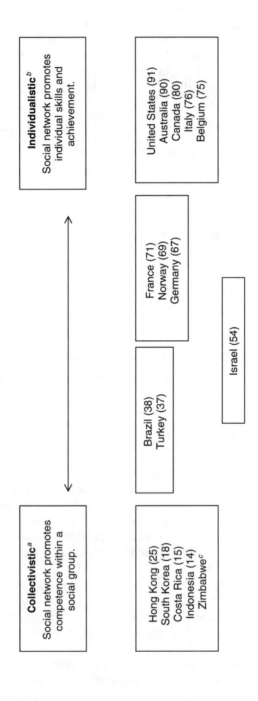

FIGURE 7.1. Placement of countries in cross-cultural studies of friendship on Hofstede's (2001) individualism index. [a] Indicates a country that received a score of 25 or lower on Hofstede's (2001) individualism index (scale = 0 to 100); [b] Indicates a country that received a score of 75 or higher on Hofstede's individualism index (scale = 0 to 100); [c] Not one of the countries included separately in Hofstede's calculations.

ian adolescents rated parents higher than friends in the support they provide even though friends were viewed as strong sources of emotional and instrumental support (Van Horn & Marques, 2000). Also showing the emphasis on family in the collectivistic, family-oriented culture of Brazil, friends and siblings were rated as comparable in their provisions of support. U.S. adolescents, in contrast, relied on friends much more than siblings to meet their support needs (Furman & Buhrmester, 1992).

French, Rianasari, Pidada, Nelwan, and Buhrmester (2001) found some of the same differences between Indonesian and U.S. children as DeRosier and Kupersmidt (1991) found between Costa Rican and U.S. children and Hortacsu (1997) found between Turkish and U.S. adolescents with regard to the role of parents and friends as providers of social support. Indonesian children generally reported equal companionship with their mothers and friends, but children in the United States ranked friends as higher in companionship. Both Indonesian and U.S. children ranked friends as their primary source of intimacy. U.S. children reported the most satisfaction with their friends, but Indonesian youth were most satisfied with their relationships with their mothers and fathers. As with the children in Costa Rica (DeRosier & Kupersmidt, 1991), instrumental aid was a particularly important provision of Indonesian children's friendships. In fact, instrumental aid appears to be a provision that differs most significantly between Indonesian and U.S. youth (French, Pidada, & Victor, 2005) and is more central in the friendships of Indonesian than U.S. youth. In contrast, children and youth in the United States rely more on their close friends for enhancement of self-worth and promotion of self-esteem than those in Indonesia (French, Pidada, & Victor, 2005).

Zimbabwean adolescents living in both traditional and modified extended families reported that their friends were a significant source of companionship, and for adolescents in traditional families, a sibling was just as important for companionship as friends (Harrison et al., 1997). In a further study of early adolescents living in rural Zimbabwe, urban Zimbabwe, and the United States, significant differences were found in the type of relationship that was associated with specific relationship provisions. In urban Zimbabwe, best friends were rated higher on conflict, instrumental help, and intimacy; mothers and teachers were rated highest on reliable alliance and affection; and fathers were rated highest on enhancement of worth, companionship, and satisfaction. Adolescents in rural Zimbabwe did not make as clear a distinction among the various types of relationships. Nevertheless, best friends and mothers were rated highest on reliable alliance; best friends and teachers were highest on companionship; best friends were rated highest on intimacy and conflict; and fathers and other relatives were rated highest on enhancement of worth. In contrast to both groups of Zimbabwean youth, adolescents in the United States rated their best friends as the most important members of their social network. Specifically, best friends received higher scores than all other network members on enhancement of worth, companionship, intimacy, and satisfaction. In direct comparisons of best friends, U.S. youth consistently rated their best friends higher on positive features and lower on conflict than did the Zimbabwean adolescents (Harrison et al., 1995).

The studies above all examine national cultures that differ significantly according to collectivism versus individualism and a host of other dimensions, but what about comparisons between national cultures that are similar in many ways? Australia and the United States, for example, are largely similar in features such as the role of the state, legal heritage, levels of suburbanization, trends in marriage and family size, adult social networks, and individualism (Shute, De Blasio, & Williamson, 2002). There is no apparent reason for hypothesizing major differences in children's assessment of social support within the two countries. Indeed, a direct comparison shows many similarities in children's satisfaction with the support provided by their mothers, fathers, siblings, best friends, and teachers (Shute et al., 2002). Nevertheless, one difference was that best friends provided almost exclusively companionship support for children in Australia, and other relationships were valued for emotional, instrumental, and informational support. In the United States, however, children rated their friends just as high in companionship as the Australian children but also as important providers of emotional and other types of support. The Australian children, then, made greater distinctions among provisions of friends and provisions of family members than did the U.S. children.

Taken together, these findings are generally consistent with Tietjen's (1989) proposal that social support networks promote competence in areas that correspond with the goals and values of that particular cultural and ecological context. The most consistent and dramatic difference is in the relative role of parents versus friends for children and adolescents in the more collectivistic and family-oriented cultures of Indonesia, Costa Rica, Brazil, and Zimbabwe, as compared to the United States. It is only in the U.S. context that friends are consistently perceived as the best provider of various types of support. This conclusion should not be interpreted as suggesting that friends are not valued by youth in other cultures as well. Friends are clearly important in the lives of all of the children and adolescents in these studies, especially as a source of intimacy, and there is some evidence that children in other cultures turn to friends as sources of specific help and aid more so than children in the United States. For example, French, Pidada, and Victor (2005) describe sharing resources and helping others as a primary way to demonstrate and strengthen social ties in Indonesia, and this appears to hold true in other collectivistic cultures as well (Tietjen, 1989). In the United States, however, friendships may be based more typically on affective, rather than instrumental, ties.

Another specific difference appears to be in the role of friends as supporting and enhancing self-worth. Sullivan (1953) and other theorists (Hartup, 1996a) describe affirming and enhancing a friend's competence and worth as one of the most important functions of friendships, particularly in preadolescence. This certainly seems to be true for youth in the United States. In Indonesia and Zimbabwe, however, this function is ascribed to parents and relatives more than to friends (French, Pidada, & Victor, 2005; Harrison et al., 1995). In part, a focus on self-esteem and promotion of one's talents and abilities is a central part of cultures that value independence and individualism, such as in the United States. Thus, enhancement of self-worth may be an important reinforcing function of best friends in individualistic societies. A preoccupation with self-esteem is not a central characteristic of many other cultures, and as French, Pidada, and Victor (2005) note, it may be viewed as antagonistic to social harmony in some cultures.

Support from Friends and Parents

Comparisons of parents versus friends as providers of intimacy, closeness, and other aspects of support should not imply a dichotomy where support comes either from parents or from friends. This latter view represents a compensation model in which children who do not receive much support from one relationship look to other relationships to provide what is missing (Cooper & Cooper, 1992; East & Rook, 1992; Stocker, 1994). Alternatively, attachment and social learning theories suggest that high-quality family relationships and high-quality friendship relationships would be correlated because positive relationships in one domain should promote the maintenance of satisfying relationships in another domain (see Lansford, 2004, for a discussion). Cross culturally, more support is generally found for this latter model than for a compensation model.

Italian adolescents, for example, who reported high levels of support and closeness in family relationships also reported having very close relationships with peers (Claes, 1998; Kirchler, Pombeni, & Palmonari, 1991). In Claes's (1998) study, adolescents in Italy, Belgium, and Canada all reported that they had the most intimate conversations with their friends, followed by mothers, siblings, and fathers. Nevertheless, when asked to name the person with whom they are the closest, Canadian adolescents named a best friend, Italian adolescents named a parent, and Belgian adolescents chose parents and friends equally often (Claes, 1998). Similarly, German and U.S. adolescents reported high levels of closeness in their friendships even though more German adolescents had very close relationships with their mothers than did U.S. adolescents (Laursen, Wilder, Noack, & Williams, 2000). In another study of German youth, support from parents and support from classmates (including friends) were not related, and high support in one domain could not compensate for low support in the other (van Aken & Asendorpf, 1997). Finally, friendship quality has been linked to adolescent romantic relationships in both China and Canada (Li, Connolly, Jiang, Pepler, & Craig, 2010), suggesting important continuity between friendships and other close relationships.

Support from Friends and Other Peers

The role of friends versus other peers in meeting social needs has also been compared. Jewish students in Israel (an individualistic culture) reported higher-quality relationships with their best friend (greater security and closeness and less conflict) than did Arab students in Israel (a collectivistic culture). In contrast, Arab students reported greater companionship and help and security and closeness with the larger peer network than did Jewish students (Scharf & Hertz-Lazarowitz, 2003). These findings may indicate that the culture with a more collectivistic orientation places greater emphasis on connectedness within the larger peer group, but the culture with a more individualistic orientation places higher priority on specific dyadic relationships, like friendships. Nevertheless, for both groups of students, intimacy was highest with their best friend, suggesting a special role of best friends even among the more collectivistic Arab culture (Scharf & Hertz-Lazarowitz, 2003).

Assessing the different provisions and functions of best friendships and the larger peer network, as Scharf and Hertz-Lazarowitz (2003) did, seems to be especially helpful in making sense of some inconsistent findings and hypotheses about the significance of friends in collectivistic and individualistic cultures. According to arguments of Triandis and others, allocentric people and collectivistic cultures are expected to emphasize highly intimate and long-lasting relationships with a few people, whereas idiocentric people and individualistic cultures are predicted to focus on many more social relationships that are not as intimate (Triandis, 1990). There is indeed some support for these predictions in collectivistic cultures. For example, college students in Hong Kong interacted with fewer people in their everyday social interactions over a 2-week period than did U.S. students, yet they reported higher levels of self-disclosure in their interactions (Wheeler, Reis, & Bond, 1989). Similarly, South Korean students reported more exclusivity and more disclosure in their interactions with friends than did U.S. students (French, Bae, et al., 2006).

Do these findings indeed suggest closer friendships in collectivistic cultures than in individualistic cultures? Studies with Indonesian and U.S. college students find the opposite—Indonesian students interacted with more others than did U.S. students, were more inclusive in their interactions, and had less close relationships (French, Pidada, & Victor, 2005). In kibbutz societies in Israel in which extensive interactions in the community are emphasized, adolescents indeed spend much of their time with peers but do not develop as much closeness and intimacy with particular friends as do other adolescents (e.g., Israeli adolescents who live in cities or Arab adolescents; Sharabany, 2006; Sharabany & Wiseman, 1993). It appears then, that the conclusion that relationships with friends are especially intimate and close in collectivistic societies is too simplistic. Rather, this may hold true in some societies, but in other collectivistic cultures, involvement and closeness with larger peer groups is important, but specific friendships are not emphasized (see also French, Pidada, & Victor, 2005).

Summary

Overall, these observed differences in the social support networks of youth living in different countries reflect major and minor variations in cultural norms, values, and practices that determine how daily life, particularly social life, is organized and experienced. There are clear differences in the relative role of friends vis-à-vis other relationships for important social provisions, and these differences should not be overlooked inasmuch as they may be predictive of different patterns of adjustment outcomes for youth in different countries and cultural contexts. At the same time, the empirical findings are overwhelmingly consistent in supporting the conclusion that close friends are salient and valued members of children's and adolescents' social networks across a variety of cultural contexts.

FRIENDSHIP FEATURES AND QUALITY

Closely related to the study of support from members of a child's social network is a more specific focus on the features and quality of individual relationships—specifically best friendships. There are three general dimensions of children's relationships with their best friend that have been examined cross culturally and that have an impact on the quality of the relationship—the time children spend with friends; the positive features of the relationship, including reciprocity and prosocial behavior;

and the negative features of the relationship, specifically conflict between friends.

Time Spent with Friends

Friendships in youth can only emerge and develop with time for peer interactions. At a very basic level, then, time with friends helps determine the features and quality of these relationships. There are cultural variations in the amount of time children and adolescents spend with peers and friends. For example, Claes (1998) found that Canadian adolescents had the most frequent and longest daily contacts with friends compared to Belgian and Italian adolescents. Italian adolescents spend a majority of their time with parents and siblings. Parents choose their children's early contacts, both in terms of the amount of emphasis placed on encouraging young children to socialize with same-age peers and on controlling the specific others with whom young children associate. Harkness and Super (1983) argued that parents' most important role in socializing young children is in assigning the children to different settings, settings that might differ greatly in the age and sex of others in that setting. For example, in Kenya, parents teach their children to distrust nonrelatives by keeping their children on the family land, limiting children's time with peers (Whiting et al., 1988). In contrast, Cuban children are expected to spend a majority of their free time with other children to build social competency and other skills necessary for the adult world (Valdivia et al., 2005). Even within nations, differences exist in the frequency of contacts between peers. Industrialized cities—such as Los Angeles, California; Seoul, Korea; and Tianjin, China—provide larger neighborhoods and more access to peer networks than rural areas, making it more commonplace for adolescents to spend substantial time with peers (Greenberger, Chen, Beam, Whang, & Dong, 2000). Despite the variations in time allotted to friends across cultures, a trend seems to be that youth spend an increasing amount of time with friends as they enter adolescence and become more independent. However, depending on the culture, this increase could be minimal or substantial.

In addition to parental influence on peer interactions and the amount of contact children and adolescents have with friends, immediate contexts also affect how much time children spend with their peers. In areas of the world where women are engaging more in the work world outside of the home, such as in Taiwan, children have more opportunities to interact with their peers (Benjamin, Schneider, Greenman, & Hum, 2001). For individuals experiencing economic hardship or deprivation, needs for economic advancement and basic sustenance outweigh the need to form friendships (Schneider, 1998). The organization of a school may restrict or expand opportunities for contact with peers and friends based on the amount of free time children have and the teaching methods employed (Schneider, Wiener, & Murphy, 1994). Thus, examining time with friends is a first step in exploring the features of friendships cross culturally.

Positive Friendship Features

Given that the quality of a friendship is defined by the relative amount of positive and negative features in the relationship, assessments of friendship quality are expected to differ cross culturally to the extent that the salient features of friendships differ from culture to culture. It perhaps makes more sense, then, to examine cross-cultural variations in friendship quality at the level of specific friendship features. Much of what we know about specific friendship features cross culturally comes from the studies reviewed above that use self-report questionnaires and Likert-style rating scales to ask children and adolescents about the amount of companionship, support, closeness and intimacy, and instrumental aid in their friendships. As discussed above, these studies reveal many similarities (especially with features such as intimacy and companionship) but also some differences (especially with features such as instrumental aid and enhancement of worth) in the positive features that define children's friendships across national boundaries. Table 7.2 summarizes the empirical studies assessing cross-cultural similarities and differences in friendship features.

Reciprocity

Hartup and Stevens (1997) describe reciprocity as an underlying condition of friendship across the lifespan (a "deep structure") and note that manifestations of reciprocity may change as a function of age. In much the same way, reciprocity may be a critical component of friendship across various cultures. Reciprocity is apparent in that both friends consent to the relationship and see themselves as more or less equals. It is also apparent in the mutual obligations friends have for one another and their commitment to mutual support. Just what these obligations are, however, may differ quite dramatically in different societies and cultures. For example, Cohen (1961) studied 65 non-Western societies and identified four types of friendships that are not all found in all societies and have very different obligations and accepted rules governing their existence. Cohen's typology of friendship ranges from inalienable friendships (e.g., "blood brothers") to expedient friendships that are based on mutual advantage (such as that between superordinates and subordinates) but not affective or emotional ties. The obligations of these relationships

TABLE 7.2. Cross-Cultural Comparisons on Friendship Features and Quality

Study	Cross-cultural comparison	Cross-cultural similarities	Cross-cultural differences
		Positive friendship features	
Benjamin, Schneider, Greenman, and Hum (2001)	Taiwan, Canada (3rd and 4th grades)	No difference between Canadian and Taiwanese children on closeness, companionship, help, or security with their best friend. Companionship predicts stability of friendships for children in both countries.	
Chen, Kaspar, Zhang, Wang, and Zheng (2004)	China, Canada[a] (3rd–7th grades)	Companionship and intimacy are the most important features of friendship for both Chinese and Canadian boys. Boys in both countries reported similar levels of intimacy in friendships. Security and protection was the least important friendship function for both groups.	Canadian boys had higher scores on companionship and enhancement of self-worth, and Chinese boys had higher scores on understanding, instrumental assistance, and security in their friendships.
French, Bae, Pidada, and Lee (2006)	Indonesia, South Korea, U.S. (college students)		Indonesian students reported less disclosure with a close friend and shorter duration friendships than did U.S. students; Korean students reported more exclusivity in friendships than U.S. and Indonesian students.
French, Pidada, and Victor (2005)	Indonesia, U.S. (5th and 8th grades)	U.S. and Indonesian adolescents rate intimacy as equally salient in their best friendships.	U.S. adolescents rated enhancement of self-worth as more prevalent and instrumental aid as less prevalent in their best friendship than Indonesian adolescents. In interviews, U.S adolescents described more companionship and reliable alliance and less instrumental aid in their best friendships than Indonesian adolescents.

244

González, Moreno, and Schneider (2004)	Cuba, Canada (7th–9th grades)	In essays about their best friends, Canadian and Cuban adolescents frequently discussed authenticity, loyalty, and acceptance.	Cuban adolescents identified reciprocity, character admiration, and intimacy as key features of friendships more than did Canadian adolescents. Canadian adolescents viewed sharing interests and having a history of social interaction as more central to their friendships than did Cuban adolescents.
Gummerum and Keller (2008)	Iceland, China, Russia, former East Germany (7, 9, 12, 15 years)	The developmental sequence in reasoning about friendship is largely consistent across the four societies.	From middle childhood into adolescence, Russian and Chinese children are more advanced in friendship reasoning than Icelandic and German youth, and these differences decrease with age. Important dimensions of friendships: Shared activities more frequently mentioned by Chinese, Russian, and German youth; friendship and moral norms and psychological functions more frequently mentioned by Russian and Chinese youth than Icelandic youth; talking mentioned more by Icelandic than Chinese youth.
Pilgrim and Rueda-Riedle (2002)	Colombia, U.S. (1st grade)	In a lab task, Colombian and U.S. children shared more with friends than with nonfriends and gave similar reasons for sharing with friends.	
Rao and Stewart (1999; India and China) and Birch and Billman (1986; U.S.)	India, China, U.S. (4 years)	Indian, Chinese, and U.S. children generally did not differ in the degree to which they shared with friends versus acquaintances (though U.S. girls shared more with friends than nonfriends and overall Asian children shared more than U.S. children but U.S. children elicited more sharing than Asian children).	

(continued)

TABLE 7.2. (*continued*)

Study	Cross-cultural comparison	Cross-cultural similarities	Cross-cultural differences
Schneider, Fonzi, Tani, and Tomada (1997)	Italy, Canada (8–9 years)	Italian and Canadian children did not differ in their reports of positive friendship features in their best friendship.	Italian children's friendships were more stable across a school year than were Canadian children's.
		Negative friendship features	
Benjamin, Schneider, Greenman, and Hum (2001)	Taiwan, Canada (3rd and 4th grades)	Conflict does not predict stability of friendships for Taiwanese or Canadian children.	Taiwanese friendships contain less conflict than Canadian children's friendships; high levels of conflict more strongly associated with low closeness, help, and security for Taiwanese than Canadian children; Taiwanese children agreed more with their friends about the presence of conflict in their relationship than did Canadian children.
French, Pidada, Denoma, McDonald, and Lawton (2005)	Indonesia, U.S. (9–11 years)	Children in both countries reported more conflict with friends than with other peers and indicated satisfaction with the outcomes of most disagreements.	Topic of conflict: Verbal aggression begins conflicts for Indonesian children more than U.S. children; arguments about facts and opinions more common for U.S. than Indonesian children. Conflict management: Indonesian children more likely to disengage or be submissive during disagreements, and U.S. children more likely to negotiate or rely on a third party for a solution.

246

Study	Countries (ages)	Findings
Haar and Krahe (1999)	Indonesia, Germany (15–17 years)	German adolescents most often use confrontation to resolve conflict with a close friend; Indonesian adolescents use confrontation, submission, and compromise equally.
Schneider, Fonzi, Tani, and Tomada (1997)	Italy, Canada (8–9 years)	Friendship quality does not predict stability in either culture. Canadian children reported more conflict with their best friend than did Italian children; Canadian children disagreed with their friend more than Italian children disagreed in their relationship more than Italian children disagreed with their friend, and for Canadian children, this disagreement predicted friendship dissolution.
Schneider, Fonzi, Tomada, and Tani (2000)	Italy, Canada (8–9 years)	Italian friends issued more sensitive counterproposals in a lab task where they had to share a desired item than did Canadian friends. Italian friends differed from nonfriends on conflict management more than did Canadian friends and nonfriends.
Schneider, Woodburn, Soteras del Toro, and Udvari (2005)	Cuba, Costa Rica, Canada (7th grade)	Conflict is associated with competition, and conflict predicts the end of best friendships similarly across cultures. Canadian adolescents' friendships continued when competition was neither very high nor very low; Costa Rican and Cuban adolescents' friendships were more likely to continue when hypercompetitiveness was low.

Note. Only studies with direct comparisons between at least two countries are included.

[a]Only boys were studied.

vary dramatically and may include physical protection, caring for one another's children, economic assistance and interdependence, sharing of property, arranging romantic liaisons, emotional support, reciprocal gift giving, or no real obligations.

In both Germany and the United States, closer friendships were characterized by higher levels of reciprocity, and less close friendships had more limited reciprocity (Laursen et al., 2000). Nevertheless, U.S. adolescents reported greater reciprocity with friends than parents, but German adolescents reported similar levels of reciprocity in relationships with their friends and their mothers. Essays about friendship written by Cuban and Canadian adolescents indicate the predominance of reciprocity as an essential feature and expectation of friendships (González, Moreno, & Schneider, 2004). However, the manifestations of reciprocity differed in the two countries. Cuban adolescents emphasized reciprocity in terms of mutual help and assistance among friends, whereas Canadian adolescents emphasized reciprocity in terms of common interests and synchronizing individual characteristics (e.g., preferences, choices) with the friend.

These different definitions and manifestations of reciprocity further support the conclusion that instrumental aid or specific help is an especially important and defining feature of high-quality friendships in collectivistic cultures. A comparison of Chinese and Canadian boys' friendships provides further evidence for this conclusion. Both Chinese and Canadian boys perceived companionship and intimacy as the primary functions of their friendships (Chen, Kaspar, Zhang, Wang, & Zheng, 2004). Thus, in both cultures friends are perceived as important for playing together and having fun and for sharing secrets, opinions, hopes, and fears. Differences between the boys in the two cultures emerged on measures of enhancement of self-worth (Canadian boys perceived it as more important), understanding and care (Chinese boys perceived it as more important), and instrumental assistance (Chinese boys perceived it as more important). These findings parallel many described above in other collectivistic cultures.

Prosocial Behavior

Prosocial behavior toward the partner is another positive feature of friendships, and this overt display is particularly important among younger children. Two studies that have specifically addressed sharing cross culturally show similarities rather than differences in this behavior. At first blush, the collectivistic versus individualistic dichotomy might again lead to hypotheses that sharing would be particularly valued in collectivistic societies, but given the importance of this type of prosocial behavior between friends in the United States and other individualistic societies, this dichotomy may be too simplistic. Indeed, in a lab-based study, young children in Colombia and the United States shared significantly more candies with friends than with other nonfriend classmates (Pilgrim & Rueda-Riedle, 2002). Importantly, the degree of difference between sharing with friends and sharing with nonfriends was consistent across the two groups of children. Even the reasons for sharing did not differ, and both Colombian and U.S. children noted that they shared because the other child was their friend. In contrast, the type of sharing differed in a comparison of U.S., Indian, and Chinese preschool children with their friends and nonfriends (Rao & Stewart, 1999). Asian children showed more spontaneous sharing than U.S. children, but U.S. children elicited more sharing than Asian children. Importantly, these differences were not specifically related to friendships. In fact, there were no cultural differences between sharing with friends versus sharing with acquaintances.

Summary

As the preceding discussion suggests, many of the positive features of children's friendships do not vary substantially across a number of cultures. Friendships grounded in reciprocity and cooperative, prosocial behavior seem to be the norm, and across a number of countries children's reasoning about friendship follows a fairly consistent developmental sequence (Gummerum & Keller, 2008). Differences appear more in how these positive features are displayed—for example, how reciprocity is shown—and in the relative importance of friends compared to others in the social network—for example, whether friends are a primary source of help and aid. An important next step is in determining whether the effects of these behaviors and characteristics of friendships differ across societies and cultures. How, for example, does the presence or absence of particular features of friendships relate to other aspects of individual adjustment? Does having a higher- versus lower-quality friendship forecast well-being differently across societies and cultures? These kinds of questions have yet to be answered, yet they are important ones because the answers would tell us about the socialization context that friendships provide. They would help us determine whether there are universal functions that friendships provide and whether the developmental significance of friendship is similar across a variety of societies and cultures.

Negative Friendship Features

Historically, in the psychological literature, the positive aspects of children's friendships have been emphasized. More recently, however, is the recognition that friendships are not all positive, and that negative features may be just as important determinants of the developmental significance of particular friendships. Conflict is the negative dimension that has received the most attention, particularly among North American samples. Along with the recognition that conflict is an inevitable aspect of any close relationship, there is some evidence that conflict may have both negative and positive effects on the children's individual development and the development of the relationship. For example, the way conflict is resolved (or not) can determine whether the relationship continues or is terminated and may provide valuable experience in skills such as negotiation and perspective taking for the children involved.

Relying again on the individualistic versus collectivistic distinction suggests some hypotheses for the role of conflict in friendships cross culturally. Given that members of collectivistic cultures strive to promote group harmony, conflict may be less apparent, and if disagreement emerges, sanctions may be higher and lead to friendship harm or even termination. In contrast, the emphasis on autonomy, self-reliance, and competition in individualistic cultures may make conflict more common (Triandis et al., 1988). At the same time, friendships may be more likely to endure disagreements. Other aspects of the cultural context in which conflict occurs are expected to influence the nature of the conflict itself, the acceptability of conflict, and strategies for managing conflict. These include availability of resources and freedom to terminate interactions (Hartup, 1992a); beliefs about whether conflict is inevitable or something to be avoided (French, Pidada, Denoma, McDonald, & Lawton, 2005); ideas about appropriate and effective strategies for resolution, including aggression and other confrontational versus nonconfrontational methods (Leung & Wu, 1990; Markus, Kitayama, & Heiman, 1996); expectations for appropriate communication during conflict situations (Corsaro & Rizzo, 1990; Schneider, Fonzi, Tomada, & Tani, 2000); and whether children are responsible for settling their own conflicts or appealing to adult intervention (Killen & Sueyoshi, 1995).

Frequency of Conflict

In terms of the presence or frequency of occurrence of conflict between friends, cross-cultural differences are somewhat consistent with the hypotheses offered above based on the individualistic versus collectivistic nature of the societies compared. Several studies provide evidence, and these are summarized in Table 7.2. In Taiwan, for example, a nation with strong collectivistic values and an emphasis on group identity, harmony, and mutual dependence based in Confucianism, children's friendships are characterized by much less conflict as compared to the friendships of Canadian children (Benjamin et al., 2001). Canada, like the United States, is strongly individualistic, and children are socialized to be independent. Conformity to the group is not a focus in Canada as it is in Taiwanese society. High levels of conflict in Taiwanese children's friendships were strongly related to low levels of positive friendship features such as closeness and security, much more so than for Canadian children. Thus, conflict seems to damage relationships to a greater degree and cannot exist in the presence of positive relationship features for Taiwanese children. For Canadian children, however, conflict is actually positively associated with closeness, suggesting that positive and negative features frequently coexist in their relationships (Schneider, Fonzi, et al., 1997).

French and colleagues have compared conflict between friends in Indonesia and the United States in several studies. Children in Indonesia and the United States both report more conflict with friends than with other peers and indicate satisfaction with the outcomes of most of these disagreements (French, Pidada, Denoma, et al., 2005). Nevertheless, U.S. students report more conflict with their friends than do Indonesian youth (French et al., 2001; French, Lee, & Pidada, 2006). Verbal aggression precipitates more of the conflicts reported by Indonesian children, and disagreements over facts or opinions are more common provocations for U.S. children (French, Pidada, Denoma, et al., 2005).

Conflict Management

Thus, there are some cross-cultural differences in the frequency and precipitants of conflict children experience in their friendships. Perhaps more telling about the experience of conflict with friends, however, are potential differences in how children manage and resolve the conflicts that do arise. For example, notable differences were found in behaviors during the conflict and in the resolution strategies employed by Indonesian and U.S. children (French, Pidada, Denoma, et al., 2005). Indonesian children reported more disengagement and submission during the disagreements and also used disengagement strategies to resolve their conflicts. In contrast, U.S. children were more likely to negotiate a solution or rely on interventions from a third party. Disengagement as a resolution strategy appears to be more acceptable among Indonesian than U.S. children as evidenced by its association with social competence in Indonesia but not in the United States. French, Pidada, Denoma, and colleagues (2005) suggest that these findings are quite consistent with a cultural script in Indonesia in which conflict is managed through avoidance and an emphasis on harmony rather than confrontation. These differences in resolution strategy echo comparisons of German versus Indonesian adolescents' responses to a hypothetical conflict situation with a close friend (Haar &

Krahe, 1999). Specifically, German adolescents predominantly endorsed confrontation as a resolution strategy, whereas Indonesian adolescents equally endorsed confrontation, submission, and compromise as likely strategies.

Conflict and Relationship Stability

To the extent that conflict occurs more or less frequently and is resolved with different strategies, there may be cross-cultural differences in the ways in which conflict predicts the stability of children's friendships. This question is particularly interesting in comparisons of Italian children's experience of conflict in their friendships and the conflict experience of children from other cultures because of the expectations Italian adults have that conflict is a common and important aspect of their relationships (Argyle, Henderson, Bond, Iizuka, & Contarello, 1986), the emphasis on encouraging children's perspective taking in social situations (New, 1994), and the extensive opportunities Italian children have to express their opinions and debate with others (Corsaro, 1994; Corsaro & Rizzo, 1990; Schneider, Fonzi, et al., 1997; Tomada et al., 2002). Italian children, then, are expected to be especially skilled in managing and negotiating conflict so that it does not negatively impact the relationship. In a short-term longitudinal study, Italian and Canadian children reported on the quality of their friendships at the beginning and end of the school year, though interestingly, friendship quality did not affect friendship stability (Schneider, Fonzi, et al., 1997). More of the Italian children's friendships continued over the course of the year than the Canadian children's. Nevertheless, initial levels of conflict in the friendships did not predict the stability of the relationship for either group. Moreover, the association between positive friendship features and stability was consistent across the two cultures as well. Higher levels of positive friendship features at the beginning of the year predicted friendship stability. Apparently, the positive features help children overcome obstacles and threats to their relationship during the course of the year so that it continues (Schneider, Fonzi, et al., 1997).

Likewise, in Benjamin and colleagues' (2001) comparison of Canadian and Taiwanese children's friendships, conflict did not predict the stability of friendships for either group, suggesting that despite the harm it might cause, particularly for Taiwanese children, the friendships are not any more likely to end because of high levels of conflict. Interestingly, it may be that conflict driven by particular forms of competition between friends may indeed predict friendship stability differentially across cultures. In samples of Cuban, Costa Rican, and Canadian early adolescents, conflict consistently predicted the end of best friendships, and conflict was strongly associated with a particular form of competition—hypercompetitiveness, an intense focus on winning with hostility toward the other person (Schneider, Woodburn, Soteras del Toro, & Udvari, 2005). However, for the Canadian youth, friendships continued most often in the context of hypercompetitiveness that was neither very high nor very low, suggesting some tolerance for the behavior, but in the Latin American samples, a linear association suggested that increases in hypercompetitiveness forecast friendship dissolution. Thus, in the more collectivistic societies of Cuba and Costa Rica (as compared to Canada), the negative effects of hypercompetitiveness within friendships were more severe.

Summary

Based on this limited evidence, then, frequency of conflict and strategies for resolving conflict may be part of cultural scripts that suggest appropriate and accepted methods for managing conflict. However, the findings from at least three studies converge to suggest that despite these differences, conflict per se does not seem to affect differentially the stability of children's friendships. It is clear that we need to consider the broader context in which conflicts occur and not focus only on discrete conflict episodes to uncover potential cultural differences in the meaning of conflict within friendships and the way particular styles of conflict are associated with individual adjustment and the functioning of the specific friendship itself. As demonstrated by Schneider and colleagues (2005), what leads to conflict between friends may differ in important ways. Likewise, the manner in which children respond to and manage conflict with friends likely reflects their level of competence at using culturally determined acceptable strategies (French, Pidada, Denoma, et al., 2005). Thus, we cannot make universal statements about the most effective strategies for managing conflicts with friends.

One limitation to the use of the individualistic versus collectivistic framework for understanding cross-cultural differences in children's understanding of conflict is that much of the research highlights similarities in children's conflict behavior. The differences, when present, are moderate and thus do not fit well with broad overarching theories that would emphasize substantial differences in the experience of and management of conflict with peers (French, Pidada, Denoma, et al., 2005). For example, teachers in Japanese preschools emphasize both independent and interdependent values when socializing children in managing peer conflicts. Furthermore, conflicts among the Japanese children over individual rights and fairness were common, and conflicts were often mutual and confrontational, involving protests from both children (Killen & Sueyoshi, 1995). These characteristics of children's conflict and adults' responses to them do not fit with the collectivistic emphasis on group harmony and interdependence rather than autonomy. In addition, characteristics of friendships are different across cultures that fall on the same side of the collectivistic versus individualistic dimension, indicating that this distinction alone does not account for all of the differences. For example, in a study of older adolescents (college students) in two collectivistic cultures—Indonesia and South Korea—and the United States, the Korean and Indonesian students differed more in the features and structural aspects of their friendships than either group did from the U.S. students (French, Bae, et al., 2006).

With the strong base of knowledge about the time children spend with friends and the positive and negative features of friendship across cultures, the field is ripe for further investigations examining how friendship quality is related to other aspects of adjustment and to experiences in other social relationships. It is with questions like these that we will be able to address more specifically whether the functions of friendship differ cross culturally and whether friendship is associated with positive and negative adjustment in similar ways across cultures. These are questions that get at the heart of the developmental significance of friendship.

SIMILARITY BETWEEN FRIENDS

To what degree is similarity, also called homophily, between friends a universal characteristic, or is this feature of friendship limited to youth in certain cultures? Resemblances between friends exist for both demographic/physical characteristics (e.g., age, gender, race) as well as psychological characteristics (e.g., competence, interests, attitudes, behaviors).

Similarity in Age and Gender

Turning first to physical or demographic concordances between friends, it is clear that contextual factors other than culture per se may determine the degree to which friends are similar on age and gender. In the United States and other industrialized countries in which the daily lives of children and adolescents are centered on school, peer groups and dyadic friendships are almost entirely age segregated. Schools are a hub of social life and feed into after-school activities (e.g., academic clubs, sports teams, dance lessons) that are also age segregated and that foster the development of same-age peer networks from which friendships form. Children and adolescents in other parts of the world often must participate in work and family activities, including caring for younger siblings, when they are not in school (Abraham, 2002; Hortacsu, 1997; Schneider, 1998). These activities are not age segregated, and youth interact and spend time with younger and older peers.

Other aspects of school organization also greatly affect the degree to which similarity in age defines children's friendships. In many studies, especially in the United States where friendship pairs are identified in school, the finding that friends are similar in age is determined by the methodological constraint of nominating a friend in the same class or grade. Thus, as Harkness and Super (1985) note, "Since school experience in American culture is closely tied to age, there is a danger ... that the structure of development may be confused with the structure of the environment" (p. 219). In contrast, in many Italian preschools, for example, government sponsored preschool classes include 3-, 4-, and 5-year-old children who stay together and with the same teachers until moving to elementary school at age 6. As a result, there is much opportunity for cross-age play and for establishing friendships with younger or older children (Corsaro, 2003). Akiyama (2001) compared a small group of adolescent boys in villages in the Central Kalahari Game Reserve of Botswana before and after relocation to a more central and larger community to attend school. After the relocation, the boys more frequently associated in same-age peer groups than they had before. In addition, those attending school associated with more same-age peers than adolescent boys who dropped out of school. Before the relocation, boys associated with their relatives, and same-age peers were scarce. This pattern of association also characterized the boys who did not attend school. As these findings illustrate, the organization of schools has a significant influence on the formation of same-age friendships even within cultures.

Perhaps the most obvious similarity between friends is gender. Around the globe, friendships among children and adolescents are overwhelmingly same-sex relationships that are embedded within same-sex peer groups (e.g., Abraham, 2002; Bukowski, Gauze, Hoza, & Newcomb, 1993; Claes, 1998; Corsaro, 2003; Edwards, 1992; French, Jansen, Riansari, & Setiono, 2003; Hartup, 1996a). In a 1963 review of over 80 ethnographic studies of diverse nonliterate cultures, Nickerson identified almost exclusively gender-segregated friend pairs and peer groups. Despite these reports, there is some evidence that gender segregation in young children's peer groups is stronger for middle-class white U.S. children than for children in other ethnic or cultural groups, even within the United States. For example, Corsaro's extensive observations of preschool and early elementary classes in various communities in the United States and Italy revealed less segregation by gender in children's play and friendships for Italian children and U.S. children in Head Start classes than for middle-class white U.S. children (Aydt & Corsaro, 2003; Corsaro, 2003).

Gender segregation in children's peer associates and friends occurs as a result of an interaction between individual development and "the culturally constructed niche" that includes settings in which children spend their daily life, parents' theories about child development (i.e., ethnotheories), and the responsibilities assigned to children (Harkness & Super, 1983, p. 223). In a small rural community in Kenya, gender segregation in children's peer associations did not emerge until children were 6 to 9 years of age (much later than in U.S. contexts), despite an extremely gender segregated adult society in this community (Harkness & Super, 1983). Gender segregation appears to emerge at this time because of a confluence of factors—adults begin to provide much less immediate supervision to children, children are assigned significant household chores, and they begin to choose their own peer companions (usually same-sex neighbor children) to share their work and play tasks.

The degree to which a culture emphasizes specific gender roles may also affect children's choice of same- versus cross-sex companions. Weisfeld, Weisfeld, and Callaghan (1984) compared Hopi and African American children in two communities in the United States. Hopi culture emphasizes peacefulness and egalitarianism. These features contrast with the greater tolerance for aggression and violence (often viewed as masculine traits) that characterized the affluent African American children from Chicago. In addition, the Hopi culture is matrilineal and collectivistic in nature with women having important economic and social power and responsibilities, whereas the African American sample was patriarchal. The Hopi children were much less likely to play in mixed-sex groups than the African American children, but in both cultures, children overwhelmingly named a same-sex peer as their best friend. In Italy, a focus on *discussione*, elaborate and extensive debates and discussions, even among young children, allows both girls and boys to be assertive, blurring more traditional gender boundaries (Corsaro, 1994; Corsaro & Rizzo, 1990). In South Africa, Alberts, Mbalo, and Ackermann (2003) found that friendships with members of the opposite sex were more important to modern Afrikaans-speaking and English-speaking adolescents than Xhosa-speaking adolescents, whose cultural experience emphasizes more traditional gender roles.

Research to date from a variety of disciplines—psychology, sociology, and anthropology—converges to indicate that some level of gender segregation in early to middle childhood appears to be nearly universal. Nevertheless, the degree of cross-sex play and friendships differs cross culturally. Furthermore, gender segregation is not simply the result of individual, ontogenetic processes but is socially negotiated, constructed by children themselves, and reflective of the values and accepted gender roles of their culture (Aydt & Corsaro, 2003). However, much of this research examines same-sex versus cross-sex play and the composition of small peer groups rather than dyadic friendships. It may be that even though children in some cultures engage more frequently and readily than others in cross-sex play, the existence of cross-sex dyadic friendships (especially cross-sex "best" friends) is still relatively rare.

Similarity in Attributes and Behaviors

In addition to the similarities between friends in demographic character-istics such as age and gender, are friends more similar in their psychologi-cal attributes and behaviors? Processes of both selection and socialization are at work here. Hartup (1996a) suggests that friends will be more simi-lar to one another on those characteristics that are most strongly associ-ated with social reputations. This "reputational salience" hypothesis has not been tested directly, but some evidence from Dutch and U.S. samples provides support. Concordances between friends in the United States and The Netherlands are stronger for aggression and antisocial behav-ior than for prosocial behavior, perhaps in part because of the strong link between aggression and social reputation (Dishion, Andrews, et al., 1995; Dishion, Capaldi, et al., 1995; Haselager, Hartup, van Lieshout, & Riksen-Walraven, 1998). Nevertheless, similarities between friends are substantial across a variety of behavioral characteristics, not just those important for social reputation—prosocial behavior, antisocial behavior, shyness, academic achievement, and peer status, for example (Dishion, Andrews, et al., 1995; Haselager et al., 1998; Kupersmidt, DeRosier, & Patterson, 1995).

To the extent that the attributes associated with social reputation differ cross culturally, the reputational salience hypothesis predicts that similarity between friends on particular characteristics also differs cross culturally. A direct test of this model in Indonesia yielded partial support. Friends were indeed highly similar in their levels of aggression and aca-demic achievement—both highly associated with social status in Indo-nesia (French et al., 2003). Social withdrawal, however, was also similar among friends, yet withdrawal is not highly associated with social status and reputation among Indonesian children. This latter finding does not fit well with the reputational salience hypothesis. It would be particu-larly interesting to examine the similarity of friends to one another on social withdrawal in China given that social withdrawal is associated with social acceptance and positive peer status in China but is associated with peer rejection in U.S. and Canadian children (Chen, DeSouza, Chen, & Wang, 2006; Chen, Rubin, & Li, 1995; Chen, Rubin, & Sun, 1992).

In addition to the reputational salience hypothesis, there are other reasons for why similarity as a feature of friendship and determinant of who one's friends are may differ cross culturally. First, similarity between friends may also be associated with the degree to which children voluntarily choose their friends. If cultures differ in the extent to which friendships are voluntary, similarity between friends may not be universal because children will not be free to choose friends to whom they are most attracted. For example, even though students in Japan and the United States value similarity with their friends equally, actual similarity with friends was lower for Japanese students because they have fewer opportunities to form new friendships (Schug, Yuki, Horikawa, & Takemura, 2009). Second, individualism versus collectivism may also relate to similarity in friendships. One hypothesis is that allocentric individuals and individuals in collectivist cultures will have a more elaborate cognitive representation of others, due to their attentiveness and sensitivity to others, than idiocentric individuals (Verkuyten & Masson, 1996). A related hypothesis is that children in individualistic cultures will be more attuned to maintaining their uniqueness and sense of individuality and will therefore report less similarity with their friends.

Using an interesting method for evaluating similarity between friends, Pinto, Bombi, and Cordioli (1997) asked children in urban and rural communities in Italy, Bolivia, and Lebanon to draw a picture of themselves with a friend "in order to show what friendship is" (p. 460). Similarity between the figures in the drawings was assessed according to a number of features—dimensions, position, physical features of the body, and attributes. Children from all of the countries depicted great similarity between themselves and their friends, yet this similarity was expressed in slightly different ways cross culturally (such as by position of the figures for some and by attributes for others). Overall, the authors note that the individualism versus collectivism of the cultures may be associated with similarity. Greater similarity between friends was demonstrated by children in the more collectivistic societies, perhaps reflecting their emphasis on group harmony and connections to others.

Similarity between friends in behavior is sometimes assumed to be a proxy for, or at least a marker of, friends' influence on one another. For example, compared to adolescents in Korea and China, the misconduct and antisocial behavior of U.S. adolescents is more highly correlated with their perceptions of their close friends' antisocial behavior (Greenberger et al., 2000). This difference may be due in part to the greater amount of time U.S. adolescents spend with their friends than Chinese and Korean youth and thus the greater opportunity for friends' to influence one another's behavior. Nevertheless, for all three groups, adolescents who participated in more misbehavior reported that their friends engaged in higher levels of misbehavior as well. The specific processes that account for friends' influence on one another (i.e., socialization effects) have not received much attention cross culturally.

Summary

Overall, then, similarity seems to be a salient feature of children's and adolescents' friendships across most cultural contexts, and the adage "birds of a feather flock together" is much more consistent with cross-cultural findings than "opposites attract." It is clear, though, that demographic similarities between friends are enhanced in contexts that limit associations to others who differ (in age or gender, for example). For homophily in personality and behavioral characteristics, there is preliminary support for the reputational salience hypothesis, but this idea demands much more study across a variety of behaviors and cultural contexts. Finally, research that investigates the relative strength of selection and socialization effects in various cultures will shed light on the ways in which friends may influence one another and on potential cultural differences in the power of friends in children's lives.

CONCLUSIONS

The time is right for further investigation of friendship and culture. A growing body of literature and interest in theoretical issues that undergird this research allow us to focus on more nuanced aspects of the role of friendship in children's lives around the globe and the ways in which friendship is itself a cultural practice. Our interest in this chapter was on two particular questions about friendship and culture—How do the characteristics and quality of friendships differ cross culturally? and How do these differences affect developmental outcomes? It is clear that research to date yields more details about the first question than the second. Across numerous cultures, the striking conclusion is that there are more similarities and consistencies in the types of interactions children and adolescents have with their friends, the features of their relationships, and the importance of friends in children's lives than there are differences. Nevertheless, converging evidence suggests that there are also compelling differences in some features—instrumental aid, enhancement of worth, and conflict, to name a few. These inconsistencies in friendships indeed highlight variations in culture as suggested by Reis et al. (2000).

Although this may be a glass-half-full versus glass-half-empty argument, it is tempting, then, to conclude that the construct of "best friend" as respected, mutual, intimate confidante is nearly universal. Nevertheless, there are certainly exceptions, which make such a conclusion premature and highlight the rich variation in friendships across cultures. Anthropologists and researchers using ethnographic methods have most readily identified exceptions. For example, Gaskins's (2006) ethnographic study of the Yucatec Maya of Mexico shows that they have a very different experience of peer relationships than has been found in the other cultures considered in this chapter. Most notably, there is no word for *friend* in the language of the Yucatec Maya, and Mayan siblings perform many of the functions and have many of the features typically ascribed to friends in European American cultures, such as companionship, intimacy, and similarity of interests. Nevertheless, siblings are typically not of the same age, and there is a strong hierarchical structure to Yucatec Maya sibling relationships that is the antithesis of the concept of friends as same-age peers who see themselves as equals. As another exception, Indians living in Teopisca, Mexico, view friendship as fragile and rare, not commonly existing beyond childhood (Aguilar, 1984). Rather than viewing friendship as a desirable relationship, Teopiscan Indians believe that friendship should be avoided. In part, this view reflects the idealization of friendship and the sense that friendship creates vulnerability. Human failures make it unlikely that true friendship can be realized, leading to "bitterness and disillusionment" (Aguilar, 1984, p. 19).

Knowledge of peoples and cultures with vastly different social lives and social experiences requires us to refocus on the definition of friendship. Does friendship mean a completely voluntary relationship (the degree of voluntariness of some friendships appears to differ culturally; Krappman, 1996)? Are only nonfamily relationships between same-age peers friendships? To what degree does mutuality, reciprocity, and intimacy define friendships? A more inclusive definition of friendship might include the sibling relationships Gaskins (2006) describes for Yucatec Mayan children, but a narrower definition as has been typically applied in studies of European American and other industrialized countries would likely not. This is more than simply an academic exercise in operationalizing a term. Rather, evaluating the developmental significance of having friends and whether friendship makes unique contributions to developmental outcomes depends on a clear understanding of the relationship and whether it is a universal experience that cannot be easily replaced by other social experiences.

Despite our growing understanding about the features of children's friendships in different cultural contexts, we have very limited evidence about the ways in which these features and characteristics might lead to different developmental outcomes cross culturally. This is not surprising given that research on how friendships contribute to individual adjustment in European American cultures is not as prevalent as research on characteristics and features of friendships. French and colleagues (2003) provide one example of a strategy for assessing friendships and developmental outcomes that is common with U.S., Canadian, and European samples—comparing Indonesian children who have a reciprocated friend (based on friendship nominations) with those who do not. Findings were quite consistent with those from North American studies. Specifically, friended children were better liked, less rejected, less aggressive, less withdrawn, and had higher academic achievement than friendless children.

Currently, we know more about associations between peer relations and developmental outcomes cross culturally in the realm of peer status than we do about dyadic friendships. Several studies have examined the predictors of and consequences of peer acceptance and rejection cross culturally and identified important differences. Shyness and social sensitivity or inhibition, for example, is positively associated with peer status in some cultures (e.g., China—Chen et al., 1992, 1995) and negatively associated with peer status in others (e.g., the United States, Canada, Italy—Casiglia, Lo Coco, & Zappulla, 1998; Newcomb et al., 1993; Schneider, Smith, Poisson, & Kwan, 1997). In contrast, peer status appears to be positively associated with academic adjustment across a number of cultural contexts. In a promising cross-cultural study including an assessment of mutual friendship as well as peer status, Chen and colleagues (2004) found that having a mutual friend was strongly associated with sociability in Brazil, Canada, China, and Italy. Aggressive children were less likely to have a mutual friend in Brazil, China, and Italy (but not Canada), and shyness was associated with being friendless in Brazil and Canada (but not in China and Italy). These findings highlight cultural differences in individual characteristics that may foster or hinder the development of close friendships. In addition, this study represents a next step in research on friendship cross culturally because it links friendship experience with aspects of individual adjustment that vary according to the sociocultural context. Clearly, the correlates and consequences of having versus not having friends, having poor-quality versus high-quality friends, and having friends with various personal characteristics (e.g., aggressive, withdrawn, socially competent) need further specification across cultures.

Future Research Directions

For further research on friendship and culture, we identify at least six issues that will be important: (1) acknowledging the strengths and limitations of the individualism versus collectivism framework, (2) including alternative dimensions along which cultures differ, (3) considering culture in terms other than national boundaries, (4) expanding the aspects of friendship that are studied, (5) incorporating multiple methodologies within individual studies, and (6) expanding the number and variety of cultures that are studied.

1. It is striking how many studies evoke the individualism versus collectivism distinction to classify cultural groups and to explain findings. This framework is useful in many circumstances, which in part explains why researchers continue to rely on it, but it clearly is not adequate for explaining all of the nuanced differences that have emerged in cross-cultural studies of children's friendships. To be fair, this framework was not intended to explain individual differences across cultures given that individualism and collectivism are not psychological constructs (Hofstede, 1994). Where the individualism versus collectivism distinction appears to run into the most difficulty in studies of friendship and culture is that it oversimplifies the complexities and differences among cultures that are presumed to be similar according to this one dimension (i.e., ignoring substantial differences between two collectivistic cultures). Relatedly, it cannot capture the wide variability of experience in friendship that exists within a particular culture. There are a variety of critiques of the individualism–collectivism model (for reviews, see Brewer & Chen, 2007; Oyserman et al., 2002). We need to look beyond this dimension as a source for explanations of cross-cultural differences and similarities in friendship experiences.

2. There are a number of alternative ways in which cultures differ that likely have a significant impact on children's relationships with peers. The structure of the school system, for example, determines whether children associate with only same-age peers, how much time children have for peer interactions outside the watchful eye of adults, how much children are exposed to others who are different than themselves, and what characteristics indicate social competence. The economic structure of the community is also important, including the extent to which children and adolescents are expected to contribute to the economic life of their families. In part, economic issues determine how much leisure time youth have and the degree to which they can participate in the peer culture (Schneider, 1998). The amount of social change occurring at a given time and the sociopolitical environment are other relevant dimensions that likely affect both directly and indirectly children's relationships with peers (Edwards et al., 2006). Chen, Wang, and De Souza (2006) reported a clear change in the association between social withdrawal and social status in China that correlates with social change in the broader culture and demonstrates the importance of a historical perspective in evaluating culture and peer relationships. As China has moved toward a market

economy and with the resulting increases in mobility, decreases in government controls, and increases in competition and more individualistic goals, shyness has become negatively associated with school adjustment and positively associated with rejection by peers and depression over time. Chen and colleagues hypothesize that inhibited behavior is no longer adaptive in an environment that emphasizes greater competition and achievement of individual goals. Similarly, Pinto and colleagues (1997) suggest that whether a country is at war or peace potentially has direct implications for peer relations to the extent that the civilian population is involved. Conditions during wartime likely restrict the opportunities that youth have to socialize with others outside of the family and may also encourage even greater focus on similarity between friends.

3. It is tempting to equate culture with national boundaries and to assume that citizenship within a particular country identifies culture. Thus, a study of children's friendships comparing a group of children in the United States and a group of children in China is taken as evidence that differences between the two groups reflect differences between U.S. and Chinese culture. National boundaries certainly provide a convenient proxy for culture, but this strategy ignores potentially great variation within countries and may lead us to attribute observed differences to cultural differences when they are better accounted for by other variables, such as social class or urban versus rural environments (see French, Pidada, & Victor, 2005, for further discussion). The value of assessing multiple samples and individuals from multiple cultures within a particular country is demonstrated in studies of Arab and Jewish adolescents living in Israel (Sharabany, 2006), Zimbabwean adolescents living in traditional and modified extended families (Harrison et al., 1995, 1997), and English-speaking and Xhosa-speaking South African adolescents' interest in cross-sex friendships (Alberts et al., 2003), to name just a few. These concerns naturally call into question the representativeness of a particular sample and thus the generalizability of the findings to other children and adolescents even within the same country. The best solution to this concern is simply to expand our database. In the same way that the generalizability of some social psychology research is questioned because of its reliance on white, middle- to upper-class college sophomores, one or a few studies of youth in a particular country obviously cannot be assumed to tell us about the experience of friendships for all youth in that country or culture.

4. With the strong (though relatively small) body of literature on cross-cultural differences in children's support networks, features of friendships, and similarities between friends, we are ready to address additional questions about friendship and culture. The progression of

friendship research in North America provides an excellent model for questions to ask from a cross-cultural framework. One area for exploration is to situate dyadic friendships within children's broader peer relationships. For example, how does friendship experience correlate with acceptance or rejection by the larger peer group, and are friendships necessarily embedded within larger peer networks? Another avenue is to consider ways in which friendships contribute to other developmental processes. For example, how does children's experience with their friends contribute to their development of emotion regulation, perspective taking, and other aspects of emotional and cognitive development? In what ways are friendships associated with the development of romantic relationships in adolescence and early adulthood? These kinds of questions have the potential to tell us much about the developmental significance of friendships cross culturally and about friendship as a context for development.

5. We need to expand the types of methodologies used to investigate friendships cross culturally. Much of the existing research, especially within psychology, relies on self-report questionnaires with rating scales. Although this strategy has the benefit of an easy administration and a great deal of control by the investigators, it is not without limitations, especially in cross-cultural research. It is unlikely that we could create an unbiased measure that could be used cross culturally and thus multiple methods, multiple measures, and whenever possible, multiple informants should be used (French, Pidada, & Victor, 2005). This point is true for studies in a single culture as well, but becomes particularly important when working cross culturally. For example, some investigators have found that youth in different countries use rating scales differently. Adolescents' endorsement of individualism or collectivism was associated with use of extreme values on the scale versus use of the midpoint, respectively (Chen, Lee, & Stevenson, 1995). This response-style bias may affect cross-cultural differences in mean ratings, especially when the differences are small. Even if corrections are made for this potential bias, such as by standardizing scores within each individual to reflect the positioning of each item or friendship dimension relative to the others for that individual (see Bond, 1988; French, Pidada, & Victor, 2005), it is difficult to be sure that questionnaire items or scores endorsed by an individual have the same meaning across cultures.

Including data from other methods along with standard questionnaire data is likely to yield a more complete and complex picture of friendships across cultures. For example, diary and experience sampling methods are helpful for gathering data about features of children's friendships such as the number of peers children are with, how much time they spend together, what friends are doing together, and where friends spend time together (e.g., Rathunde & Csikszentmihalyi, 2005; Sandstrom & Cillessen, 2003). Structured observational assessments have been used successfully with U.S. samples to examine many features of friendship. For example, studying conflict between friends in a closed-field situation allows investigators to examine carefully the process of conflict as well as its resolution (e.g., Bagwell & Coie, 2004; Hartup et al., 1988, 1993). Rarely have lab-based observational studies been used cross culturally. One notable exception is a lab-based comparison of Italian and Canadian children in which dyads of friends participated in two tasks, a sharing task and a competitive task, that required conflict management (Schneider et al., 2000).

Sociologists, anthropologists, and communications researchers rely on observation and qualitative approaches much more commonly than psychologists. The study of conflict between friends again offers examples. Corsaro (2003) provides detailed and rich accounts of children's strategies in conflicts with friends from observations of Italian and U.S. nursery school children. Also, French and colleagues' studies of Indonesian children's friendships provide examples of the benefits of using more qualitative approaches that allow children to describe their relationships or conflicts with friends in open-ended interviews. Of course, this method requires careful development and application of "scoring" systems to code the interviews and identify comparable categories for examining cross-cultural differences and similarities.

Most of the existing empirical research assessing specific dyadic friendships of children across cultures is cross sectional in design with a few studies following children over a short term, such as one school year. Longer-term longitudinal studies will be essential for identifying the influence of particular friendships on children's later adjustment. Overall, the integration of qualitative and quantitative methods and the use of longitudinal designs offer much promise for cross-cultural research and for incorporating findings from various disciplines—psychology, sociology, and anthropology, for example.

6. Last is a call for more—the study of friendships in additional cultures and further investigation of friendships in the cultures that have been studied to date. It is important to acknowledge that studies that directly compare youth from two or more cultures and studies of friendships within single cultures are both necessary. In these efforts, we need to look to cultures that differ wildly from the cultures in the United States, Canada, and Western Europe and in understudied areas of the world such as Africa and South America. It is likely that the most significant differences in friendships will emerge here. For example, small hunter–

gatherer societies are unlikely to encourage exclusive interactions among same-age peers (Gaskins, 2006; Konner, 1981), and cultures with strong hierarchical social orders may encourage friendships that do not depend on reciprocity or equality (Cole, Walker, & Lama-Tamang, 2006).

The implications of studying friendship and culture are significant. It can tell us the extent to which our theoretical ideas and understanding of this relationship are specific to children and adolescents in only certain portions of the globe or are nearly universal. It can highlight rich variations in the experience of friendships and in their importance for children's lives that might account for their role in adaptive adjustment. And, it can help foster the development of theories about social development that integrate perspectives from psychology, sociology, and anthropology.

Chapter 8

Friendship Intervention

Besides their theoretical significance, questions about the influences of friends' characteristics when friendships differ in quality are of great practical significance. Consider a plan for an intervention with adolescents who are at high risk of dropping out of high school. Suppose that the intervention includes enjoyable activities for small groups of these adolescents, and one result of these activities is that the adolescents in each group become good friends with one another. Are those good friendships desirable or undesirable?
—THOMAS BERNDT AND LONNA MURPHY (2002, p. 300)

Here, we will highlight a research paradigm that has been particularly neglected in prior studies; namely interventions designed to better understand fundamental processes while simultaneously helping children who have friendship problems. There is still considerable wisdom in Kurt Lewin's dictum that one of the best ways to understand a phenomenon is to try to change it. We recommend intervention research not only for humanitarian reasons, but also because such research can provide experimental tests of hypotheses that heretofore have only been studied correlationally.
—STEVEN ASHER AND KRISTINA MCDONALD (2004, p. 16)

In the preceding chapters we have argued that friendships are developmentally significant. A logical next step, then, is to ask whether and how we can help children who have difficulty establishing and maintaining good friendships. Friendships matter to children. If we are able to intervene successfully and assist children who are having trouble in this important area of their lives, it could be viewed as a social and ethical responsibility to do so. Given what we know about the developmental significance of friendship, successful friendship interventions may have wide-ranging effects. With improved friendships, children may be better adjusted at school. They may do better academically and be more likely to make successful school transitions. They may be better equipped to cope with stress. They may be less lonely, less likely to suffer depression, and less vulnerable to peer victimization. They may be better prepared for establishing positive romantic relationships in adolescence. And, overall, they may be happier and more satisfied with their lives. To be sure, friendship is no magic potion, but the empirical research and the reports of school-based applications of interventions we have are strong enough to suggest at least the *possibility* that an effective friendship intervention could lead to a host of changes for children and adolescents. The specific effects, of course, can only be ascertained by rigorous empirical long-term evaluation of any particular intervention program—something we are sorely lacking for the most part.

In addition to the primary goal of helping children, the successful implementation of friendship interventions also has the potential to inform our understanding of the causal processes involved in friendship. As Asher and McDonald (2004) describe in the quotation at the beginning of this chapter, evaluating such interventions may have the added bonus of providing empirical tests of hypotheses about friendship that are difficult to study without experimental manipulation. If we randomly assign children to intervention and control groups, we can, for example, teach a particular set of skills to the intervention group and observe whether changes in those skills lead to changes in friendship participation and friendship quality. By doing so, we can test specific hypotheses about what skills and competencies are important in friendship formation and maintenance. In addition, interventions may allow us to test hypotheses about the effects of friendship on various other domains. For example, one frequently asked question is whether friendships contribute to children's self-esteem in ways that Sullivan (1953) and others have suggested. As we discuss in Chapters 4 and 6, evidence from correlational studies shows links between participation in friendships (and participation in high-quality friendships) and self-esteem. Longitudinal studies, in contrast, call into question the idea that friendships contribute to self-esteem (e.g., Berndt & Murphy, 2002). Interventions provide an additional way to test this hypothesis. Stated simply, if improving children's friendships directly relates to increases in self-esteem, we have additional evidence that self-esteem enhancement is an important provision of friendship.

A third reason to encourage the development and implementation of friendship interventions is to the extent that friendships may be implicated in a variety of outcomes and causal processes, friendship interventions may play a role in combating some of the most vexing problems facing children and schools today—youth violence, delinquency, and bullying; depression and loneliness; and school dropout. For example, it is difficult to go more than a week without seeing an article or commentary about bullying in a major U.S. newspaper or magazine. Almost uniformly, these articles convey the message that bullying has serious, detrimental consequences for the victims (as well as the perpetrators). Importantly, bullying is now being recognized not only by researchers but also by parents, teachers, school officials, medical doctors, and the mass media not as "kids will be kids" but as a significant problem and one that can and should be prevented. In the most dire cases, there are reports of associations between peer victimization and committing suicide (Kim & Leventhal, 2008). A recent essay by a pediatrician in the *New York Times* (Klass, 2009) notes the importance of a policy statement by the American Academy of Pediatrics on how pediatricians can assist in the identification of victims and the prevention of bullying. States across the country are mandating antibullying programs in school, and there are also laws under consideration in the United States to provide specific enumeration of categories of protection, including race, sex, sexual orientation, religion, and so on. (Engels & Sandstrom, 2010; Russell, Kosciw, Horn, & Saewyc, 2010). There are well-established antibullying programs, primarily the Olweus Bullying Prevention Program (e.g., Olweus, 1993, 2004) designed to prevent bullying, make schools more positive environments for children, and improve peer relationships at school (see Espelage & Swearer, 2011, for a review).

We mention bullying here for two reasons. First, in the same way that programs emanating from the Olweus (1993, 2004) model are based on a solid foundation of empirical research and have caught the attention of many beyond the research community, we would hope that friendship interventions could someday achieve the same level of success and recognition—namely the recognition that problems with friendships can have serious consequences to children and adolescents and should not be brushed off lightly as a normal challenge of childhood. Second, there has been considerable attention recently to the possible protective role of friendships in the face of bullying. There is mounting evidence that children with good friends are less likely to be victimized than children without (e.g., Bukowski et al., 1995; Mouttapa, Valente, Gallaher, Rohrbach, & Unger, 2004) and that having high-quality friendships can protect children against the internalizing distress associated with peer victimization (Schmidt & Bagwell, 2007). Thus, a successful friendship intervention might also be a tool in reducing the harmful effects of bullying.

Two questions we must ask before developing a friendship intervention are (1) What are the goals of the intervention, or in other words, what are we trying to change? and (2) What is the best way to intervene to achieve those particular goals? The first question implies that there are multiple ways in which children and adolescents might experience friendship problems. Imagine four children. Luke has just entered kindergarten at age 5. Although he was in a part-time preschool setting last year, he is having trouble making friends in his new class and often seems awkward and disruptive when he tries to interact with other boys in his class. Sarah and Maggie, both in the fourth grade, have been best friends for the last 3 years. Their relationship is tumultuous and strained. Despite the fact that they want to spend every minute together, their interactions frequently involve relationally aggressive behavior (e.g., one saying "I am not going to be your friend today because . . ." or talking about the other behind her back to another peer) and trying to "one up" the other. Often one or the other of them ends up feeling hurt and left out. Jake is 12 years old. He is impulsive and aggressive and highly disliked by his classmates, yet he has formed a close friendship with the 15-year-old boy who lives next door to him. They spend time together after school and often get into minor trouble together. The particular problems these children face seem to correspond to different dimensions of the relationship and may necessitate different intervention strategies. Luke's difficulty appears to be establishing a friendship at all. Sarah and Maggie have a long-standing relationship of questionable quality. And a concern with Jake is the identity or characteristics of his friend. Thus, at a most basic level, friendship interventions can be designed to focus on at least three different goals—having a friend, improving the quality of the relationship, and making friends with the "right" friend. The specific kinds of interventions that might be effective for each of these goals may be quite different.

In this chapter, we also consider the second question—how could we intervene? We evaluate several major approaches for intervention and highlight the implications of these models for friendship interventions. We then suggest guiding principles for the future development of friendship interventions.

PEER RELATIONS INTERVENTIONS AS MODELS FOR FRIENDSHIP INTERVENTIONS

Although there is a long history of intervention research aimed at improving children's peer relationships, these programs focus almost exclusively on promoting peer acceptance (reducing peer rejection) rather than on helping children make and keep friends. This is surprising given the critical distinctions between peer acceptance and rejection and friendship (see Chapter 1). Although some interventions might improve both peer status and children's friendship experiences, few of these peer status interventions have directly assessed friendship. In addition, we expect that there are skills and competencies unique to positive friendship experiences that are not typically addressed in interventions focused on peer acceptance. A major theme of this chapter, then, is that relatively little research has been done specifically on teaching children how to make and maintain friendships, either in combination with improving social acceptance or as a goal in its own right (see also Asher et al., 1996; La Greca, 1993).

More than a decade ago, Asher and his colleagues (1996) published a comprehensive review of 16 "sociometrically oriented social skills training studies." They determined that few evaluations of interventions to promote social competence included measures of friendship, making it very difficult to evaluate the impact of these programs on dyadic friendship experiences. In fact, none of the 16 studies Asher and colleagues reviewed used reciprocal friendship nominations as an outcome of the intervention. To our knowledge, there are still no studies using reciprocal friendship nominations as a measure of intervention success. The three studies in Asher's review that used unilateral friendship nominations pre- and postintervention provided some evidence of positive changes in the friendship domain. These effects suggest that the skills taught in the context of improving peer acceptance are not completely independent of those skills necessary for forming and maintaining friendships (Asher et al., 1996). Unfortunately, the past decade has not seen a tremendous influx of work on the development and evaluation of specific friendship interventions (La Greca, 1993), and many of Asher and colleagues' conclusions from a decade ago continue to hold true today.

Below we review three general types of intervention that have been used largely to address problems with peer acceptance and rejection; however, we believe they may also contain components that could improve friendship difficulties as well. The three approaches are social skills training, social-cognitive programs, and peer-pairing interventions. We also provide an overview of several other programs that might guide friendship intervention techniques but that do not fit neatly into one of these three general types of intervention. These include traditional therapy approaches, school-based techniques, and ideas from popular press books. Wherever possible, we emphasize programs that specifically target friendships.

Social Skills Coaching Programs

The idea underlying social skills training is that by improving competencies such as social knowledge, social skills, and skill monitoring, children will improve their behavior with peers, and this change will, in turn, lead to improved peer relations—greater acceptance, less rejection, and better friendships (see Ladd, 1985; La Greca, 1993; Malik & Furman, 1993). In other words, once we identify the skills that distinguish children who have good peer relations from those with poor peer relations, we can teach those skills to the latter group and promote their acceptance in the group and their relationships with others. Although there is evidence of a few programs in the 1930s and 1940s (see Bierman, 2004; Renshaw, 1981), social skills training programs were developed primarily in the 1970s and 1980s to address the social problems of rejected and neglected children (Frankel, 2005; Mrug, Hoza, & Gerdes, 2001). This form of intervention has been used with preschool, elementary, and preadoles- cent children who have low social status within their peer group (Mize & Ladd, 1990).

Although not all studies have shown that children's peer relations improve significantly as a result of social skills training programs (e.g., Tiffen & Spence, 1986), most early studies of social skills coaching demonstrated that coaching efforts may lead to improved social status and behavior (e.g., Berler, Gross, & Drabman, 1982; Bierman, 1986; Bierman, Miller, & Stabb, 1987; Gresham & Nagle, 1980; Ladd, 1981; Oden & Asher, 1977). Nevertheless, in these studies, changes in behavior emerged more consistently than did changes in sociometric ratings. It is not surprising that changes in behaviors of children after social skills coaching are easier to achieve than changes in social status. Changes in social status require not only that children make success- ful behavior changes (e.g., more sharing and taking turns or fewer failed attempts to initiate an interaction) but also that those changes are noticed by their peers and translate into peers perceiving target children as more fun to play with, better liked, less disliked, and so on. Children's social standing based on reputation-based measures, such as nominations for being most liked and least liked, is notoriously dif- ficult to modify.

Specific Social Skills Training Programs and Friendship

Although the majority of social skills coaching programs focus on improving social standing in the larger peer group, there are also a hand- ful of studies that consider how social skills training can improve friend- ships. Oden and Asher's (1977) evaluation of their social skills training program over 30 years ago is one of the few programs to recognize and assess friendship separately from peer acceptance. It is noteworthy that the title of their article focuses specifically on friendship—"Coaching Children in Social Skills for Friendship Making." Oden and Asher's program targeted children with low peer acceptance, taught them social skills related to playing individually with a peer in one-on-one coaching sessions, provided opportunities for practicing these skills in play sessions with another classmate, and then included time to review the play session with their coach. Thus, the intervention itself focused on dyadic play and skills that might be especially relevant for friendship interactions. In the evaluation of their program, Oden and Asher considered pre- and postintervention assessments of not only peer acceptance but also the number of nominations children received as a best friend. In this way, the authors recognized the distinction between being liked and having a best friend. Small (but not statistically significant) improvements in best friend nominations were seen for the intervention group relative to the control group. Some children even "went from having no friends to having one friend" (p. 504). We highlight this program because it demonstrates how interventions can focus both on friendship and more general peer competence, uses friendship nominations as an outcome measure, and shows some support (though limited) for social skills training as a means for making improvements in the friendship domain of "having friends."

The University of California–Los Angeles (UCLA) Children's Friendship Program is the largest study of a specific friendship intervention to date (e.g., Frankel, 2005; Frankel & Myatt, 2003). Begun in the early 1990s, the program is designed to teach skills for social interaction both in the larger peer group and in dyadic friendships (Frankel, 2005). In addition to working directly with the children on social skills, the program also includes a significant parent component. To date, more than 1,000 children and their parents have participated in the program. One report of the UCLA program describes a study of 7- to 12-year-old boys who were having problems making or keeping friends and who were experiencing peer rejection (Frankel, Cantwell, & Myatt, 1996). The group of boys participated in a 12-session "parent-assisted" social skills training program, which used homework, didactic presentations, behavioral rehearsal, and coaching with the children. Parents were involved in reviewing homework assignments and receiving informational handouts aimed to help them better understand their children.

Boys who received the intervention improved their social skills (e.g., Frankel et al., 1996; Frankel, Myatt, Cantwell, & Fineberg, 1997). Surprisingly, although part of the purpose of the UCLA program was to directly affect friendships, the authors did not assess whether the ability to make lasting friendships changed with the intervention. The authors only concluded that the intervention techniques—parent-assisted social skills training sessions in areas such as how to have a play date, praising others, being a good winner, meeting friends; coached play sessions in

which children were talked through the social skills lessons in real settings; child socialization homework assignments that included children
practicing on their own what they learned in the social skills sessions—
"offer promise in changing peer status and chumships in socially rejected
children" (Frankel et al., 1996, p. 613).

A more recently developed social skills program called S. S. Grin
aims to improve peer relationships (and friendship indirectly) in children
with a variety of peer problems—peer rejection, peer victimization, or
social anxiety. In contrast to the UCLA program, which takes place in a
clinic setting, the S. S. Grin program has been implemented in schools in
North Carolina. An initial evaluation after the intervention showed that
children with peer problems who received social skills training weekly
over an 8-week period showed improvement in being liked, self-esteem
and self-efficacy, and social anxiety (DeRosier, 2004). There was one
effect specific to friendship. Children in the intervention group demonstrated a decrease in affiliations with antisocial peers compared to the
control group, suggesting that they make "better choices about friendships" (DeRosier & Marcus, 2005, p. 148). Thus, social skills training
may have an effect on the identity of children's friends. One possibility is
that the intervention fostered greater acceptance in the peer group overall, allowing for the establishment of peer interactions and even friendships with more prosocial peers. One year later, children in the intervention group were less disliked by peers than those in the control group, but
the difference between the treatment and control groups on the degree to
which they reported hanging out with others who get in trouble was no
longer statistically significant (DeRosier & Marcus, 2005). The S. S. Grin
program is particularly interesting because it demonstrates the benefits
of a generic social skills training program for children with a variety of
peer problems.

Social Skills Training as Part of a Comprehensive Intervention Program

Social skills training, or social competence interventions, have also been
used as one component of comprehensive intervention programs. One
example is the "friendship group" component of the Fast Track preventive intervention program, and we highlight it here because it is a key
example of a theoretically grounded, well-researched social skills training program. The Fast Track program was begun in the early 1990s to
prevent serious conduct problems in adolescence. High-risk children
were identified at the end of their kindergarten year based on aggressive and disruptive behaviors (Conduct Problems Prevention Research
Group, 2002a). Families were part of the Fast Track program from the

time the children were enrolled in the program at the beginning of first grade through the tenth-grade year, with more effort concentrated in the first 2 years of the program and at the time of transition to middle school. This comprehensive program addresses child needs (e.g., academic competency, self-regulation, social skills) as well as parent and family needs (e.g., discipline issues, parental response to conflict and frustration) while also promoting communication between the child's home and school (e.g., parent involvement in school, parental monitoring of child's activities). It includes a school-based universal prevention component as well as more intense targeted interventions with the at-risk children and their families.

Most relevant to our discussion are components of the Fast Track program that address peer relations and friendship. The program uses friendship groups to teach children skills that are developmentally appropriate for establishing and maintaining friendships (see Bierman, Greenberg, & Conduct Problems Prevention Research Group, 1996). In grades one through three, teachers assist with teaching lessons on friendship, with lessons in areas such as participation, cooperation, fair play, and negotiation. During grades one and two, children meet in small groups for friendship groups at evening and weekend sessions. Discussion, role plays, and modeling are used to teach skills, and there are opportunities for children to engage with their groups to practice various skills and get feedback. In an attempt to help children generalize their learned friendship skills, children are subsequently observed at play with "peer pairs" in the classroom. These sessions are intended to help children make friends with peers in their classroom.

Reports of the Fast Track program indicate success in numerous areas. Several reports to date have outlined how the children have progressed through Fast Track at each grade level (e.g., Conduct Problems Prevention Research Group, 2002a, 2002b, 2011; Lavallee, Bierman, Nix, & Conduct Problems Prevention Research Group, 2005). At the end of grade one, observations in classrooms and on the playground showed higher levels of positive exchanges with peers for the intervention children than for children in the control group. Notably, children who received the intervention also had higher social preference scores according to sociometric nominations (Bierman, 2004; Conduct Problems Prevention Research Group, 1999). Interestingly, one report of the "friendship groups" component of the Fast Track program considered how much of the change in the intervention group, measured at the end of grade one, was related to variations in behavior during the friendship group sessions carried out during that school year (Lavallee et al., 2005). Results showed that positive behavior in the friendship groups was associated with improvement in problem solving, emotion recognition, prosocial behavior, and positive peer interactions, and with decreases in hostile attributions and aggressive and disruptive behaviors.

Another report of the program described outcomes at the end of grade three (Conduct Problems Prevention Research Group, 2002a). The improvements in social status that were seen at the end of grade one (Conduct Problems Prevention Research Group, 1999a) were not similarly found at the end of grade three, perhaps because of a change in the intensity of the intervention. Friendship groups met monthly as opposed to weekly or biweekly as in earlier grades, and peer pairing was discontinued by the third grade. Children, therefore, had fewer formal opportunities to practice what they learned in their regular classroom setting. Nevertheless, the findings show limited long-term effects for the kinds of peer measures assessed, and notably, specific friendship measures are not among those that were reported. At the end of grade four (Conduct Problems Prevention Research Group, 2002b), however, there were a number of significant improvements in peer relations distinguishing the intervention and control groups—higher acceptance and less rejection, fewer associations with substance-using peers, and greater teacher-rated social competence. Thus, although no specific assessments of dyadic friendship were evaluated, the comprehensive Fast Track intervention, of which social skills training was a significant component, showed improvements in general peer relations and in the degree to which children associate with friends who use drugs. It is difficult to argue, however, that these changes were due specifically to the friendship groups component of the intervention because that was just one piece of a multifaceted comprehensive intervention.

Interestingly, at least two of these social skills training interventions (Fast Track and S. S. Grin) show promise in reducing children's affiliations with deviant peers. Importantly, however, it is unclear whether children were reporting on true friends or acquaintances or both when they indicated how much they "hang out with children who get in trouble a lot or engage in antisocial activities" in the assessment of S. S. Grin (DeRosier & Marcus, 2005, p. 143) or whether none, some, or most of their friends had used drugs in the last year in the assessment of Fast Track (Conduct Problems Prevention Research Group, 2002b). We need to know more about this process—what components of the intervention are responsible for this effect? How does it happen? Does it encourage the formation of friendships with more prosocial peers? Can these effects be maintained over longer periods of time?

Evaluation of Social Skills Training Approaches

Although there are many precursors to difficulty in friendships and low peer acceptance, poor social skills is one well-documented antecedent.

Social skills training thus has high face validity as a method for improving peer relations. Unfortunately, and somewhat surprisingly, the existing literature on social skills training suffers from a number of limitations. The most significant is that we have no rigorous, carefully controlled and implemented studies with specific measures of friendship as outcomes, particularly having friends or friendship quality. The most promising finding is the glimmer of evidence that social skills training approaches may help reduce children's association with deviant peers. As mentioned above, however, these effects are probably not due solely to social skills training in the Fast Track program, and we need to know more about the association between these measures of deviant peers and children's actual friendships.

A second concern with the existing social skills interventions is that they do not focus specifically on the skills and competencies that might promote making and maintaining a friendship. To be sure, there is overlap between the skills required for being a well-liked peer and for being a good friend, but we should not assume they are identical. Children who cooperate, share, and communicate well with others are likely to be well liked and have friends, for example. But, other skills, including knowing how to engage in appropriate self-disclosure, understanding and respecting reciprocity and equality, and being a loyal and reliable partner are expected to forecast friendship success rather than peer acceptance (see Asher et al., 1996). To our knowledge, none of the existing social skills programs focus specifically on these kinds of skills and competencies. Instead, any positive effect the programs have on friendship stem from the fact that there is indeed overlap in some of the skills important for both types of positive peer relations—friendship and acceptance by the group. Improvements in friendship are thus incidental to the other peer-related outcomes the programs are designed to address.

As a result, we can discuss the overall effectiveness of social skills training programs on social competence, social behavior, and social adjustment, but the answer to the question of whether social skills training is effective for helping children without friends or with low-quality or other problematic friendships is simply unknown. Several meta-analyses summarize the utility of social skills training approaches for improving children's behavior and social competence and reveal small to moderate posttreatment effect sizes but weaker long-term effects (Beelmann, Pfingsten, & Losel, 1994; Quinn, Kavale, Mathur, Rutherford, & Forness, 1999; Schneider, 1992). Notably, some of the programs included in these meta-analyses are better described as social-cognitive interventions because they focus on cognitive processes, such as perspective taking, that are linked to social competence. We describe these in the next section. In general, the programs are effective for changing specific behaviors and social-cognitive skills. Smaller effects are found for measures of social adjustment, such as popularity and peer acceptance (Beelman et al., 1994). Again, friendship has not been adequately assessed.

There are at least four potential reasons why significant improvement in peer relations from social skills training might not occur. First, the lack of significant improvement could be attributable to a failure to train children on socially valid target behaviors (Frankel, 2005). As a result of the poor selection of content in the intervention, the learned behaviors cannot be applied easily in the child's social environment outside of the treatment group or setting. Generalization to everyday social settings is clearly a sticking point for the success of many social skills interventions. Although there may be positive changes in behavior during treatment, the changes do not always carry over to the larger social environment (Beelman et al., 1994; Bierman, 1989). Second, some children may not be significantly deficient in social skills to begin with and thus are not likely to improve substantially on their already adequate social skills (Malik & Furman, 1993). For these children, their poor peer relations stem from something other than a lack of skills. Third, social skills training may not work for youth of all ages. There is evidence that social skills training programs work better with those under 10 years old (Furman, 1984). Fourth, social skills training programs may not work equally well in all environments. Frankel (2005) notes that social skills training in outpatient clinic settings has shown limited effectiveness (e.g., Yu, Harris, Solovitz, & Franklin, 1986).

Substantial additional research is needed to test various social skills models and applications. We need rigorously controlled studies with large sample sizes, outcome measures specifically focused on friendship, and longer-term follow-up periods to determine how long positive changes persist. There is much heterogeneity in existing social skills training models, including variability in the criteria used for selecting participants (e.g., children with minor vs. severe peer problems), variability in the strategies used to implement the interventions (e.g. direct instruction by an adult, teaching within dyads or small groups, role plays with other children), variability in the content of the intervention programs (e.g., broad: participation, communication, and cooperation; specific: how to ask questions, how to offer suggestions), variability in the settings for the intervention (e.g., clinical settings vs. schools), variability in the duration of the intervention, and variability in the outcomes assessed to test the success of the intervention (e.g., specific observed behaviors, peer nominations for being liked, global ratings of social skills) (see also Asher et al., 1996). The various programs and models have not been directly pitted against one another, so we have little evidence for recommending particular strategies over others. In addition, given the lack of overwhelmingly positive effects of social skills training, careful analyses of the situations in which they are and are not successful are warranted. Furthermore, even when the programs show positive effects, we are generally left with only assumptions about the mechanisms of change. Specific analysis of what behavioral changes relate to improved peer relations would tell us a lot about peer relations processes and about the specific components of the intervention that are responsible for their effects.

Implications of Social Skills Training for Friendship Intervention

Although most social skills training programs are designed with a focus on positive outcomes in the area of peer acceptance and rejection, we think these programs have strong implications for friendship interventions as well. At the most basic conceptual level, we know that social skills and friendship are linked in multiple areas: quantity of friends (e.g., Fox & Boulton, 2006), quality of friendships (e.g., Greco & Morris, 2005), and choice of friends (e.g., Lansford et al., 2006). From an empirical perspective, then, we could reasonably expect that social skills training programs might be effective in assuaging children's friendship difficulties, including making friends, maintaining high-quality relationships, and making good choices about friends.

There are three aspects of social skills interventions that we believe to be important for helping children with friendships. First, there is some evidence that social skills programs that have been applied at the classroom level, with the teacher assisting with the intervention process, have been successful (e.g., the Fast Track program; see also Tierney & Dowd, 2000). This approach is important because the teacher knows the classroom peer dynamic better than an outsider. The teacher can effectively identify friendships and peer groups and holds a unique position in which he or she can work with children both during direct intervention efforts (e.g., discussion of what makes a good friend) and in the times in-between those sessions. Obviously, the difficulty here is that not all teachers would be effective in working on interventions at the classroom level. Nevertheless, in those classrooms where the teachers are committed and capable, a classroom approach to teaching social skills (e.g., speaking and listening effectively) with a friendship component (e.g., how to get to know each other better) may create a more positive overall social context.

We have been struck in our own work by the significant impact a teacher can have on the friendship environment in a particular classroom. In the course of data collection in numerous elementary school classrooms, we have run across several classrooms in which almost all of the children maintain that everyone in their class is a friend. In response to the question "How many kids in your class are your friends?" many of the children in these classes raise their hand to ask, "How many kids are in our class?" and diligently enter that number in response. Do these teachers' efforts translate into more reciprocal friendships or higher-quality friendships among the students in their classroom? Do children experience fewer rejection experiences in these classrooms? What is it that teachers do to create an environment in which positive friendships flourish? These are all empirical questions, and the answers may provide helpful information for designing specific friendship interventions. In the least, it is clear that teachers can play an important role in implementing the interventions.

Second, particularly with younger children, we suggest that efforts to improve social skills with the assistance of parents could be an effective approach for children with friendship difficulties. Although the UCLA program focused on 7- to 12-year-olds, it may be the case that using parents in interventions with even younger children could help with social skill and friendship improvements. With younger children, parents are in a unique position to initiate and oversee play dates, for example, which may provide the opportunity to promote friendships and teach social skills on the spot. This would be particularly effective with the UCLA model of teaching parents how to understand their children. In other words, parents would be "trained" and then would serve as the "interveners."

Third, the Fast Track program uses small friendship groups that meet in the evenings and weekends. These groups use role plays and modeling, as well as other activities, and provide children with direct feedback. The children are then observed in the classroom in pairs in order to see how well they have generalized what was taught to them and to provide opportunities for positive interactions with classmates one at a time. Friendship interventions that include observation, feedback, and follow-up are expected to be most successful. To simply provide social skills training in isolation and believe that children will naturally take those skills and behave appropriately as a result is naïve.

The social skills model of intervention might be effective with Luke, the 5-year-old introduced at the beginning of the chapter. Luke is having trouble making friends in a new class and often seems awkward and disruptive when he tries to interact with other kids. A long-term (over the course of months, starting at the beginning of the school year when the problems are identified), multicontext (home and school), and multi-intervener (parents and teacher) approach to social skills training could potentially help Luke to overcome his difficulties before they grow into bigger problems. In this case, ideally the approach would be more of a preventive intervention. Although beginning school is a stressful time because it is a marked time of transition, it also affords those around the child an opportunity to assist with the transition and create rules and guidelines for appropriate behavior in the new setting.

For Luke, the social skills training approach might be especially appropriate, given his age, period of development, and school and home situations. We would argue, however, that the biggest difficulty in intervention (social skills or any other) is that one size does not fit all. Some teachers are capable of teaching social skills and helping children with their friendships; some parents are capable of this. But, put simply, not all of these individuals will be able to produce the same results. Additionally, without follow-through and a long-term view of friendship intervention, efforts will likely be unsuccessful.

Social-Cognitive Interventions

Whereas social skills coaching involves training in overt skills, social-cognitive training focuses as well on the underlying cognitive processes that interfere with successful peer relations (Malik & Furman, 1993). Indeed, there is a fine line between these two approaches, and most recent intervention programs use a social-cognitive approach that includes both a specific behavioral component and a cognitive component. Social cognition includes several dimensions (see Shantz, 1983): (1) conceptions of other people and oneself as psychological organisms; (2) conceptions of the relations between people; and (3) conceptions of social groups, rules, and roles. Thus, social-cognitive skills include skills in perspective taking, social problem solving and conflict management, and understanding social goals. Clearly, these skills are relevant to interacting successfully in the larger peer group and to making and keeping friendships.

One hallmark of social-cognitive models is the assumption that it is not the event itself that provokes a problem behavior; instead, it is the cognitive processing of the event that influences a behavioral outcome. Dodge's social information processing model (Crick & Dodge, 1994; Dodge, 1993) is one example of a social-cognitive model that has been particularly influential in describing the problems of aggressive children. The steps of this model include noticing and encoding social cues, interpreting and making attributions about those social cues, forming social goals, generating potential solutions to the problem at hand, evaluating those solutions and deciding upon one, and carrying out the selected response. Cognitive distortions at the interpretation stage might include a hostile attribution bias in which one interprets another's ambiguous behavior as having an aggressive intent. For example, in a game of tag at recess, John trips over Alex's foot and assumes Alex stuck out his foot on purpose to make him fall. Cognitive deficiencies at the problem solution phase, in contrast, might underlie a child's inability to think of only aggressive solutions when in conflict with another about who gets to play the harmonica in music class. Social-cognitive models such as this one provide a host of possibilities for intervention (e.g., Lochman & Wells, 2002a). Because aggressive children have significant problems with peers (e.g., rejection) and because their social-cognitive deficits and aggressive behavior are often displayed in the peer context, peer relations are a key target of intervention. Here we describe two recent and ongoing intervention programs based on social-cognitive models of aggression that illustrate the central place of peer relations as risk factors for aggressive and delinquent behavior and as a primary focus for intervention.

Anger Coping or Coping Power Program

The Anger Coping program or Coping Power program was developed by John Lochman and his colleagues, primarily as an intervention for aggressive boys (Lochman, Dunn, & Klimes-Dougan, 1993; Lochman & Lenhart, 1993; Lochman & Wells, 1996, 2002a, 2002b, 2004). Early reports of the program with aggressive school-age boys revealed decreased aggression and increased time on task (Lochman, Burch, Curry, & Lampron, 1984; Lochman, Nelson, & Sims, 1981) and higher perceived social competence (Lochman, Lampron, Gemmer, Harris, & Wyckoff, 1989). Some of the positive gains in social problem solving were maintained over a 3-year period (Lochman, 1992).

A more recent report of the Coping Power program describes a 15-month intervention effort including a substantial focus on peer relations with aggressive and disruptive boys during fourth and fifth grades (Lochman & Wells, 2002a). The program included both a child component and a parent component. Group sessions with the boys focused primarily on peer problems with lessons on perspective taking and attribution retraining, social problem-solving skills, skills in avoiding peer pressure, and relaxation techniques for dealing with anger. The potential importance of these particular intervention goals for friendship can be seen in Lochman and Wells' (2002a) description of the process of improving hostile attributions: "As children ... begin to have more tolerant and accurate perceptions of others' intentions during social encounters, they are likely to respond less angrily, emit more prosocial behaviors, and have increased possibilities for developing satisfying social relationships over time" (p. 963).

After 15 months of intervention, the Coping Power program produced a number of key changes that supported the social-cognitive model (Lochman & Wells, 2002a). Changes in the ways that the boys perceived and processed information in their social world coupled with increases in the consistency of parents' responses to them contributed to lower levels of delinquent behavior at follow-up. Boys who improved the most showed reduced hostile attribution biases. Across the transition to middle school, the Coping Power program has produced noteworthy improvements in boys' social competence and social behavior, including greater perceived social competence, improved social skills, and increased social problem-solving skills (Lochman & Wells, 2002b). Although the Coping Power program does not specifically address friendship, improvements in the accuracy of perceptions of others should ultimately improve social relations and reduce isolation from prosocial, competent peers. In addition, children who are less aggressive in the peer group make more attractive friendship partners, and more socially competent children are less likely to be negatively influenced by deviant peer groups and aggressive friends.

Social Cognitive Intervention Program

Most recently, the Social Cognitive Intervention Program (SCIP) was developed to help 8- to 13-year-old children diagnosed with oppositional defiant disorder and conduct disorder (van Manen, Prins, & Emmelkamp, 2004). Designed according to Dodge's social information processing model, the program was structured to change deficits and distortions in social information processing that are common in children with disruptive behavior problems. The program focused as well on problem-solving skills and self-control skills.

In one evaluation of the program, children were randomly assigned to SCIP, social skills training, or a wait-list control group. In the social skills group, children learned skills such as how to join a group, how to negotiate, and how to be helpful and supportive. Results indicated that both the SCIP and the social skills training were effective at posttest and at a follow-up 1 year later in a number of areas compared to the control condition. Boys in the two treatment groups showed significant improvement in aggressive and disruptive behavior, self-control, social-cognitive skills, and appropriate social skills and social behavior. Direct comparisons of the SCIP and social skills training showed that the positive effects of the SCIP were more robust than the positive effects of social skills training. This analysis suggests that focusing on broader social-cognitive and social information processing deficits rather than social skills only may be more efficacious. For the purposes of the discussion in this chapter, however, we note that the measure of appropriate social behavior is a global measure of positive social behaviors and overall social skills but does not focus specifically on friendship. As we discuss above, however, these kinds of behaviors are expected to be a necessary precursor to initiating and maintaining high-quality friendships.

Another group of researchers tested the effectiveness of the SCIP in a group of early adolescents with disruptive behavior problems (Muris, Meesters, Vincken, & Eijkelenboom, 2005). The authors indicate that in their intervention "children learn to solve various social problem situations, such as how to make friends, how to help and support others, how to negotiate ... and so on" (p. 20). The SCIP intervention produced a decrease in disruptive behaviors along with an increase in social-cognitive skills, and the effects were maintained over a 3-month period. Most relevant to peer relations outcomes were the composite measures of adolescents' "difficulties" (which included assessments of peer problems) and "strengths" (i.e., prosocial behavior). Interestingly, the intervention yielded significant decreases in difficulties but no significant increase in prosocial behavior.

Evaluation of Social-Cognitive Interventions

Social-cognitive interventions have been used primarily to address aggressive behavior in boys. This strategy is believed to reduce aggressive behavior by changing the individual's interpersonal problem solving and understanding (e.g., Kennedy, 1982). Some evidence suggests that these programs may provide better results than social skills programs for aggressive and other problem social behavior (e.g., van Manen et al., 2004), and other evidence suggests that they may not be as effective as social skills programs involving modeling and direct coaching (e.g., Schneider, 1992). Despite this disagreement, in 2000, the Centers for Disease Control and Prevention named school-based social-cognitive approaches as "best practices" for preventing aggression (Thornton, Craft, Dahlberg, Lynch, & Baer, 2000). Because peer interactions provide a context in which much aggressive and disruptive behavior takes place and because poor peer relations are one of the most significant risk factors for aggression and delinquency, most comprehensive social-cognitive approaches target peer problems in the intervention. To evaluate their effectiveness in improving peer relations and friendships, we need additional research comparing the approaches directly to social skills coaching programs as well as more research with specific outcome measures associated with peer relations, and especially friendships.

Implications of Social-Cognitive Approaches for Friendship Intervention

There is evidence for the effectiveness of social-cognitive interventions in the peer setting, yet how does this approach to intervention inform the development of specific interventions for friendship? The case of 12-year-old Jake presented at the beginning of the chapter provides an example of how social-cognitive interventions may enhance friendships. Although we recognize that Jake is only an example of the type of child who can potentially benefit from social-cognitive intervention, his experiences show how we might apply this kind of intervention to a particular type of friendship difficulty. To review, Jake is impulsive and aggressive and highly disliked by his classmates. Although Jake has formed a close friendship with the 15-year-old boy who lives next door to him and they spend time together after school, they often get into minor trouble together. Jake serves as our example of an early adolescent who has difficulty making friends and also making the "right friends." The social-cognitive model of intervention can offer several strategies for helping Jake to make friends at school and to make better choices about his friends and his behavior within his friendships.

A major focus of social-cognitive intervention is to change cognitive distortions. We can divide Jake's relevant problems into at least two categories: being impulsive and aggressive at school and making bad choices with his older, neighborhood friend. A program like the Coping Power program focuses on teaching skills such as perspective taking and attribution retraining, as well as social problem-solving skills, including skills to avoid peer pressure—all are skills that relate to both of Jake's problem areas. By helping Jake notice appropriate social cues, interpret those cues appropriately, and devise and implement effective nonaggressive solutions to social problems, he will be more successful with his peers, including friends. He may be better able to establish a friendship with a same-age, nonaggressive peer at school, and he may be better equipped to make good choices with his older neighborhood friend. As Lochman and Wells (2002a) indicated, improving behavior and perceptions of others *should* improve social relations. If Jake were more appropriate and less aggressive in his behaviors, he would be expected to attract other adolescents who engage in more prosocial behavior.

Again, we offer the example of Jake as, just that, an example of a scenario in which we believe a child with friendship difficulties can benefit from a particular type of intervention that is traditionally more oriented toward increasing peer acceptance and reducing peer rejection. For children and adolescents with friendship difficulties, it is likely that their distortions in processing social information interfere with their ability to engage in healthy friendships. Cognitive retraining, with a specific focus on the level of the dyad, should be further investigated.

Peer-Pairing Interventions

The hallmark of peer-pairing interventions is that the intervention occurs at the level of the dyad. At first blush, then, these techniques seem particularly well suited for friendship interventions. Peer pairing has a rich history (e.g., Lieberman & Smith, 1991; Selman & Schultz, 1990), and practitioners are enthusiastic about its effectiveness. However, these kinds of programs are often employed in school and clinical settings—not in a research-based context. As a result, there are few rigorously designed and implemented empirical evaluations of the efficacy and effectiveness of peer-pairing approaches.

Advocates of this form of intervention contend that its primary advantage is the emphasis on creating an ongoing close relationship rather than on developing general relationship patterns or prosocial skills like those fostered in social skills training and social-cognitive programs. Pair therapies fall between individual therapy and group therapy; pair therapy takes the child further into the peer world than individual therapy does but it avoids overwhelming the child who does not have the social repertoire necessary for a larger group setting. Although it works at the dyadic level, pair therapy typically uses a social-cognitive strategy, much like that described in the last section (Dykeman, 1995).

Pair Therapy

Some of the earliest work on pair therapy (also called pairing or pair counseling) was done by Robert Selman and his colleagues in the late 1970s and early 1980s (e.g., Lyman & Selman, 1985; Selman, 1989; Selman & Demorest, 1984; Selman & Schultz, 1990; Selman et al., 1992). Selman developed the pair therapy approach in concert with his theoretical and empirical work on the development of interpersonal understanding. This clinical approach is strongly grounded in developmental theory and involves pairing together two children, usually in pre- or early adolescence, with "contrasting, but equally ineffective, relational approaches to friendship" (Selman, 1997, p. 10). The two children meet together regularly with a therapist with the goal of using peer conflict in a therapeutic way in order to understand, and subsequently teach, conflict negotiation skills. The pair therapy program builds directly on Sullivan's (1953) ideas about the "psychotherapeutic possibilities" of friendships for those whose interpersonal functioning is immature; specifically, its goal is to "help troubled children develop the capacity to establish and maintain close friendships" (Selman, Schultz, Caplan, & Schantz, 1989, p. 60).

Pair therapy seeks to improve children's capacity for *intimacy* (i.e., to learn to trust another child, to give and receive support, and to share personal experiences) and *autonomy* (i.e., to stand up for oneself by negotiating one's needs) (e.g., Selman, 1989) with the ultimate goal of helping children form and maintain good relationships. With close adult supervision, children should develop social knowledge, social skills, and social values, which should foster intimacy and autonomy. The therapist creates opportunities for conflict in a safe environment, mediates the conflict by setting limits and providing incentives, and teaches the pair to reflect on their behavior during the conflict situation (Lyman & Selman, 1985). Through these sessions, children should cultivate a more mature understanding of the friendship experience and learn constructive ways to resolve conflict. In particular, the therapy involves three aims: (1) an *individual* goal of creating a context for the child to learn mutual and collaborative behaviors when dealing with another person in a one-on-one relationship, (2) a *dyadic* goal of improving the dyad's regulation of social interactions without external help, and (3) a *systems* goal of teaching the child how to reach synchrony in relationships with more than one person at a time (Selman et al., 1989). It is important to note that the point of pair therapy is *not* to establish a friendship between the two children in the pair (though that sometimes happens). Rather, the children should develop the capacity for getting along with peers, understanding friendships, and making friends with others (Selman & Schultz, 1990).

Evidence of the effectiveness of peer-pairing programs has been largely based on clinical process notes kept by therapists and on case studies. Selman notes that rigorous empirical evaluation has not been a priority for his research and clinical group (Selman & Schultz, 1990), and the majority of his work has been done with children who have severe emotional and behavioral disorders. There are several small-scale reports and case studies that describe some positive outcomes for children involved in peer pairing, including those described in the book *Making a Friend in Youth* (Selman & Schultz, 1990) and other case reports (Karcher, 1997; Lyman & Selman, 1985; Schultz, 1997). At a minimum, these case studies suggest that those who undergo pair therapy become more aware of techniques for interacting with a friend. But whether or not children's experiences change in the "real world" following this type of intervention is a critical, and largely unanswered, question.

Several researchers have also used quantitative measures in combination with qualitative measures to assess children's progress through pair therapy, but these reports still include only a few children. For example, an 8-month study of six pairs of emotionally disordered 8- to 11-year-olds found that friendship competencies, including negotiation behavior, quality of communication, interpersonal understanding of friendship, and knowledge of strategies to deal with friendship dilemmas, increased with pair therapy (see Lyman & Selman, 1985). A second study (Yeates, Schultz, & Selman, 1991) found that pair therapy helped to decrease impulsive and aggressive behaviors over a 12-week period among public-school students. Finally, in another 12-week study of pair therapy with 4 eighth-grade boys diagnosed with conduct disorder, participants reduced their level and expression of outward anger, decreased their aggression in the classroom, and increased their control of anger (Dykeman, 1995). These latter two studies focus on outcomes other than friendship and suggest that pair therapy may be effective in reducing problem behaviors as well as in encouraging the formation of positive relationships. It is important to note, however, that we cannot draw conclusions about what mechanisms were responsible for the changes these investigators and clinicians observed following pair therapy, and larger-scale studies with rigorous assessments are needed to evaluate the effectiveness of pair therapy.

The Buddy System

Children with ADHD have significant problems in friendship and peer relations. Hoza and colleagues developed a "buddy system" intervention specifically to help children with ADHD establish and maintain friendships (Hoza, Mrug, Pelham, Greiner, & Gnagy, 2003; Mrug et al., 2001). The buddy system is one component of an intense 8-week summer treatment program (STP) for children with ADHD. It uses a dyadic approach for several reasons. First, improvements in friendships may enhance other outcomes as well (e.g., social competence, academic performance, social behavior). Second, dyadic intervention may be easier to conduct and more likely to show positive effects than interventions targeting peer acceptance, where a child's negative reputation is a significant hurdle to overcome. As we discussed above with social skills training, for peer status to improve, children's positive behavior changes must be noticed by many in the peer group and translated to likability. But friendships may improve if social interactions become more positive between the target child and only one or two particular children. Because of its dyadic nature, the buddy system is similar to other peer-pairing approaches.

In the STP for ADHD (Pelham & Hoza, 1996) in which the buddy system was developed, teachers and counselors implement a behavior modification system, with peer-oriented interventions such as social skills training and problem-solving assistance, as well as sports skills training and academic remediation. In the buddy system component, children were paired with a "buddy" during the third week of the 8-week program. They spent more time with their buddy than with other children (e.g., being partners in sports activities, sitting together on the bus). Buddies were also given privileges that emphasized sharing with their buddy, such as sharing the points they accumulated in the token economy system and being recognized by daily "best buddies" awards. In addition, pairs worked both individually and jointly with a "buddy coach." Parents were encouraged to get the buddies together on a weekly basis outside of the STP (e.g., coming over to one buddy's house to play or going on an outing together).

The results of the buddy system intervention with ADHD children can be used to guide friendship intervention efforts. The main finding related to friendship was that the quality of the friendship (according to the STP counselors and the children themselves) at the end of the intervention was predicted by the number of times parents arranged a meeting of the dyad. Thus, the effectiveness of the intervention was related to the parents' investment and compliance with the treatment program. Overall, the buddy system provides promising initial results for dealing specifically with friendship problems within a particular group of children known to have significant peer problems. Cautious enthusiasm about the buddy system is necessary until further evaluation of the program is completed, especially including a comparison of children randomly assigned to the buddy system versus a control group that does not receive the intervention.

Evaluation of Peer-Pairing Approaches

Various types of pair therapy and the buddy system are interventions that work with children at the dyadic level over an extended period of time with the goal of improving how children relate to one another and form friendships. Of all the interventions we discuss, peer-pairing approaches are the only ones systematically focused on friendship rather than other aspects of peer relations. These interventions are used with different populations (e.g., emotionally disturbed, aggressive, ADHD), in different settings (e.g., residential, clinical, school, summer camp), and with different facilitators (e.g., clinicians, counselors). The use of peers as treatment partners has also been incorporated in social skills coaching programs. Often, target children are paired with more socially competent children, for example, well-accepted children have been paired with unpopular children (e.g., Bierman, 1986; Bierman & Furman, 1984; Oden & Asher, 1977). Evaluations of these techniques suggest that improvements are more likely to be made when the pairs (or triads in some cases) receive coaching but not when the children are simply given the experience of playing with more socially competent peers.

Additional research is necessary to understand the degree to which the results of peer pairing interventions are generalizable and whether the results are maintained after the intervention has stopped. In addition, these approaches, unlike the social skills training and social-cognitive interventions described above, have generally not been subject to rigorous systematic study with carefully designed control conditions and random assignment to treatment or intervention. The relative lack of empirical evaluation makes it difficult to consider the effectiveness of these approaches in the same way that we can evaluate social skills training and social-cognitive interventions.

Implications of Peer-Pairing Programs for Friendship Intervention

Clearly, there are lessons to be learned from nearly four decades of research on some form of peer-pairing technique. The most promising part of peer-pairing programs for friendship intervention is that these programs focus on the level of the dyad. Whereas social skills and social-cognitive interventions are primarily interested in the larger peer group and social functioning, most peer-pairing programs have within their set of goals to establish and maintain close friendships and to improve the dyad's regulation of social interaction (Selman et al., 1989). Capacities such as intimacy coupled with autonomy are important building blocks for this type of program.

In further investigating peer-pairing interventions, it is important to keep in mind the particular goals of each program. Is the goal to improve a friendship or create a friendship between the two children involved, or is it to improve children's friendship-building skills more generally so that they can be applied to establishing friendships in other contexts? In reality, successful interventions may lead to both outcomes. For example, Hoza and colleagues' (2003) buddy system focuses on building a relationship between two particular children. If this approach is successful, however, it is also likely to increase the children's ability to form and maintain other friendships as well. Selman's pair therapy approach is not explicitly focused on "matchmaking" between the two children involved (Selman & Schultz, 1990, p. 134), yet in some cases specific friendships do develop. Thus, although these goals are different from the outset, it is likely that approaches that involve working with specific dyads might lead to similar outcomes in many cases.

Other Intervention Programs

There are several other commonly used approaches for dealing with friendship difficulties and for promoting the formation and maintenance of friendship. In general, these programs use a variety of intervention approaches, are conducted in school or clinic settings, and do not have rigorous empirical research to document their effectiveness, despite the frequency with which they are used. These are the kinds of interventions that are used "in the trenches"—at home by parents or in classrooms and schools; implemented by parents, teachers, school counselors, and occasionally psychologists; and evaluated primarily by case studies, anecdotal reports, and occasionally small-scale qualitative or quantitative research designs. They are discussed and debated in teacher lunchrooms and other venues far away from the research lab, and the findings tend to be published in the educational psychology literature and in journals and newsletters devoted to education and clinical practice.

Traditional Therapy Approaches

Individual and group therapy have been used with the goal of enhancing children's friendships. These approaches may target social skills or social-cognitive skills, but they are typically eclectic and difficult to tie to a particular intervention approach. First, individual treatment programs focus on the therapist as a coach for the child who has difficulties. Although this type of therapy is likely used quite a bit, research into its effectiveness has not been promising. For example, Bierman and Furman (1984) compared individual coaching in skills with a peer group experience (with and without coaching) in which children worked toward a superordinate goal of making films. The coaching was helpful in improving some skills, but changes in children's acceptance by peers only occurred when the coaching took place during a peer group experience. Similarly, the peer group experience led to more positive changes in children's social self-perceptions. Other studies have found that training sessions between a child and a therapist do not generalize well to peer interactions (e.g., Berler et al., 1982; Malik & Furman, 1993).

In contrast to individual treatment, group therapy programs bring together multiple children or adolescents for intervention purposes, usually in school settings. According to one recent analysis of these programs, 40% are psychoeducational (general population of students, focus on skills training, led by a paraprofessional), 50% are counseling oriented (students with social or emotional needs, growth oriented, conducted by a mental health professional), and 10% are psychotherapy oriented (students with emotional or social disorders, remedial treatment, very small groups led by an expert in therapy) (Shechtman, Freidman, Kashti, & Sharabany, 2002). The thinking here is that group sessions are appropriate for dealing with friendship difficulties because the group environment focuses on creating trust and cohesion between members and on establishing comfortable levels of self-expression and self-disclosure (Corey, 1990). These are the kinds of processes that are necessary for close friendships, too, and may generalize from positive group experiences to dyadic friendships.

In one test of the effectiveness of school-based group counseling, Shechtman and colleagues (2002) attempted to improve adolescents' intimacy with a close friend during 15 weeks of classroom-based group sessions. Group sessions centered on developing a language of feelings; improving self-acceptance and self-awareness; and discussing perceptions of friendship, difficulties in establishing and maintaining friendships, and fears about close relationships. In contrast to the control group, adolescents in the intervention reported increases in intimacy with their best friend from pre- to postintervention to a follow-up 6 months later (Shechtman et al., 2002). Although individual and group therapy may be commonly used to target peer problems in school settings, there is not enough structured research done to draw conclusions about the effectiveness of these approaches.

The "Circle of Friends" Program

One peer-based intervention program, Circle of Friends, was first developed to help children and adolescents with disabilities better connect with their peer group (Frederickson, Warren, & Turner, 2005; see James & Leyden, 2010, for a review). Subsequently applied to students with special educational needs (e.g., Falvey, Forest, & Pearpoint, 2002), emotional, behavioral, and social difficulties (e.g., Newton, Taylor, & Wilson, 1996), and autism spectrum disorders (Greenway, 2000; Gus, 2000; Kalyva & Avramidis, 2005), the intervention creates a circle of friends from the target child's classroom that, in cooperation with an adult facilitator, helps to develop and monitor a program of support for the child who is having problems (Frederickson et al., 2005). The goals of the intervention are to help the child change his or her behavior, improve social relations and friendships, and simultaneously change peers' behaviors and feelings toward the child. The Circle of Friends seeks to help children by using their immediate peer group as part of the intervention (Newton et al., 1996). In order to achieve this, the facilitator asks the class about the target child's behavioral strengths and weaknesses, and then discusses with the class the feelings and difficulties that come with a lack of friendship and support (Frederickson et al., 2005). A group of six to eight children is then recruited to serve as the "circle of friends." A very limited amount of evaluative research has been done on the Circle of Friends intervention program. Positive outcomes, including the development of empathy, problem-solving skills, and listening skills as well as improvements in social acceptance, have been reported using qualitative case study methodologies (Frederickson & Turner, 2003; Newton et al., 1996; Pearpoint, Forest, & O'Brien, 1996).

Several modifications of the Circle of Friends program have appeared in the educational psychology literature. In one, the focus is on the whole class needing to be more effective at establishing and maintaining friendships (although ultimately a subgroup of students is still chosen as the circle of friends for intervention purposes; Shotton, 1998). After 6 weeks, the participants reported feeling happier because they had made friends through the group. Teachers also reported that the target child seemed happier and less isolated after the group sessions. In a second modification of Circle of Friends, several circles were set up within the classroom, each to benefit an isolated child (Barratt & Randall, 2004). Another case study demonstrated that using the whole-class approach to teach about friendship (i.e., what children do and say to show they are friends) for the benefit of a low-accepted child helped to improve the social situation of the at-risk child (Smith & Cooke, 2000).

Overall, it is nearly impossible to determine the extent to which changes in behavior are attributable to the Circle of Friends intervention. Despite the lack of hard data to support the effectiveness of the program, there are several things to be learned from this intervention model. First, a classroom-based approach may be beneficial for both the target student and the other students in the class. Universal interventions that target whole populations, regardless of at-risk status or diagnosis, can make recruiting, screening, and attrition less problematic, enhance peer support, reduce stigmatization, and reach a broad range of children (e.g., Evans, 1999; Kubiszyn, 1999). Second, the intervention program may empower teachers by making them a part of the intervention process. Third, from an ecological perspective, helping children within the environments in which they are having difficulty may be an effective way to teach them the skills and behaviors that are necessary in that context. In this regard, it is important to note that friendship interventions are rarely classroom based. Future intervention models should consider how the classroom can be used as the context for intervention.

Popular Press Books for Parents

Outside of the research and academic arena, there are popular press books marketed to parents and teachers who wish to help children with friendship problems. These books demonstrate the growing recognition that peer relations, especially friendships, are not only valued by children but are developmentally significant, and that friendship problems should not be ignored. In addition, these books suggest that successful intervention is possible and that parents can and should play a central role in helping children develop social competence. The subtext of these books is that just as a parent would be concerned and would work to help their child who is struggling with learning and academics, parents should work to help a child with social difficulties. Two recent examples of this kind of book are Michele Borba's (2005) *Nobody Likes Me, Everybody*

Hates Me and Natalie Elman and Eileen Kennedy-Moore's (2003) *The Unwritten Rules of Friendship*. Both books have subtitles emphasizing a problem-focused orientation—Borba's *The Top 25 Friendship Problems and How to Solve Them* and Elman and Kennedy-Moore's *Simple Strategies to Help Your Child Make Friends*. The books are marketed primarily to parents and possibly to teachers.

In the first section of Borba's book, she briefly discusses why friends matter, why children have friendship problems, and how to evaluate a child's friendship skills. She also gives an overview of 25 friendship issues and the 10 worst things parents can do. The second section of the book is a "how to" for parents. Parents are instructed on how to organize a playgroup, how to get their older children teamed up with other children, and how parents and children can be good "hosts" when others come to their house to play. The third and lengthiest part of the book presents the top 25 friendship problems (e.g., argues, bad friends, bad reputation, bossy, bullied, and harassed). For each, there is an overview of the problem, reasons for the problem, examples of what parents can say to their children to help with the problem, strategies to help parents themselves deal with their children's problems, and a list of resources that parents can consult for additional assistance.

Elman and Kennedy-Moore's book begins with an overview of "unwritten rules" that underlie and govern social interactions. According to the authors, understanding these rules is necessary for knowing how to interpret social situations and how to act in appropriate and expected ways. Their view is that many children suffer social problems because they lack these important pieces of social knowledge. Thus, a child may have adequate social skills but without understanding of the "unwritten rules," he or she will not know how or in what situations to display those skills effectively. The book then proceeds to discuss nine children with particular characteristics that make it difficult for them to get along well in the peer group and to make friends, including "the shy child," "the short-fused child," "the vulnerable child," and "the intimidating child." For each one, the authors list the particular unwritten rules with which that child struggles and give specific concrete suggestions for parents to help their children learn those rules.

Although these authors use some existing research to guide the intervention ideas and the books may be useful resources in some situations, intervention is not likely to be as simple as Borba and Elman and Kennedy-Moore make it out to be. There is no empirical evidence provided to suggest that the approach or information in the books has been successful with children who have friendship difficulties. Although promises of "solv[ing] these problems and boost[ing] your child's social competence" (Borba, 2005) are likely overstated, the potential benefits of this type of book are that it gives parents some information about their children's problems, acknowledges that friendship problems are worthy of intervention, and tries to empower parents to help their children. These books are also reminders of the need for researchers and clinicians to translate their intervention work into usable ideas for parents and teachers. Much of the intervention work that has been conducted to date has not resulted in information that is easily digested and applied by those who spend their days with children and adolescents who experience friendship difficulties.

Implications of These Programs for Friendship Intervention

Like the peer-pairing programs introduced in the previous section of the chapter, the Circle of Friends program and the interventions described in popular press books speak more directly to friendship than the social skills and social-cognitive models. Therefore, it is important to ask, How can the Circle of Friends and popular books guide friendship interventions, more generally?

The Circle of Friends model would be most useful for those children who have difficulty making friends. It has been used with children who need to better connect with their peers and specifically focuses on creating a group of children who can become "friends" of the child with difficulties. The benefit of this approach is that it uses the peer group, guided by the teacher, to try to understand and reach out to the troubled child. Although we realize that this can certainly backfire if not implemented and overseen in an effective and productive way, the overall model is a good one. This technique has been used selectively in elementary schools in the school district of the second author (with parental permission), and based on anecdotal evidence, it has been used successfully to help some children with friendship difficulties. It awaits more thorough evaluation.

Popular media books can serve a purpose as well. Put simply, they serve as resources for parents (and possibly teachers) who see their children having trouble. Many parents describe a feeling of helplessness when they see their children struggling, particularly with problems such as friendship and peer problems. These books can empower parents, teachers, and others to help their children—they give them a toolbox with which they can experiment, presumably in the best interest of the child. Nevertheless, these approaches have never been tested empirically so we have no research evidence to support their effectiveness. There is perhaps an opportunity here for researchers and authors of these books to establish partnerships to evaluate these programs thoroughly, and if effective, to disseminate them widely through these more accessible books (rather than, or in addition to, academic journals).

GUIDING PRINCIPLES
FOR FRIENDSHIP INTERVENTION

So what can we take away from the variety of programs we have reviewed to guide the future development of friendship interventions? There is not one intervention program or technique that is overwhelmingly success-ful or that clearly outshines the others. This can be frustrating as we are far from being able to identify a set of "best practices" for friend-ship intervention or to publicize one or several programs that can be implemented on a larger scale and recommended to schools, teachers, or others who are simply looking for a way to help particular children in need. At the same time, having several different kinds of interventions that work would allow individuals to select a particular program that meets their specific goals. As we discuss at the beginning of the chap-ter, there are multiple ways that children might experience friendship problems—some struggle with establishing a friendship at all and are friendless; others have trouble maintaining a high-quality relationship; still others have friends but only form relationships with peers who have questionable characteristics (e.g., aggressive or antisocial youth or peers who bully them). Targeting any of these problems could be a worthwhile goal for intervention, and additional research evaluating friendship out-comes from the various interventions discussed should help clarify which programs are most effective for which goals.

The existing literature suggests that there are multiple ways to inter-vene. Unfortunately, the existing literature suffers from two primary limi-tations. First, many of the programs with strong empirical evaluation, including social skills training and social-cognitive interventions, do not focus directly on friendship. Rather, they focus on improving peer accep-tance and reducing peer rejection, and in the evaluations of the programs, friendship is not an outcome that has been assessed. As a result, we are confident in the effectiveness or ineffectiveness of various programs for these peer problems, but not in their ability to tackle friendship prob-lems directly. Second, many of the programs that *do* specifically target friendship development and friendship problems, including peer-pairing approaches and classroom-based interventions such as the "circle of friends" programs have not been tested using large sample sizes, control groups, empirically supported outcome measures, and other hallmarks that we look for in empirically supported treatments where the gold standard is a randomized controlled trial. In many ways, this limitation represents a larger issue—the gap between research and practice—that is certainly not unique to the study of friendships. Nevertheless, in bridging this gap and in developing interventions that specifically target children's friendships, we offer several guiding principles and raise questions to help focus research in this area.

1. Intervention efforts need to be firmly grounded in what we know about friendship. In particular, it is clear that friendship is multidimensional, and there may be unique intervention components that are most effective for these various dimensions. For example, it is likely that children who are having difficulty making and maintaining even one friendship might require different kinds of intervention than children whose difficulty is in achieving high-quality friendships or forming friendships with prosocial positive peers and avoiding affiliations with deviant peers. Over a decade ago, Asher and colleagues (1996) identified 10 specific skills children needed for success in friendships. These include skills in initiating contact; being fun, resourceful, and enjoyable companions; achieving equality in friendship; engaging in self-disclosure; expressing caring, concern, and admiration appropriately; helping friends in need; being a reliable partner; managing and resolving disagreements; learning to forgive; and learning that friendships exist within a larger social network. The focus on these particular skills comes from basic research on friendship (e.g., comparisons of friends vs. nonfriends) and from research distinguishing friendship from peer group acceptance. Thus, in addition to focusing intervention efforts on multiple aspects of friendship (e.g., having friends vs. friendship quality), we need to focus on what we know is necessary for friendship specifically (and not only on peer relations more generally).

A related point is that components of different intervention approaches may need to be combined in order to create the most effective interventions. Teaching children socially appropriate behavior, while also working to change the underlying flawed cognitive processes is critical (e.g., van Manen et al., 2004). Nevertheless, before taking a "kitchen sink" approach to intervention with the idea that more is better, we need careful analyses of which aspects of existing interventions are responsible for their positive effects. In other words, what processes are involved?

2. Particularly with younger children, parent involvement should be included in intervention efforts. Parents of young children are gatekeepers for their children, and parents' choices in terms of social opportunities can influence their children's peer and friendship outcomes. Parents determine what peer contact young children have. They enroll them (or

not) in particular preschools. They invite (or not) other children to their house to play. Where parents are included in intervention, research has demonstrated benefits to the target children (e.g., Hoza et al., 2003; Parke & Ladd, 1992; Lochman & Wells, 2002b). For example, there is preliminary support for training parents to be their child's "friendship coach" in an intervention for children with ADHD. Children of trained parents showed positive changes in social skills and friendship quality (as assessed by parents) and in peer acceptance and rejection (reported by teachers) compared to a control group (Mikami, Lerner, Griggs, McGrath, & Calhoun, 2010). In addition, we are seeing the emergence of various self-help books for parents (e.g., Borba, 2005; Elman & Kennedy-Moore, 2003; Rubin & Thompson, 2002; Thompson, Grace, & Cohen, 2001) aimed at educating parents about their child's peer world and teaching them how to help their children solve friendship problems. Clearly, many parents want to be involved and can be involved successfully in friendship interventions.

This recommendation raises the broader question of who should be involved in the intervention in order to achieve maximum results. Is it most effective to work only with troubled youth? Should special populations or general populations be targeted (keeping in mind that a large portion of the literature to date has been done on children with externalizing difficulties)? Should peers be involved? Depending on the population under investigation, these questions should be thoughtfully considered in order to design the best approach. Questions about who should be included also need to be considered from an ethical standpoint. Asher and McDonald (2004) report that only some children say they would like help with their peer relations when asked. These findings beg the question of whether friendship interventions should be available to everyone as part of the school curriculum, for example, or whether children should be involved only if they are interested. Is friendship more important for some children than for others? Children's own varying levels of motivation for having friends is likely to affect the degree to which any friendship intervention is successful (e.g., Asher & McDonald, 2004; Bukowski, 2004; Rubin, 2004)

3. Intervention efforts should be focused on working directly with children to improve social and cognitive processes, but opportunities to practice what is learned in natural settings must also be part of the program. Interventions should phase out over time so that children begin to generalize what they learn in the intervention program to their natural environment. Perhaps the most obvious conclusion from the programs reviewed above is that maintaining improvements in behavior and social-

cognitive processes is quite difficult once intervention ends and children are back in their everyday social world with peers. Nevertheless, in this regard, interventions with the goal of helping children form a friendship may have greater success than interventions aimed at improving children's status in the peer group (see Hoza et al., 2003). Success from a friendship intervention might require "only" forming a positive and reciprocal bond with one other child in the classroom, whereas success from a peer-status intervention requires overcoming a child's negative reputation and getting many peers in the class to like (or at least not strongly dislike) the child.

The broader research question here is how generalizable are the results of any intervention approach? One of the biggest challenges for intervention is to change behavior not only in the short term but in the long term as well. According to Elliott and Busse (1991), generalization may be more likely when (1) we teach behaviors that are valued and are likely to be reinforced when they naturally occur, (2) we train the child in different settings with different people, (3) we fade training over time until the child is in a natural environment, (4) we reinforce behavior when it occurs in new situations, and (5) we include peers in the training process. Specific challenges to generalization include preexisting friendship networks, social status, and negative interaction with peers (Pellegrini & Urbain, 1985). This is where social-cognitive training may be effective in cooperation with social skills training to change perceptions of and judgments by peers (Frederickson & Turner, 2003). Generalization is a problem in all of the existing intervention approaches and needs to be a primary consideration in further development of any particular program.

4. Universal or classroom-based interventions for friendship development should be considered as standard practice in elementary schools. A naturalistic approach to intervention, perhaps better termed *preventive intervention,* can potentially teach all children in a school or classroom the necessary skills for friendship development (e.g., Evans, 1999; Kubiszyn, 1999). This approach would place social competence at the forefront of what teachers and schools aim to accomplish and would recognize the value of positive friendships for contributing to the primary academic goals of scholastic achievement and school adjustment. Classroom-based interventions also allow teachers or others to guide children in their "natural" context and may help to avoid problems with generalization discussed above. Particularly promising are approaches that combine a universal classroom-based intervention and a more specific individual intervention (called an indicated intervention) for children showing peer

and friendship problems. Theoretically, the universal component creates a more accepting classroom context and would enable high-risk children to generalize the skills they learn in the indicated intervention component more easily. As one example, van Lier, Vuijk, and Crijnen (2005) found that their intervention to decrease antisocial behavior and affiliation with deviant friends helped both those children in need of intervention and those who were not the targets of the intervention.

5. A developmental approach should be taken when designing friendship interventions. As we describe in Chapters 3 and 4, the nature of friendships changes throughout the school years and during adolescence. An approach for those in the early grade school years is likely not appropriate or meaningful for adolescent populations. This is one example of the importance of thoroughly grounding intervention programs in developmental research on friendship and carefully describing the models of friendship on which interventions are based—something that is done extensively in several of the successful comprehensive interventions described here (e.g., the Fast Track and Coping Power programs, for example).

6. In designing friendship interventions, we need to give careful consideration to some of the challenges that potentially arise when targeting specific friendships per se. First, many specific friendships may be fleeting. Some may last for years, but many others are much more fickle. In that sense, improving skills in making new friendships may be just as important as improving skills that are important for maintaining relationships over time.

Second, we need to be concerned about possible iatrogenic effects. Many of the interventions described here bring together target children in small groups or even in pairs. Intuitively, this approach makes sense as it provides a setting like the child's social world in the classroom, and it allows children to practice and try out the skills they are learning. As we describe in detail in Chapter 5, however, this approach may have critical costs. Specifically, to the extent that bringing children with aggressive or other problems together creates a deviant peer group and allows for deviancy training, such interventions may have iatrogenic effects. This problem has been thoroughly described by Dishion and colleagues (1999) and more recently by Dodge, Lansford, and Dishion (2006) and Prinstein and Dodge (2008), and potential solutions for this problem are garnering significant attention. A related point is that some parents may not be enthusiastic about promoting a close friendship between their son or daughter and a less socially competent or more aggressive or disruptive peer. Parental involvement in arranging opportunities for the buddies to get together was crucial to the success of Hoza and colleagues' (2003) buddy program, yet careful parental monitoring and/or adult supervision of these get-togethers would be important for avoiding iatrogenic effects.

In fact, anecdotal evidence from some school and summer camp personnel about friendship interventions reveals considerable concern about negative influence from friends. A recent news article describes some educators actually discouraging children from forming best friendships altogether (Stout, 2010). This approach is surprising and seems to illustrate well problems captured by the adage "throwing the baby out with the bathwater." What we know about the developmental significance of friendship clearly advocates against this kind of intervention and highlights the need for researchers and practitioners—educators, clinicians, and others—to work together to design, implement, and evaluate effective friendship interventions.

7. A nagging question remains about how to evaluate existing interventions and ones we hope will soon be developed. What kind of evidence is good enough to demonstrate that an intervention is worthwhile? The existing evaluations range from case notes to anecdotal evidence to pre- and postintervention quantitative analyses. Which results are good enough? Are moderate effect sizes strong enough? Do case notes matter? Does it have to be quantitative to be deemed rigorous? If a child reports "feeling better," is that enough? Does anecdotal evidence from school-based implementations speak loudly enough to the validity of a particular intervention? The extent to which intervention programs are evaluated vary widely, making it difficult to draw conclusions based on a comparison of intervention programs. Ideally, we could develop interventions that show efficacy with randomized controlled trials. Clearly, some of the interventions described above have been subjected to these rigorous scientific tests. Others have not, and we need to decide what we will judge to be "effective." What will we allow to "count?" A related question is how long do positive effects need to last in order to be called a successful intervention? Short-term follow-ups of a few months to a couple of years later have been published, but they are not enough to suggest that short-term gains will necessarily carry forward for extended periods of time. More longitudinal analysis is needed to determine the long-term effects of intervention. Thus, our final guiding principle is that evaluation plans need to be developed hand in hand with the intervention itself and whenever possible should include rigorous tests of improvements in multiple dimensions of friendship—reciprocal friendship nominations, friendship quality assessments, and information about the characteristics of children's friends—and long-term follow-up.

CONCLUSIONS

Each of the chapters in Parts II and III of this book addressed the question, What do we know about the developmental significance of friendship? Unfortunately, the intervention research to date does not allow us to draw conclusions about that question. Overall, this is perhaps the most striking direction for future research, and the developmental psychopathology model is critical here. Specifically, this model suggests that our basic research in developmental psychology about friendships should be used to inform the development of intervention programs. This point is not surprising. As we describe in this chapter, this would include addressing multiple dimensions of friendships, such as having friends and keeping friends, establishing friendships of high quality, and maintaining friendships with children who have desirable characteristics; paying attention to developmental changes in friendship; and focusing directly on skills and competencies most important to friendship (as opposed to popularity or acceptance). Likewise, however, implementing and evaluating friendship interventions would allow us to test hypotheses about friendship in a unique and valuable way, and might even provide direct evidence of the developmental significance of friendship. Stated simply, if we design effective interventions that successfully modify friendships—helping friendless children make and keep a friend; improving the quality of poor-quality friendships; or encouraging the development of friendships with prosocial, positive others, for example—and those changes do (or do not) in turn have a positive impact on children's adjustment and well-being, that tells us something about the significance of friendships and the differential significance of having a friend, the quality of the friendship, and the characteristics of the friend.

Here is one recent example of how interventions can help evaluate the significance of friendship. A randomized controlled trial of the Good Behavior Game, a universal classroom-based intervention designed to reduce externalizing behavior and promote prosocial behavior, demonstrated that children in the intervention condition showed a significant reduction in externalizing behavior from kindergarten to the end of second grade compared to the control group, who showed an increase in externalizing problems (Witvliet, van Lier, Cuijpers, & Koot, 2009). The Good Behavior Game also had a significant positive effect on children's number of mutual friends, peer acceptance, and proximity to others in their friendship network over this time period. Importantly, these three peer variables partially mediated the link between the intervention and improvements in externalizing behavior. When considered simultaneously, peer acceptance was the only unique mediator, perhaps because of the young age of the children—friendships may be more important than peer acceptance at older ages. Nevertheless, what these findings tell us about models of the development of externalizing behavior problems is that positive peer relations are not merely incidental to the development of problem behavior but are mediators of this process. Testing the importance of friendship and hypotheses about different dimensions of friendship through intervention is a critical direction for future research that has not yet been realized.

Change is not necessarily easy and it generally takes time. We see friendship intervention in that light. Researchers have published their work on peer relations and friendship interventions, and some teachers and counselors have done hands-on work with children "in the field." There has not, however, been a "movement" or a clear and universal commitment to help children who have friendship difficulties, whether it be making friends (or the right friends) or keeping friends. As we mention at the beginning of this chapter, the most common peer-oriented efforts in schools today are antibullying programs (e.g., Olweus & Limber, 2010). Many schools have committed significant resources to decrease the amount and degree of bullying in their classrooms and on their playgrounds, and for better and for worse, some school districts and states mandate these programs. With knowledge of the pernicious effects on both victims and perpetrators of bullying that came from years of basic research, attention turned to intervention and prevention. This commitment, however, did not take place over a short period of time—it was at least two decades in the making. Just like bullying, friendship problems can have devastating effects on children and adolescents. And just like prevention programs for bullying and aggressive behavior have gained prominence, we hope friendship interventions will, too.

We must begin a movement, a movement that includes researchers, clinicians, teachers, counselors, parents, mentors, and others who are significant in children's lives and that is designed to improve children's social and emotional health through friendship training and intervention. If we think about the fact that 39% of children live in families with low incomes (Fass, Briggs, & Cauthen, 2008), 21% of children live in families in poverty (Wight, Chan, & Aratani, 2011), 25% of children live with a single parent, and 12 out of every 1,000 children are maltreated (Federal Interagency Forum on Child and Family Statistics, 2008), then it should be common sense that many children need to *learn* how to have healthy and rewarding relationships, including and perhaps especially, friendships. We challenge those in the research arena and those in applied settings to make a commitment to addressing the needs of children who experience compromised friendship abilities. As Gary Ladd so eloquently asked at the 2009 biennial meetings of the Society for Research on Child Development, "Do we have research to give back?" He said that we are research rich but practically poor. He called for a "fourth r"—relationships; that is, in addition to reading, 'riting [writing], and 'rithmetic [arithmetic], we need to make efforts to teach children about relationships. We second his call for the fourth r as well as his call for more policy-oriented papers and training for teachers, school personnel, and anyone working closely with children on the importance of relationships with peers. In closing this chapter, we quote Ladd—"As resources diminish, our worth as a discipline is likely to be judged in terms of its utility." Using what we know about friendship to develop effective interventions for children having trouble in this domain; working closely with those who can actually implement those interventions effectively; and educating parents, teachers, school administrators, pediatricians, and policy makers about the significance of friendship and the value of helping children develop social competence would go a long way toward demonstrating this utility.

Chapter 9

The Significance
of Friendship

Wherever you are, it is your friends who make your world.
—WILLIAM JAMES

A friend may well be reckoned the masterpiece of nature.
—RALPH WALDO EMERSON

The better part of one's life consists of his friendships.
—ABRAHAM LINCOLN

James, Emerson, and Lincoln clearly suggest that friendship plays a unique and significant role in life. These pithy quotes echo most people's understanding of ideal friendships and the potential for friendships to contribute in valuable ways to a well-lived life. Nevertheless, most people also recognize that some are not so lucky in their friendships and that not all relationships fulfill these ideals.

In this last chapter, we discuss two issues. First, we present a conceptual framework for thinking about the developmental significance of friendship. This framework incorporates the multidimensional nature of these relationships and considers both positive and negative effects on children's adjustment. We propose that including both a nomothetic and an ideographic approach provides a more complete assessment of friendship's developmental significance. In describing this framework, the chapter summarizes the major conclusions that can be drawn about the importance of friendship in the lives of children and adolescents. Second,

305

the chapter ends with a discussion of 10 directions for future research on friendships and their developmental significance.

CONCEPTUAL FRAMEWORK

Figure 9.1 shows one framework for thinking about children's experience in friendships and the developmental significance of this relationship. This framework has seven key components. First, it recognizes what children bring with them to a friendship, including individual characteristics (such as temperament/personality and social behavior), experiences in other relationships (such as family relationships and other experiences), and demographic characteristics (such as sex and age). Not surprisingly, and as we discuss particularly in Chapters 5 and 6, these individual-level variables have a significant effect on friendship—children's likelihood of participating in a friendship at all and the quality of that relationship. We know much less about how individual characteristics influence the stability or developmental course of friendships, but we expect that they do.

To summarize some of what we know about the effects of the characteristics of the friends, we draw these conclusions. On attachment history: The quality of children's early attachment with their primary caregiver predicts their success in forming and maintaining friendships in early childhood, in part by the association of attachment and sociability and emotional and behavioral regulation skills, but also because of specific experiences and interactions within intimate family relationships. Secure attachment history is associated with having friends and having higher-quality friendships, and these associations continue well beyond early childhood. Finally, friendship quality and attachment to friends may moderate the association between parent–child attachment and psychosocial adjustment, but this research is too limited to make that claim too strongly.

On aggression and peer rejection: Although aggressive and rejected children are more likely to be friendless than nonaggressive/nonrejected youth, most still have a reciprocal friend. According to their own reports, aggressive and/or rejected children do not have consistently lower-quality friendships. Nevertheless, observations and reports of others note distinct differences and lower-quality friendships for aggressive/antisocial children and adolescents. Aggressive and rejected youth are also less likely to share their perspective on the quality of the relationship with their friend than are other youth. Deviancy training is a powerful process within the friendships of aggressive and antisocial youth and predicts a host of indicators of poor adjustment, including delinquency, drug use, and violence.

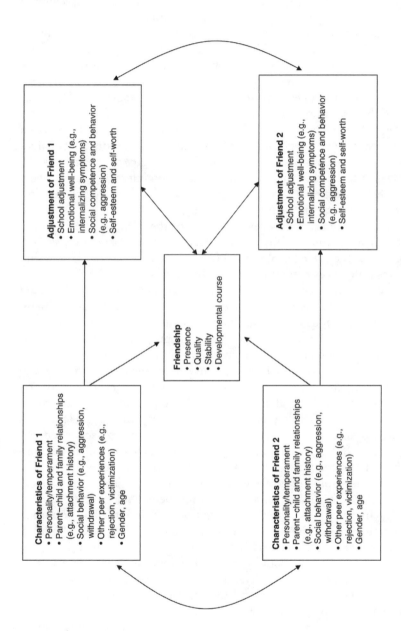

FIGURE 9.1. Conceptual framework for the developmental significance of friendship.

307

On peer victimization: Children who are victims of peer-directed aggression have lower-quality friends, yet friendship protects children against victimization. Having friends also buffers against the negative outcomes, such as loneliness and depression, associated with victimization. Unfortunately, then, children who may be most in need of high-quality, supportive friendships may be least likely to have them. Thus, many individual characteristics of children and adolescents have substantial effects on their likelihood of participating in friendships and on features of their relationships.

Second, we know from extensive research on similarity between friends that friends are often similar on many of these individual characteristics (see Chapters 3 and 4). Although some degree of similarity is due to socialization within the relationship, selection effects operate as well. Thus, the bidirectional arrow on the far left side of Figure 9.1 captures this similarity between friends.

Third, there are a number of aspects of the friendship relationship itself that have implications for its effects on adjustment. At the most basic level is the presence of mutual friendship. This aspect of friendship captures differences between children with and without friends. Here we see the normative significance of friendship, beginning in early childhood and continuing through adolescence and beyond. As we discuss in Chapters 3 and 4, friends differ from nonfriends in numerous ways—in the characteristic of their interactions and in the properties of their relationships. Although longitudinal evidence remains limited, having versus not having friends is associated with positive adjustment concurrently and into adolescence and early adulthood. The evidence generally supports hypothesized functions of friendship including promoting social skills and competencies, serving as sources of support, staving off loneliness and promoting adjustment during times of transition (e.g., school adjustment), and offering a foundation for the development of other relationships. At the same time, it is clear from the extensive research that the effects of friendship are rarely as large or as consistent as a simple model of friendship as necessary for adaptive adjustment would predict. A much more nuanced view is essential. In addition, research highlights normative developmental changes in friendship across childhood and adolescence. As Hartup and Stevens (1997) describe, the underlying structure of reciprocity within a relationship between two equals is fairly constant across developmental periods, yet interactions between friends, the most salient features of friendship, and the complexity of and manifestations of the relationship change with development.

As we discuss in Chapter 6, the quality of the friendship is another critical dimension to assess. Friendship quality is predicted by family relationships—the quality of parents' own relationships, parental behaviors, and parenting style. As discussed above, many individual characteristics of children relate to the quality of their friendships. There are mean-level gender differences in particular dimensions of friendship quality—girls typically report greater intimacy and closeness in their friendships—yet the effects of friendship quality seem to be more consistent than different for boys and girls. Friendship quality is concurrently associated with many dimensions of adjustment. High levels of positive friendship features are correlated with high self-worth and social competence and with low anxiety, loneliness, and depression. Critically, though, the expectation that high friendship quality promotes increased self-esteem over time has not been supported empirically. Finally, the stability and developmental course of the relationship have received far less attention but may have important implications for how relationships influence the participants.

Fourth, the separate arrows in Figure 9.1 leading from the friendship experience to the adjustment of the individual friends recognizes that the same relationship may not have the same effects on each friend. These arrows are bidirectional to capture the fact that the friendship itself is not static but changes as a function of the individual friends—their own development and adjustment and their interactions with one another.

Despite the recognition that a friendship may influence the two participants in unique ways, the fifth point is that in the same way the characteristics of the friends are similar, the adjustment outcomes associated with friendship are likely to be similar (represented by the arrow between adjustment of Friend 1 and adjustment of Friend 2 in Figure 9.1). As is clear from previous chapters, a number of adjustment domains have been shown to be related to the friendship experience—school adjustment, emotional well-being (including loneliness and internalizing symptoms such as depression), social competence and behavior (including aggression and delinquency), and self-worth and self-esteem.

Sixth, arrows directly from characteristics of the individual children to their adjustment outcomes in Figure 9.1 reflect the recognition that although friendship has important implications for children's adaptation, we should not overstate its importance.

Seventh, it must be acknowledged that the influences and effects depicted in this framework occur in a larger context. Many of these contextual factors have been considered in earlier chapters. They include the cultural context and the domains and physical context in which the friends interact, such as at school or in their neighborhood. In addition, friendships exist in a dynamic developmental context. The individuals change and develop over time as does the relationship itself. This recognition of context is consistent with Bronfenbrenner's (1979) ecological theory.

Conceptualizing friendship as depicted in Figure 9.1 accomplishes several important goals. It allows for both a nomothetic and an idiographic perspective on friendships. For example, most children have a mutual friend and thus the normative significance of this relationship is captured in part by the presence of friendship. In addition, the normative significance of friendship is realized to the extent that these relationships accomplish the functions of offering opportunities for learning social skills and competencies, serving as emotional and cognitive resources, and providing templates for future relationships (Hartup, 1992b, 1996a). Nevertheless, an equally important way of thinking about the developmental significance is to consider individual differences in the experience of friendship and in the outcomes associated with that experience. This idiographic approach is captured in the proposed framework by considering (1) the characteristics that children bring to the relationship and the effect of those characteristics on the friendship and on the friend; and (2) variations in friendship, such as the variations in friendship quality that have been studied extensively, and the effects of those variations on the children's adjustment.

Inherent in this view is the recognition that there may be tradeoffs in children's experience of friendship. Take, for example, a highly aggressive child. As we discuss in Chapter 5, this child may establish a high-quality relationship full of companionship, positive affect, and closeness, yet through deviancy training that same relationship may provide a training ground and reinforcement for increased delinquent and antisocial behavior. Does the aggressive child receive the positive benefits of a high-quality, satisfying friendship we might expect and at the same time find reinforcement for deviant behavior? If so, how do we conceptualize this tradeoff, and what does it mean for the developmental significance of the relationship? Rose and Rudolph (2006) describe tradeoffs in developmental outcomes from peer relationship processes that are associated with sex differences. For example, peer relationship processes such as corumination may affect girls and boys differently and thus predict adjustment in different ways. Corumination involves excessive discussion of problems and focusing on negative affect with another, especially a friend (Rose, 2002). For girls, but not boys, corumination is associated both with greater closeness in friendships and with higher levels of depression and anxiety symptoms (Rose, 2002; Rose & Rudolph, 2006). We propose that an idiographic approach to the developmental significance of friendship lends itself to identifying these kinds of tradeoffs— situations or relationships in which certain processes or features (mutuality, closeness, self-disclosure, etc.) are not monolithic in their effect on adjustment and well-being but contribute to both positive outcomes (e.g., companionship, lower feelings of loneliness) and negative outcomes (e.g., increased delinquency). These kinds of questions have not yet been answered adequately. Finally, the proposed framework embraces a multidimensional perspective on friendship including having a friend, the quality of the relationship, and the characteristics of friends (e.g., Hartup & Stevens, 1997).

FUTURE RESEARCH DIRECTIONS

As the preceding chapters demonstrate, there is a considerable amount of research on friendships in childhood and adolescence—according to a PsycInfo search, literally thousands of studies. As a result, we know a lot about the time children spend with their friends, the characteristics of their interactions, their expectations for the relationship, how friendships fit with other experiences in the peer group, how friendships differ from one another, and ways in which friendship is associated with adjustment and well-being. At the same time, there is no shortage of questions about friendships in childhood and adolescence, and we are part of an exciting field of research where new findings yield additional questions. Though there are probably countless directions for future research, we suggest 10 that seem particularly likely to contribute in valuable ways to our understanding of the significance of friendship.

1. One of the important developments in the last 10 years has been the more widespread use of statistical models and procedures that enable researchers to model and evaluate bidirectional patterns of influence, particularly in longitudinal and dyadic data. These statistical models allow data analyses to more closely mirror theoretical understandings of transactional and reciprocal influences in friendships and peer relations in general. One very promising approach for research questions about friendship is the actor–partner interdependence model (APIM) developed by Kenny and colleagues (Kashy & Kenny, 2000; Kenny, 1996; Kenny, Kashy, & Cook, 2006; Kenny, Mohr, & Levesque, 2001; see also Laursen, 2005). The APIM recognizes that dyadic relationships, such as friendships, are inherently interdependent. In other words, friends affect one another. Statistical models that assume nonindependence may thus not be appropriate for data from friends, and the APIM provides the statistical techniques for measuring this interdependence.

The APIM allows for estimations of actor effects and partner effects in friendship dyads. Actor effects indicate associations between a child's own score on an independent variable and his or her own score on a dependent variable. Partner effects indicate associations between a child's own score on an independent variable and his or her friend's score on the dependent variable. These effects take into account the association between friends' scores on the independent variable, and the APIM also allows for estimation of actor–partner interaction effects. As an example, the APIM can be used to examine actor and partner effects of individual behaviors, such as aggression, on friendship quality (see Cillessen, Jiang, West, & Laszkowski, 2005, for an example). The actor effect would describe the association between a child's aggression and his or her perception of the quality of the friendship. The partner effect would describe the association between a child's aggression and his or her friend's perception of the friendship quality. Two actor and two partner effects are modeled. For two friends, Noah and Will, we would estimate the effect of Noah's behavior on Noah's rating of the quality of their friendship and the effect of Will's behavior on Will's rating of the quality of their friendship (actor effects) as well as the effect of Noah's behavior on Will's rating of friendship quality and the effect of Will's behavior on Noah's rating of friendship quality (partner effects).

Additional use of statistical techniques such as structural equation modeling, hierarchical linear modeling, and survival curve analyses and specific models such as the APIM hold considerable promise for friendship researchers. In particular, they allow our statistical analyses to catch up with the rich and complicated data, full of correlations and nested effects, that necessarily arise when we test theories of development involving reciprocal influences and interdependencies.

2. Questions about the importance of friendship quality as a key determinant of individual differences in friendships and thus in outcomes associated with participating in a particular relationship have been investigated most extensively in the last 15 years. As we describe in Chapter 2 and also Chapter 6, there are a number of methodological questions and inconsistencies that make it difficult to compare findings across studies. Additional research is needed on two questions in particular. First, although assessments of positive friendship features and negative friendship features are correlated, the correlations are often relatively low, suggesting that these two dimensions should be considered separately. One problem, however, is that we have not identified what the most important positive and negative features are, and this is particularly true for negative features. Most studies assess conflict, but few studies include negative features other than conflict. Additional research focused on identifying other friendship features that contribute to low friendship quality is essential. Some possibilities include rivalry and competition, social aggression and exclusiveness, and imbalance and/or dominance.

Second, with statistical models such as the APIM described above, we are in a better position to evaluate the significance of concordance between friends on perceptions of the features and quality of their inter-actions. Further research on the implications of agreeing or disagreeing with a friend about the relationship might help explain the lack of con-sistent longitudinal predictions between friendship quality and outcome measures. In addition, there is some evidence that discordance in percep-tions about the relationship is an indicator of problems—either ways in which individuals have difficulty with friendships or ways in which the relationship may be a weak one. Further investigation of these possibili-ties is warranted.

3. We know a lot about friendship among elementary, middle, and high school students in the United States and some about friendships among students in Canada and western Europe. Beyond that, we have a hand-ful of studies from other countries—Indonesia (e.g., French et al., 2003; French, Pidada, & Victor, 2005), China (e.g., Chen et al., 1992, 2004), and Latin American countries (Costa Rica [DeRosier & Kupersmidt, 1991] and Cuba [González et al., 2004]), for example. Recent friendship research focuses extensively on context, both the context that friendship provides for development and the ways in which friendships are situ-ated within broader contexts. Cultural context, including norms and val-ues within particular cultures, clearly has an impact on children's social competence and the development and significance of peer relationships. Additional studies of friendship experiences and processes of children and adolescents in a variety of cultural contexts (especially if "culture" is not defined merely by national boundaries) will tell us much about the impact of culture and about culturally specific and universal processes and outcomes associated with friendship. In addition, such research will contribute to a greater understanding of the ways in which children's peer and friendship relations transmit culture (Corsaro, 2003).

4. There are two ways to think about intervention associated with friendship. First, are there systematic and effective ways to improve chil-dren's friendships? As we discuss in detail in Chapter 8, a number of dif-ferent approaches to intervention have been tried, with varying levels of success. Overall, however, interventions to help children having difficulty with friendships should not be identical to those designed to improve children's acceptance by peers or reduce peer rejection. One significant problem with interventions to reduce peer rejection is that rejection is a reputation-based construct. As a result, social skills-based or other pro-grams that aim to change a child's behavior might be very effective in altering undesirable behaviors and improving social skills, but rejection is resistant to change. Even when children return to the classroom con-text with improvements in their behavior and other skills, peers may not recognize these changes and are likely to continue to reject the child.

Preliminary evidence suggests that changing the classroom context rather than, or in addition to, changing individual child competencies has the potential to decrease peer rejection. For friendship, however, improving a child's experiences with a friend does not require changing the views of all classmates or the context of the classroom. Rather, children need to find that one other with whom to establish and maintain a friendship. Rather than adopting intervention programs aimed at improving peer relations more generally, we now know much about friendship specifically that would allow for the development of programs specifically geared to children who are having difficulty establishing and maintaining a high-quality friendship.

A second way of thinking about friendship and intervention is to examine ways in which friendship may serve as an intervention for other challenges children and adolescents face. For example, there is preliminary evidence to suggest that focusing on friendship (teaching parents how to help their children form good friendships and using friendship "buddy" pairs as a form of intervention) is helpful for children with ADHD (Hoza et al., 2003; Mikami, Lerner, et al., 2010). Research showing that friendship serves as a buffer or moderates the association between some risk factor and negative outcomes offers suggestions for other ways to consider friendship itself as an intervention—for example, for children who experience victimization by peers or for children who have less than ideal family relationships. This idea fits directly with Sullivan's (1953) proposals about the therapeutic possibilities of friendship and has been considered in only limited ways thus far.

5. Many of the early studies of friendship compared pairs of children who are friends and pairs of children who are not friends (e.g., acquaintances, strangers, and even disliked peers), and often these studies relied on observations, typically in lab settings but also in natural settings. In more recent years, however, the focus has shifted to larger-scale questionnaire-based studies in which hundreds of children (and sometimes their teachers or parents) complete various measures assessing their friendships and individual behavior and adjustment. The contributions of these "large n" studies are substantial. At the same time, we should not forget the value of often smaller-scale observational assessments. These studies offer the possibility for identifying friendship processes and thus complement questionnaire-based studies focused on predictors and outcomes. For example, we know a good bit about the strength and direction of associations between friendship quality and adjustment, but we are left only with theory and speculation about what processes undergird these associations. Observational studies can be particularly beneficial here. Regardless of what methods we use, a focus on understanding friendship

processes is essential. For example, what happens in friends' interactions that is responsible for links between friendship and well-being?

6. In several writings in the mid- to late 1990s, Hartup (1996a; Hartup & Stevens, 1997) was instrumental in focusing our attention on the multidimensional nature of friendships and particularly the distinctions between having friends, friendship quality, and the identity or characteristics of a child's friends. Researchers have responded to Hartup's call to examine more specifically these various aspects of friendship. Conceptually, examining multiple dimensions of friendship as well as other peer relations simultaneously (social status, peer victimization, social networks) is important for identifying the unique effects of particular aspects of friendship on adjustment and well-being. Statistical procedures, such as structural equation modeling, allow for the examination of complex models that identify links between various aspects of peer relations and can compare competing models.

To date, this goal has been accomplished by examining various ways that friendship and peer acceptance are associated with particular outcomes. For example, Bukowski, Hoza, and Boivin (1993) considered links between friendship quality, having friends, popularity, and belongingness and loneliness. Specifically, they examined whether popularity and friendship are directly and uniquely associated with adjustment, whether popularity and friendship are associated with different indicators of adjustment, or whether friendship mediates the association between popularity and adjustment. Bukowski and colleagues identified both direct and indirect associations between peer relations and adjustment. Thus, specifying pathways and trajectories through which various dimensions of peer relations and friendship exert their effects is an important direction for future research. An improved understanding of these pathways in normal development also has the potential to inform our understanding and identification of maladaptive pathways and offer suggestions for intervention.

7. What factors moderate the experience of and outcomes associated with friendship? The two factors that have been addressed most thoroughly as determinants of differences in friendship experiences are gender and age. We know most about these two factors as main effects. In other words, we know about mean-level differences in friendship for boys versus girls and for older versus younger children. We know less about how variables such as gender and age moderate the association between other variables—individual characteristics, for example—and participation in friendship or friendship quality or any other friendship variable. In addition, we need more systematic study of the ways in which the significance of friendship or the outcomes associated with

friendship may differ according to variables such as gender, age, ethnicity, and culture.

The role of friendship as a moderator between other aspects of development and outcomes has been considered surprisingly infrequently, especially given the importance Sullivan (1953), Hartup (1996a), and other theorists placed on the role of friends as emotional and cognitive resources. As we discuss in previous chapters, there is strong evidence that friendship serves as a buffer against the negative effects of peer victimization (e.g., Hodges et al., 1999; Schmidt & Bagwell, 2007). In what other ways might friendship be an important protective factor? Alternatively, how might friendship serve as a risk factor and perhaps contribute in problematic ways to developmental outcomes? The idea of friendship as a risk and a protective factor, moderating the association between other factors and developmental outcomes, fits within the framework of developmental psychopathology. In particular, friendships are important for studying normal development and for studying the development of psychopathology and maladjustment—the central tenet of the developmental psychopathology approach (see Bukowski & Adams, 2005; Masten, 2005). Thus, although this integrative approach has clearly influenced the way we think about friendships in recent years, we have only scratched the surface of understanding the potentially complex ways in which friendship moderates links between other experiences and outcomes. It is likely that friendship both attenuates or protects against other negative experiences, such as in protecting against depression associated with peer victimization or externalizing problems associated with family adversity, and amplifies internalizing (such as through corumination) and externalizing (such as through deviancy training) symptoms.

8. Although it is intuitively obvious that friendships develop over time as youth progress from "hitting it off" and acquaintances to close and even best friends, we know very little about the developmental course of friendships and even less about the dissolution or end of friendships. This is in contrast to research on adult friendships where there is considerable focus on the stages of the relationship and factors that influence the development of friendships over time (e.g., Fehr, 1996; Levinger, 1983). Understanding the temporal aspect of friendships in childhood and adolescence, including the processes involved in making, maintaining, and losing friendships (but see Chapters 3 and 4) would go a long way in underscoring the dynamic nature of friendship and might help in intervention planning if we can then identify children who are having difficulty with the different stages of friendship—moving from acquaintanceship to friendship versus maintaining established relationships, for example.

Closely related to the idea of learning more about the temporal nature of friendship is understanding the importance of friendship stability. Some longitudinal studies examine the stability of the relationship as a predictor of various outcomes with the idea that stable friends are likely to have greater influence than unstable friends. The findings, though, about the importance of stability and what predicts friendship stability are not consistent. For example, Berndt and colleagues (1986) found that reports of lower intimacy and lower frequency of interaction in the fall identified friendships that would not remain close over the course of the school year. In contrast, Bowker (2004) found that positive and negative friendship features did not predict the stability of the relationship from fall to spring. There is some evidence that similarity predicts the stability of friendships and that stable (but not unstable) friends become more similar over the course of the school year (Newcomb et al., 1999). In addition, adolescents who failed to maintain satisfying and high-quality relationships over the course of the school year experienced lower self-competence in some areas over time (Keefe & Berndt, 1996). Overall, then, there is much to learn about the development of friendships over time and whether the stability of particular friendships helps to account for their developmental significance.

9. With the popularity of new technologies, including e-mail, instant messaging, text messaging, and online social network applications (e.g., Facebook), children, and especially adolescents, conduct many of their peer interactions online and without face-to-face contact. Online communication with existing friends is quite common, and youth who communicate frequently with their friends online feel closer to them (Valkenburg & Peter, 2007). For many children and adolescents, the Internet is simply a new medium for engaging in the same level of socially competent interactions as offline (Mikami, Szwedo, Allen, Evans, & Hare, 2010). For example, measures of positive and negative interactions with friends at ages 13 and 14 predicted the number of friends on their social network website (e.g., Facebook, MySpace) in young adulthood, and those with more positive interactions in adolescence had more connections with friends on their webpage in young adulthood. For other children and adolescents, online communication may provide an opportunity to strengthen existing relationships by engaging in self-disclosure in ways that are more comfortable to them than face-to-face interactions. This social compensation hypothesis suggests that socially anxious youth may turn to online communication to help them overcome the inhibition they experience in interactions with friends in real life, and socially anxious youth do perceive the Internet as particularly valuable for self-disclosure with friends (Valkenburg & Peter, 2007). Similarly, for adolescents with

low friendship quality, but not high friendship quality, using the Internet for social communication was associated with less depression over time, supporting the social compensation hypothesis (Selfhout, Branje, Delsing, ter Bogt, & Meeus, 2009). Although most youth use the Internet to participate in, strengthen, and maintain their existing friends and social network (Gross, 2004), some also form new relationships with others they have never met in person (Wolak, Mitchell, & Finkelhor, 2003).

Research has not yet caught up with these trends in children's peer relations, yet given the amount of time children spend in their online worlds and the extent to which peer interactions dominate these interactions, we would be remiss if we did not take them seriously. Basic questions such as how much time children spend online with friends, how those interactions complement or work against face-to-face interactions, how the features, norms, and quality of online interactions compare to typical physical interactions, and the impact of these kinds of interactions on the relationship and on individual friends are important places to start.

10. Finally, given the recognition that the importance of friendship needs to be addressed from both a nomothetic and idiographic perspective, future research that integrates these perspectives is warranted. This integration would involve, for example, considering processes within friendships that contribute to desired outcomes for most children and adolescents, and at the same time, examining how those processes may be particularly beneficial or, alternatively, problematic for some children or in some relationships. This approach accomplishes three goals. First, it recognizes that the context in which friendships occur may help to determine their developmental significance. A single friendship may have different significance for a child who is victimized by peers and has difficulty making friends than for a child who has very positive peer relationships and easily establishes relationships. A close friendship with a peer in the neighborhood may have different implications for a child who spends lots of unsupervised time with this peer and gets into trouble than for a child whose parents know the other child well and monitor the pair's activities closely and appropriately. Second, this perspective assumes that friendships do not have exclusively positive developmental implications and that there are potential tradeoffs that make it difficult to define a particular relationship as either positive or negative. Third, simultaneously embracing a nomothetic and idiographic perspective fits with a focus on the two individuals within a friendship as well as the relationship itself. In other words, the context a friendship provides for development depends on the individual characteristics both children bring to the relationship and on features and characteristics of the relationship itself that are not

simply a function of the characteristics of any individual child. In the simplest terms, the individual friends affect the relationship, but the relationship influences the children as well, and all of this occurs in a dynamic way over time as the children develop and the relationship develops.

In sum, friendships are developmentally significant. They provide rich contexts for social, emotional, and cognitive development; they are considerable sources of support; and they have important implications for socioemotional adjustment and well-being. Most children and adolescents interact with friends every day, many times each day—in person, on the phone, through e-mails, text messages, and other Internet communications. Friends and relationships with friends are highly valued by children and adolescents (and, in fact, across the lifespan). These are reason enough to continue to study friendships with the hope of understanding even more completely the nature, the nuances, and the effects of this powerful relationship in children's lives.

References

Aboud, F. E., Mendelson, M. J., & Purdy, K. T. (2003). Cross-race peer relations and friendship quality. *International Journal of Behavioral Development, 27*(2), 165–173.

Abraham, L. (2002). Bhai-behen, true love, time pass: Friendships and sexual partnerships among youth in an Indian metropolis. *Culture, Health and Sexuality, 4,* 337–353.

Adams, R. E., Bukowski, W. M., & Bagwell, C. L. (2005). Stability of aggression during early adolescence as moderated by reciprocated friendship status and friend's aggression. *International Journal of Behavioral Development, 29,* 139–145.

Adler, P. A., & Adler, P. (1995). Dynamics of inclusion and exclusion in preadolescent cliques. *Social Psychology Quarterly, 58,* 145–162.

Adler, P. A., & Adler, P. (1998). *Peer power: Preadolescent culture and identity.* New Brunswick, NJ: Rutgers University Press.

Aguilar, J. L. (1984). Trust and exchange: Expressive and instrumental dimensions of reciprocity in a peasant community. *Ethos, 12,* 3–29.

Aikins, J. W., Bierman, K. L., & Parker, J. G. (2005). Navigating the transition to junior high school: The influence of pre-transition friendship and self-system characteristics. *Social Development, 14,* 42–60.

Akiyama, H. (2001). The influence of schooling and relocation on the G/UI pupil companionship. *African Study Monographs, 26,* 197–208.

Alberts, C., Mbalo, N. F., & Ackermann, C. J. (2003). Adolescents' perceptions of the relevance of domains of identity formation: A South African cross-cultural study. *Journal of Youth and Adolescence, 32,* 169–184.

Allan, G. (1989). *Friendship: Developing a sociological perspective.* San Francisco: Westview Press.

Allen, J. P., & Land, D. (1999). Attachment in adolescence. In J. Cassidy & P. R. Shaver (Eds.), *Handbook of attachment: Theory, research, and clinical applications* (pp. 319–335). New York: Guilford Press.

Allen, J. P., Porter, M., McFarland, C., McElhaney, K. B., & Marsh, P. (2007). The relation of attachment security to adolescents' paternal and peer relationships, depression, and externalizing behavior. *Child Development, 78,* 1222–1239.

Argyle, M., Henderson, M., Bond, M., Iizuka, Y., & Contarello, A. (1986). Cross-cultural variations in relationship rules. *International Journal of Psychology, 21,* 287–315.

Arnett, J. J. (2000). Emerging adulthood: A theory of development from the late teens through the twenties. *American Psychologist, 55,* 469–480.

Arnett, J. J. (2007). Socialization in emerging adulthood: From the family to the wider world, from socialization to self-socialization. In J. E. Grusec & P. D. Hastings (Eds.), *Handbook of socialization: Theory and research* (pp. 208–230). New York: Guilford Press.

Asher, S. R., & Coie, J. D. (1990). *Peer rejection in childhood.* New York: Cambridge University Press.

Asher, S. R., & McDonald, K. L. (2004). Intervening to promote friendship: Experimental tests of hypotheses about fundamental skills and processes [Commentary]. *International Society for the Study of Behavioural Development Newsletter* (Serial No. 46).

Asher, S. R., & Paquette, J. A. (2003). Loneliness and peer relations in childhood. *Current Directions in Psychological Science, 12,* 75–78.

Asher, S. R., Parker, J. G., & Walker, D. L. (1996). Distinguishing friendship from acceptance: Implications for intervention and assessment. In W. M. Bukowski, A. F. Newcomb, & W. W. Hartup (Eds.), *The company they keep: Friendship in childhood and adolescence* (pp. 366–405). New York: Cambridge University Press.

Asher, S. R., & Rose, A. J. (1997). Promoting children's social-emotional adjustment with peers. In P. Salovey & D. J. Sluyter (Eds.), *Emotional development and emotional intelligence: Educational implications* (pp. 196–230). New York: Basic Books.

Asher, S. R., Zellis, K. M., Parker, J. G., & Bruene, C. M. (1991, April). *Self-referral for peer relations problems among aggressive and withdrawn low-accepted children.* Paper presented at the biennial meeting of the Society for Research in Child Development, Seattle, WA.

Aydt, H., & Corsaro, W. A. (2003). Differences in children's construction of gender across culture. *American Behavioral Scientist, 46,* 1306–1325.

Azmitia, M., Ittel, A., & Radmacher, K. A. (2005). Narratives of friendship and self in adolescence. In N. Way & J. V. Hamm (Eds.), *The experience of close friendships in adolescence. New Directions for Child and Adolescent Development, 107,* 23–39.

Azmitia, M., & Montgomery, R. (1993). Friendship, transactive dialogues, and the development of scientific reasoning. *Social Development, 2,* 202–221.

Azmitia, M., & Perlmutter, M. (1989). Social influences on children's cognition:

State of the art and future directions. *Advances in Child Development and Behavior, 22,* 89–144.

Bagwell, C. L., Bender, S. E., Andreassi, C. L., Kinoshita, T. L., Montarello, S. A., & Muller, J. G. (2005). Friendship quality and perceived relationship changes predict psychosocial adjustment in early adulthood. *Journal of Social and Personal Relationships, 22,* 235–254.

Bagwell, C. L., & Coie, J. D. (1999, April). Social influence in the friendship relations of aggressive boys. In J. D. Coie (Chair), *A closer look at deviant peer influences on delinquent activity.* Paper symposium presented at the biennial meeting of the Society for Research in Child Development, Albuquerque, NM.

Bagwell, C. L., & Coie, J. D. (2004). The best friendships of aggressive boys: Relationship quality, conflict management, and rule-breaking behavior. *Journal of Experimental Child Psychology, 88,* 5–24.

Bagwell, C. L., Coie, J. D., Terry, R. A., & Lochman, J. E. (2000). Peer clique participation and social status in preadolescence. *Merrill-Palmer Quarterly, 46,* 280–305.

Bagwell, C. L., Newcomb, A. F., & Bukowski, W. M. (1998). Preadolescent friendship and peer rejection as predictors of adult adjustment. *Child Development, 69,* 140–153.

Bagwell, C. L., Schmidt, M. E., Newcomb, A. F., & Bukowski, W. M. (2001). Friendship and peer rejection as predictors of adult adjustment. In D. W. Nangle & C. A. Erdley (Eds.), *The role of friendship in psychological adjustment* (pp. 25–49). San Francisco: Jossey-Bass.

Baldwin, M. W. (1995). Relational schemas and cognition in close relationships. *Journal of Social and Personal Relationships, 12,* 547–552.

Banton, M. (1966). *The social anthropology of complex societies.* London: Tavistock.

Barber, B. L., Stone, M. R., Hunt, J. E., & Eccles, J. S. (2005). Benefits of activity participation: The roles of identity affirmation and peer group norm sharing. In J. L. Mahoney, R. W. Larson, & J. S. Eccles (Eds.), *Organized activities as contexts of development: Extracurricular activities, after-school and community programs* (pp. 185–210). Mahwah, NJ: Erlbaum.

Barratt, W., & Randall, L. (2004). Investigating the circle of friends approach: Adaptations and implications for practice. *Educational Psychology in Practice, 20,* 354–368.

Baumeister, R. F., Bratslavsky, E., Finkenauer, C., & Vohs, K. D. (2001). Bad is stronger than good. *Review of General Psychology, 5,* 323–370.

Baumeister, R. F., Smart, L., & Boden, J. M. (1996). Relation of threatened egotism to violence and aggression: The dark side of high self-esteem. *Psychological Review, 103,* 5–33.

Bauminger, N., Finzi-Dottan, R., Chason, S., & Har-Even, D. (2008). Intimacy in adolescent friendship: The roles of attachment, coherence, and self-disclosure. *Journal of Social and Personal Relationships, 25,* 409–428.

Beelmann, A., Pfingsten, U., & Losel, F. (1994). Effects of training social competence in children: A meta-analysis of recent evaluation studies. *Journal of Clinical Child Psychology, 23,* 260–271.

Bell, S., & Coleman, S. (Eds.). (1999). *The anthropology of friendship*. New York: Berg.

Belsky, J., & Cassidy, J. (1994). Attachment and close relationships: An individual-difference perspective. *Psychological Inquiry, 5,* 27–30.

Benenson, J. F., & Christakos, A. (2003). The greater fragility of females' versus males' closest same-sex friendships. *Child Development, 74,* 1123–1129.

Bengtson, V. L., Biblarz, T. J., & Roberts, R. E. L. (2002). *How families still matter: A longitudinal study of youth in two generations*. New York: Cambridge University Press.

Benjamin, W. J., Schneider, B. H., Greenman, P. S., & Hum, M. (2001). Conflict and childhood friendship in Taiwan and Canada. *Canadian Journal of Behavioural Science, 33,* 203–211.

Benner, A., & Graham, S. (2007). Navigating the transition to multi-ethnic urban high schools: Changing racial/ethnic congruence and adolescents' school-related affect. *Journal of Research on Adolescence, 17,* 207–220.

Bennett, D. S., Bendersky, M., & Lewis, M. (2002). Facial expressivity at 4 months: A context by expression analysis. *Infancy, 3,* 97–113.

Bennett, D. S., Bendersky, M., & Lewis, M. (2004). On specifying specificity: Facial expressions at 4 months. *Infancy, 6,* 425–429.

Berkowitz, M. W., & Gibbs, J. C. (1983). Measuring the developmental features of moral discussion. *Merrill-Palmer Quarterly, 29,* 399–410.

Berkowitz, M. W., & Gibbs, J. C. (1985). The process of moral conflict resolution and moral development. *New Directions for Child Development, 29,* 71–84.

Berler, E. S., Gross, A. M., & Drabman, R. S. (1982). Social skills training with children: Proceed with caution. *Journal of Applied Behavior Analysis, 15,* 41–53.

Berlin, L. J., & Cassidy, J. (2003). Mothers' self-reported control of their preschool children's emotional expressiveness: A longitudinal study of associations with infant–mother attachment and children's emotion regulation. *Social Development, 12,* 477–495.

Berndt, T. J. (1981a). Age changes and changes over time in prosocial intentions and behavior between friends. *Developmental Psychology, 17,* 408–416.

Berndt, T. J. (1981b). Effects of friendship on prosocial intentions and behavior. *Child Development, 52,* 636–643.

Berndt, T. J. (1982). The features and effects of friendship in early adolescence. *Child Development, 53,* 1447–1460.

Berndt, T. J. (1986). Children's comments about their friendships. In M. Perlmutter (Ed.), *Cognitive perspectives on children's social and behavioral development. The Minnesota Symposia on Child Psychology* (Vol. 18, pp. 189–211). Hillsdale, NJ: Erlbaum.

Berndt, T. J. (1989). Obtaining support from friends during childhood and adolescence. In D. Belle (Ed.), *Children's social networks and social supports* (pp. 308–331). New York: Wiley.

Berndt, T. J. (1996). Exploring the effects of friendship quality on social development. In W. M. Bukowski, A. F. Newcomb, & W. W. Hartup (Eds.), *The company they keep: Friendship in childhood and adolescence* (pp. 346–365). New York: Cambridge University Press.

Berndt, T. J. (1999). Friends' influence on students' adjustment to school. *Educational Psychologist, 34,* 15–28.

Berndt, T. J. (2002). Friendship quality and social development. *Current Directions in Psychological Science, 11,* 7–10.

Berndt, T. J. (2004). Children's friendships: Shifts over a half-century in perspectives on their development and their effects. *Merrill-Palmer Quarterly, 50,* 206–223.

Berndt, T. J., & Das, R. (1987). Effects of popularity and friendship on perceptions of the personality and social behavior of peers. *Journal of Early Adolescence, 7,* 429–439.

Berndt, T. J., & Hanna, N. A. (1995). Intimacy and self-disclosure in friendships. In K. J. Rotenberg (Ed.), *Disclosure processes in children and adolescents* (pp. 57–77). New York: Cambridge University Press.

Berndt, T. J., Hawkins, J. A., & Hoyle, S. G. (1986). Changes in friendship during a school year: Effects on children's and adolescents' impressions of friendship and sharing with friends. *Child Development, 57,* 1284–1297.

Berndt, T. J., Hawkins, J. A., & Jiao, Z. (1999). Influences of friends and friendships on adjustment to junior high school. *Merrill-Palmer Quarterly, 45,* 13–41.

Berndt, T. J., & Hoyle, S. G. (1985). Stability and change in childhood and adolescent friendships. *Developmental Psychology, 21,* 1007–1015.

Berndt, T. J., & Keefe, K. A. (1995). Friends' influence on adolescents' adjustment to school. *Child Development, 66,* 1312–1329.

Berndt, T. J., & Murphy, L. M. (2002). Influences of friends and friendships: Myths, truths, and research recommendations. In R. V. Kail (Ed.), *Advances in child development and behavior* (Vol. 30, pp. 275–310). New York: Academic Press.

Berndt, T. J., & Perry, T. B. (1986). Children's perceptions of friendships as supportive relationships. *Developmental Psychology, 22,* 640–648.

Berndt, T. J., & Perry, T. B. (1990). Distinctive features and effects of early adolescent friendships. In R. Montemayor, G. R. Adams, & T. P. Gullotta (Eds.), *From childhood to adolescence: A transitional period?* (pp. 269–287). Thousand Oaks, CA: Sage.

Berndt, T. J., Perry, T., & Miller, K. E. (1988). Friends' and classmates' interactions on academic tasks. *Journal of Educational Psychology, 80,* 506–513.

Berndt, T. J., & Savin-Williams, R. C. (1993). Peer relations and friendships. In P. H. Tolan & B. J. Cohler (Eds.), *Handbook of clinical research and practice with adolescents* (pp. 203–219). Oxford, UK: Wiley.

Berscheid, E., Snyder, M., & Omoto, A. M. (1989). Issues in studying close relationships: Conceptualizing and measuring closeness. In C. Hendrick (Ed.), *Close relationships* (pp. 63–91). Newbury Park, CA: Sage.

Bersheid, E., & Walster, E. (1969). *Interpersonal attraction.* Reading, MA: Addison-Wesley.

Bierman, K. L. (1986). Process of change during social skills training with preadolescents and its relation to treatment outcome. *Child Development, 57,* 230–240.

Bierman, K. L. (1989). Improving the peer relationships of peer rejected children. In B. Lahey & A. Kazdin (Eds.), *Advances in clinical child psychology* (Vol. 12, pp. 53–84). New York: Plenum Press.

Bierman, K. L. (2004). *Peer rejection: Developmental processes and intervention strategies.* New York: Guilford Press.

Bierman, K. L., & Furman, W. (1984). The effects of social skills training and peer involvement on the social adjustment of preadolescents. *Child Development, 55,* 151–162.

Bierman, K. L., Greenberg, M. T., & Conduct Problems Prevention Research Group. (1996). Social skills training in the fast track program. In R. D. Peters & R. J. McMahon (Eds.), *Preventing childhood disorders, substance abuse, and delinquency* (pp. 65–89). Thousand Oaks, CA: Sage.

Bierman, K. L., Miller, C. L., & Stabb, S. D. (1987). Improving the social behavior and peer acceptance of rejected boys: Effects of social skills training with instructions and prohibitions. *Journal of Consulting and Clinical Psychology, 55,* 194–200.

Bigelow, B. J. (1977). Children's friendship expectations: A cognitive-developmental study. *Child Development, 48,* 246–253.

Bigelow, B. J., & La Gaipa, J. (1975). Children's written descriptions of friendship: A multidimensional analysis. *Developmental Psychology, 11,* 857–858.

Bigelow, B. J., & La Gaipa, J. (1980). The development of friendship values and choice. In H. C. Foote, A. J. Chapman, & J. Smith (Eds.), *Friendship and social relations in children* (pp. 15–44). New York: Wiley.

Billy, J. O. G., Rodgers, J. L., & Udry, J. R. (1984). Adolescent sexual behavior and friendship choice. *Social Forces, 62,* 653–678.

Billy, J. O. G., & Udry, J. R. (1985). Patterns of adolescent friendship and effects on sexual behavior. *Social Psychology Quarterly, 48,* 27–41.

Bluebond-Langner, M., & Korbin, J. E. (2007). Challenges and opportunities in the anthropology of childhoods: An introduction to "children, childhoods, and childhood studies." *American Anthropologist, 109,* 241–246.

Blyth, D. A., Hill, J. P., & Thiel, K. S. (1982). Early adolescents' significant others: Grade and gender differences in perceived relationships with familial and nonfamilial adults and young people. *Journal of Youth and Adolescence, 11,* 425–450.

Bohnert, A. M., Aikins, J. W., & Edidin, J. (2007). The role of organized activities in facilitating social adaptation across the transition to college. *Journal of Adolescent Research, 22,* 189–208.

Boivin, M., Hymel, S., & Bukowski, W. M. (1995). The roles of social withdrawal, peer rejection, and victimization by peers in predicting loneliness and depressed mood in childhood. *Development and Psychopathology, 7,* 765–785.

Boivin, M., Thomassin, L., & Alain, M. (1989). Peer rejection and self-perceptions among early elementary school children: Aggressive rejectees vs. withdrawn rejectees. In B. H. Schneider, G. Attili, J. Nadel, & R. P. Weissberg (Eds.), *Social competence in developmental perspective* (pp. 392–393). Boston: Kluwer.

Bokhorst, C. L., Sumter, S. R., & Westenberg, P. M. (2010). Social support from parents, friends, classmates, and teachers in children and adolescents aged 9 to 18 years: Who is perceived as most supportive. *Social Development, 19,* 417–426.

Bollmer, J. M., Milich, R., Harris, M. J., & Maras, M. A. (2005). A friend in need: The role of friendship quality as a protective factor in peer victimization and bullying. *Journal of Interpersonal Violence, 20,* 701–712.

Bond, M. H. (1988). Finding universal dimensions of individual variation in multicultural studies of values: The Rokeach and Chinese value surveys. *Journal of Personality and Social Psychology, 55,* 1009–1015.

Booth, C. L., Rubin, K. H., & Rose-Krasnor, L. (1998). Perceptions of emotional support from mother and friend in middle childhood: Links with social-emotional adaptation and preschool attachment security. *Child Development, 69,* 427–442.

Booth-LaForce, C., Rubin, K. H., Rose-Krasnor, L., & Burgess, K. B. (2005). Attachment and friendship predictors of psychosocial functioning in middle childhood and the mediating roles of social support and self-worth. In K. A. Kerns & R. A. Richardson (Eds.), *Attachment in middle childhood* (pp. 161–188). New York: Guilford Press.

Borba, M. (2005). *Nobody likes me, everybody hates me: The top 25 friendship problems and how to solve them.* San Francisco: Jossey-Bass.

Bosma, H., & Kunnen, E. (Eds.). (2001). *Identity and emotion: Development through self-organization.* New York: Cambridge University Press.

Boulton, M. J., & Smith, P. K. (1994). Bully/victim problems in middle-school children: Stability, self-perceived competence, peer perceptions and peer acceptance. *British Journal of Developmental Psychology, 12,* 315–329.

Bowker, A. (2004). Predicting friendship stability during early adolescence. *Journal of Early Adolescence, 24,* 85–112.

Bowker, J. C. W., Rubin, K. H., Burgess, K. B., Booth-LaForce, C., & Rose-Krasnor, L. (2006). Behavioral characteristics associated with stable and fluid best friendship patterns in middle childhood. *Merrill-Palmer Quarterly, 52,* 671–693.

Bowlby, J. (1969). *Attachment and loss: Vol. 1. Attachment.* New York: Basic Books.

Bowlby, J. (1973). *Attachment and loss: Vol. 2. Separation: Anxiety and anger.* New York: Basic Books.

Bowlby, J. (1980). *Attachment and Loss: Vol. 3. Loss: Sadness and depression.* London: Hogarth Press.

Bowlby, J. (1982). Attachment and loss: Retrospect and prospect. *American Journal of Orthopsychiatry, 52*(4), 664–678.

Bowlby, J. (1988). *A secure base: Parent–child attachment and healthy human development.* London: Routledge.

Brendgen, M., Lamarche, V., Wanner, B., & Vitaro, F. (2010). Links between friendship relations and early adolescents' trajectories of depressed mood. *Developmental Psychology, 46,* 491–501.

Brendgen, M., Little, T. D., & Krappmann, L. (2000). Rejected children and their friends: A shared evaluation of friendship quality. *Merrill-Palmer Quarterly, 46,* 45–70.

Brendgen, M., Markiewicz, D., Doyle, A. B., & Bukowski, W. M. (2001). The relations between friendship quality, ranked-friendship preference, and adolescents' behavior with their friends. *Merrill-Palmer Quarterly, 47,* 395–415.

Brendgen, M., Vitaro, F., & Bukowski, W. M. (2000). Deviant friends and early adolescents' emotional and behavioral adjustment. *Journal of Research on Adolescence, 10,* 173–189.

Brendgen, M., Vitaro, F., Turgeon, L., & Poulin, F. (2002). Assessing aggressive and depressed children's social relations with classmates and friends: A matter of perspective. *Journal of Abnormal Child Psychology, 30,* 609–624.

Brendgen, M., Vitaro, F., Turgeon, L., Poulin, F., & Wanner, B. (2004). Is there a dark side of positive illusions?: Overestimation of social competence and subsequent adjustment in aggressive and nonaggressive children. *Journal of Abnormal Child Psychology, 32,* 305–320.

Bretherton, I. (1985). Attachment theory: Retrospect and prospect. *Monographs of the Society for Research in Child Development, 50*(1/2), 3–35.

Bretherton, I. (1992). The origins of attachment theory: John Bowlby and Mary Ainsworth. *Developmental Psychology, 28,* 759–775.

Brewer, M. B., & Chen, Y. (2007). Where (who) are collectives in collectivism? Toward conceptual clarification of individualism and collectivism. *Psychological Review, 114,* 133–151.

Bridges, L. J., Denham, S. A., & Ganiban, J. M. (2004). Definitional issues in emotion regulation research. *Child Development, 75,* 340–345.

Brody, G. (1998). Sibling relationship quality: Its causes and consequences. *Annual Review of Psychology, 49,* 1–24.

Bronfenbrenner, U. (1979). *The ecology of human development: Experiments by nature and design.* Cambridge, MA: Harvard University Press.

Bronfenbrenner, U. (Ed.). (2005). *Making human beings human: Bioecological perspectives on human development.* Thousand Oaks, CA: Sage.

Brown, B., & Klute, C. (2003). Friendships, cliques, and crowds. In G. R. Adams & M. D. Berzonsky (Eds.), *Blackwell handbook of adolescence* (pp. 330–348). Malden, MA: Blackwell.

Brown, B. B. (1990). Peer groups and peer cultures. In S. S. Feldman & G. R. Elliott (Eds.), *At the threshold: The developing adolescent* (pp. 171–196). Cambridge, MA: Harvard University Press.

Brown, B. B., Eicher, S. A., & Petrie, S. (1986). The importance of peer group ("crowd") affiliation in adolescence. *Journal of Adolescence, 9,* 73–96.

Brown, B. B., & Lohr, M. J. (1987). Peer-group affiliation and adolescent self-esteem: An integration of ego-identity and symbolic-interaction theories. *Journal of Personality and Social Psychology, 52,* 47–55.

Brown, J. R., Donelan-McCall, N., & Dunn, J. (1996). Why talk about mental states? The significance of children's conversations with friends, siblings, and mothers. *Child Development, 67*, 836–849.

Brownell, C. A., & Kopp, C. B. (Eds.). (2007). *Socioemotional development in the toddler years: Transitions and transformations.* New York: Guilford Press.

Browning, C., Cohen, R., & Warman, D. M. (2003). Peer social competence and the stability of victimization. *Child Study Journal, 33*, 73–90.

Buehler, C., Franck, K. L., & Cook, E. C. (2009). Adolescents' triangulation in marital conflict and peer relations. *Journal of Research on Adolescence, 19*, 669–689.

Bugental, D., & Goodnow, J. J. (1998). Socialization processes. In N. Eisenberg, W. Damon, & N. Eisenberg (Eds.), *Handbook of child psychology: Vol 3. Social, emotional, and personality development* (5th ed., pp. 389–462). Hoboken, NJ: Wiley.

Buhrmester, D. (1990). Intimacy of friendship, interpersonal competence, and adjustment during preadolescence and adolescence. *Child Development, 61*, 1101–1111.

Buhrmester, D. (1996). Need fulfillment, interpersonal competence, and the developmental contexts of early adolescent friendship. In W. M. Bukowski, A. F. Newcomb, & W. W. Hartup (Eds.), *The company they keep: Friendships in childhood and adolescence* (pp. 158–185). New York: Cambridge University Press.

Buhrmester, D., & Furman, W. (1986). The changing functions of friends in childhood: A neo-Sullivanian perspective. In V. G. Derlega & B. A. Winstead (Eds.), *Friendship and social interaction* (pp. 41–62). New York: Springer-Verlag.

Buhrmester, D., & Furman, W. (1987). The development of companionship and intimacy. *Child Development, 58*, 1101–1113.

Buhrmester, D., & Prager, K. (1995). Patterns and functions of self-disclosure during childhood and adolescence. In K. J. Rotenberg (Ed.), *Disclosure processes in children and adolescents* (pp. 10–56). New York: Cambridge University Press.

Bukowski, W. M. (2004, November). Research on children's and adolescents' friendships: Four old and new questions that deserve our attention. *International Society for the Study of Behavioural Development Newsletter* (Serial No. 46), 7–10.

Bukowski, W. M., & Adams, R. (2005). Peer relationships and psychopathology: Markers, moderators, mediators, mechanisms, and meanings. *Journal of Clinical Child and Adolescent Psychology, 34*, 3–10.

Bukowski, W. M., Gauze, C., Hoza, B., & Newcomb, A. F. (1993). Differences and consistency between same-sex and other-sex peer relationships during early adolescence. *Developmental Psychology, 29*, 255–263.

Bukowski, W. M., & Hoza, B. (1989). Popularity and friendship: Issues in theory, measurement, and outcome. In T. J. Berndt & G. W. Ladd (Eds.), *Peer relationships in child development* (pp. 15–45). Oxford, UK: Wiley.

Bukowski, W. M., Hoza, B., & Boivin, M. (1993). Popularity, friendship, and emotional adjustment during early adolescence. In B. Laursen (Ed.), *Close friendships in adolescence. New Directions for Child Development, 60,* 23–37.

Bukowski, W. M., Hoza, B., & Boivin, M. (1994). Measuring friendship quality during pre- and early adolescence: The development and psychometric properties of the friendship qualities scale. *Journal of Social and Personal Relationships, 11,* 471–484.

Bukowski, W. M., & Kramer, T. L. (1986). Judgments of the features of friendship among early adolescent boys and girls. *Journal of Early Adolescence, 6,* 331–338.

Bukowski, W. M., Newcomb, A. F., & Hartup, W. W. (Eds.). (1996). *The company they keep: Friendship in childhood and adolescence.* New York: Cambridge University Press.

Bukowski, W. M., Pizzamiglio, T., Newcomb, A. F., & Hoza, B. (1996). Popularity as an affordance for friendship: The link between group and dyadic experience. *Social Development, 5,* 189–202.

Bukowski, W. M., Sippola, L. K., & Boivin, M. (1995, March). Friendship protects "at risk" children from victimization from peers. In J. M. Price (Chair), *The role of friendship in children's developmental risk and resilience.* Symposium at the biennial meeting of the Society for Research in Child Development, Indianapolis, IN.

Bukowski, W. M., Sippola, L. K., & Hoza, B. (1999). Same and other: Interdependency between participation in same- and other-sex friendships. *Journal of Youth and Adolescence, 28*(4), 439–459.

Burk, W. J., & Laursen, B. (2005). Adolescent perceptions of friendship and their associations with individual adjustment. *International Journal of Behavioral Development, 29,* 156–164.

Buss, D. M. (2005). Sex differences in the design features of socially contingent mating adaptations. *Behavioral and Brain Sciences, 28,* 278–279.

Byrne, D., & Nelson, D. (1965). Attraction as a linear function of proportion of positive reinforcements. *Journal of Personality and Social Psychology, 1,* 659–663.

Cairns, R., Xie, H., & Leung, M. (1998). The popularity of friendship and the neglect of social networks: Toward a new balance. In W. M. Bukowski & A. H. N. Cillessen (Eds.), *Sociometry then and now: Building on six decades of measuring children's experiences with the peer group* (pp. 25–53). San Francisco: Jossey-Bass.

Cairns, R. B., & Cairns, B. D. (1994). *Lifelines and risks: Pathways of youth in our time.* New York: Cambridge University Press.

Cairns, R. B., Cairns, B. D., Neckerman, H. J., Gest, S. D., & Gariepy, J. (1988). Social networks and aggressive behavior: Peer support or peer rejection? *Developmental Psychology, 24,* 815–823.

Cairns, R. B., Leung, M-C., Buchanan, L., & Cairns, B. D. (1995). Friendships and social networks in childhood and adolescence: Fluidity, reliability, and interrelations. *Child Development, 66,* 1330–1345.

Calkins, S. D., Gill, K. L., Johnson, M. C., & Smith, C. L. (1999). Emotional reactivity and emotional regulation strategies as predictors of social behavior with peers during toddlerhood. *Social Development, 8,* 310–334.

Call, K., & Mortimer, J. T. (2001). *Arenas of comfort in adolescence: A study of adjustment in context.* Mahwah, NJ: Erlbaum.

Camarena, P. M., Sarigiani, P. A., & Petersen, A. C. (1990). Gender-specific pathways to intimacy in early adolescence. *Journal of Youth and Adolescence, 19,* 19–32.

Campos, J. J., Frankel, C. B., & Camras, L. (2004). On the nature of emotion regulation. *Child Development, 75,* 377–394.

Camras, L. A., & Fatani, S. S. (2008). The development of facial expressions: Current perspectives on infant emotions. In M. Lewis, J. M. Haviland-Jones, & L. F. Barrett (Eds.), *Handbook of emotions* (3rd ed., pp. 291–303). New York: Guilford Press.

Camras, L. A., Oster, H., Bakeman, R., Meng, Z., Ujiie, T., & Campos, J. J. (2007). Do infants show distinct negative facial expressions for fear and anger?: Emotional expression in 11-month-old European American, Chinese, and Japanese infants. *Infancy, 11,* 131–155.

Capaldi, D. M., Dishion, T. J., Stoolmiller, M., & Yoerger, K. (2001). Aggression toward female partners by at-risk young men: The contribution of male adolescent friendships. *Developmental Psychology, 37,* 61–73.

Caplan, M., Vespo, J., Pedersen, J., & Hay, D. F. (1991). Conflict and its resolution in small groups of one- and two-year-olds. *Child Development, 62,* 1513–1524.

Card, N. A. (2010). Antipathetic relationships in child and adolescent development: A meta-analytic review and recommendations for an emerging area of study. *Developmental Psychology, 46,* 516–529.

Card, N. A., & Hodges, E. E. (2007). Victimization within mutually antipathetic peer relationships. *Social Development, 16,* 479–496.

Card, N. A., Isaacs, J., & Hodges, E. E. (2009). Aggression and victimization in children's peer groups: A relationship perspective. In A. L. Vangelisti (Ed.), *Feeling hurt in close relationships* (pp. 235–259). New York: Cambridge University Press.

Carlson, S. M. (2003). Executive function in context: Development, measurement, theory, and experience. *Monographs of the Society for Research in Child Development, 68*(3), 138–151.

Carlson, S. M. (2005). Developmentally sensitive measures of executive function in preschool children. *Developmental Neuropsychology, 28,* 595–616.

Carrier, J. G. (1999). People who can be friends: Selves and social relationships. In S. Bell & S. Coleman (Eds.), *The anthropology of friendship* (pp. 21–38). New York: Berg.

Casiglia, A. C., Lo Coco, A., & Zappulla, C. (1998). Aspects of social reputation and peer relationships in Italian children: A cross-cultural perspective. *Developmental Psychology, 34,* 723–730.

Challman, R. C. (1932). Factors influencing friendships among preschool children. *Child Development, 3,* 146–158.

Champion, K., Vernberg, E., & Shipman, K. (2003). Nonbullying victims of bullies: Aggression, social skills, and friendship characteristics. *Applied Developmental Psychology, 24,* 535–551.

Chan, A., & Poulin, F. (2009). Monthly instability in early adolescent friendship networks and depressive symptoms. *Social Development, 18,* 1–23.

Chen, C., Lee, S., & Stevenson, H. W. (1995). Response style and cross-cultural comparisons of rating scales among East Asian and North American students. *Psychological Science, 6,* 170–175.

Chen, X., DeSouza, A. T., Chen, H., & Wang, L. (2006). Reticent behavior and experiences in peer interactions in Chinese and Canadian children. *Developmental Psychology, 42,* 656–665.

Chen, X., & French, D. C. (2008). Children's social competence in cultural context. *Annual Review of Psychology, 59,* 591–616.

Chen, X., French, D. C., & Schnedier, B. H. (2006). *Peer relationships in cultural context.* New York: Cambridge University Press.

Chen, X., Kaspar, V., Zhang, Y., Wang, L., & Zheng, S. (2004). Peer relationships among Chinese boys. In N. Way & J. Y. Chu (Eds.), *Adolescent boys: Exploring diverse cultures of boyhood* (pp. 197–218). New York: New York University Press.

Chen, X., Rubin, K. H., & Li, Z. (1995). Social functioning and adjustment in Chinese children: A longitudinal study. *Developmental Psychology, 31,* 532–539.

Chen, X., Rubin, K. H., & Sun, Y. (1992). Social reputation and peer relationships in Chinese and Canadian children: A cross-cultural study. *Child Development, 63,* 1336–1343.

Chen, X., Wang, L., & DeSouza, A. (2006). Temperament, socioemotional functioning, and peer relationships in Chinese and North American children. In X. Chen, D. C. French, & B. H. Schneider (Eds.), *Peer relationships in cultural context* (pp. 123–147). New York: Cambridge University Press.

Chipuer, H. M. (2001). Dyadic attachments and community connectedness: Links with youths' loneliness experiences. *Journal of Community Psychology, 29*(4), 429–446.

Ciairano, S., Rabaglietti, E., Roggero, A., Bonino, S., & Beyers, W. (2007). Patterns of adolescent friendships, psychological adjustment and antisocial behavior: The moderating role of family stress and friendship reciprocity. *International Journal of Behavioral Development, 31,* 539–548.

Cillessen, A. H. N., Jiang, X. L., West, T. V., & Laszkowski, D. K. (2005). Predictors of dyadic friendship quality in adolescence. *International Journal of Behavioral Development, 29,* 165–172.

Claes, M. (1998). Adolescents' closeness with parents, siblings, and friends in three countries: Canada, Belgium, and Italy. *Journal of Youth and Adolescence, 27,* 165–187.

Claes, M. E. (1992). Friendship and personal adjustment during adolescence. *Journal of Adolescence, 15,* 39–55.

Clark, M. L., & Ayers, M. (1992). Friendship similarity during early adolescence: Gender and racial patterns. *Journal of Psychology, 126,* 393–405.

Clark, M. L., & Ayers, M. (1993). Friendship expectations and friendship evaluations: Reciprocity and gender effects. *Youth and Society, 24,* 299–313.

Clark, M. L., & Bittle, M. L. (1992). Friendship expectations and the evaluation of present friendships in middle childhood and early adolescence. *Child Study Journal, 22,* 115–135.

Clore, G. L., & Byrne, D. (1974). A reinforcement–affect model of attraction. In T. L. Huston (Ed.), *Foundations of interpersonal attraction* (pp. 143–169). New York: Academic Press.

Cohen, Y. A. (1961). Patterns of friendship. In Y. A. Cohen (Ed.), *Social structure and personality: A casebook* (pp. 351–386). New York: Holt, Rinehart & Winston.

Cohn, D. A. (1990). Child–mother attachment of six-year-olds and social competence at school. *Child Development, 61,* 152.

Coie, J. D., Cillessen, A. H. N., Dodge, K. A., Hubbard, J. A., Schwartz, D., Lemerise, E. A., et al. (1999). It takes two to fight: A test of relational factors and a method for assessing aggressive dyads. *Developmental Psychology, 35,* 1179–1188.

Coie, J. D., Dodge, K. A., & Coppotelli, H. (1982). Dimensions and types of social status: A cross-age perspective. *Developmental Psychology, 18,* 557–570.

Coie, J. D., Lochman, J. E., Terry, R., & Hyman, C. (1992). Predicting early adolescent disorder from childhood aggression and peer rejection. *Journal of Consulting and Clinical Psychology, 60,* 783–792.

Coie, J. D., Terry, R., Lenox, K., Lochman, J. E., & Hyman, C. (1995). Childhood peer rejection and aggression as predictors of stable patterns of adolescent disorder. *Development and Psychopathology, 7,* 697–714.

Cole, P. M., Martin, S. E., & Dennis, T. A. (2004). Emotion regulation as a scientific construct: Methodological challenges and directions for child development research. *Child Development, 75,* 317–333.

Cole, P. M., & Tan, P. Z. (2007). Emotion socialization from a cultural perspective. In J. E. Grusec & P. D. Hastings (Eds.), *Handbook of socialization: Theory and research* (pp. 516–542). New York: Guilford Press.

Cole, P. M., Walker, A.R., & Lama-Tamang, M. S. (2006). Emotional aspects of peer relations among children in rural Nepal. In X. Chen, D. C. French, & B. H. Schneider (Eds.), *Peer relationships in cultural context* (pp. 148–169). New York: Cambridge University Press.

Collins, W., & Steinberg, L. (2006). Adolescent development in interpersonal context. In N. Eisenberg, W. Damon, & R. M. Lerner (Eds.), *Handbook of child psychology: Vol. 3. Social, emotional, and personality development* (6th ed., pp. 1003–1067). Hoboken, NJ: Wiley.

Colvin, C. R., Block, J., & Funder, D. C. (1995). Overly positive self-evaluations and personality: Negative implications for mental health. *Journal of Personality and Social Psychology, 68,* 1152–1162.

Conduct Problems Prevention Research Group. (1999). Initial impact of the fast track prevention trial for conduct problems: I. The high-risk sample. *Journal of Consulting and Clinical Psychology, 67,* 631–647.

Conduct Problems Prevention Research Group. (2002a). Evaluation of the first 3 years of the fast track prevention trial with children at high risk for adolescent conduct problems. *Journal of Abnormal Child Psychology, 30,* 19–35.

Conduct Problems Prevention Research Group. (2002b). Using the fast track randomized prevention trial to test the early-starter model of the development of serious conduct problems. *Development and Psychopathology, 14,* 925–943.

Conduct Problems Prevention Research Group. (2011). The effects of the fast track preventive intervention on the development of conduct disorder across childhood. *Child Development, 82,* 331–345.

Connolly, J., Craig, W., Goldberg, A., & Pepler, D. (1999). Conceptions of cross-sex friendships and romantic relationships in early adolescence. *Journal of Youth and Adolescence, 28,* 481–494.

Connolly, J., Craig, W., Goldberg, A., & Pepler, D. (2004). Mixed-gender groups, dating, and romantic relationships in early adolescence. *Journal of Research on Adolescence, 14,* 185–207.

Connolly, J., Furman, W., & Konarski, R. (2000). The role of peers in the emergence of heterosexual romantic relationships in adolescence. *Child Development, 71*(5), 1395–1408.

Connolly, J., & Johnson, A. M. (1996). Adolescents' romantic relationships and the structure and quality of their close interpersonal ties. *Personal Relationships, 3* 185–195.

Cooley, C. H. (1902). *Human nature and the social order.* New York: Charles Scribner's Sons.

Cooper, C. R., & Cooper, R. G. (1992). Links between adolescents' relationships with their parents and peers: Models, evidence, and mechanisms. In R. D. Parke & G. W. Ladd (Eds.), *Family–peer relationships: Modes of linkage* (pp. 135–158). Hillsdale, NJ: Erlbaum.

Corey, G. (1990). *Theory and practice of group counseling* (3rd ed.). Belmont, CA: Thomson Brooks/Cole.

Corsaro, W. A. (1985). *Friendship and peer culture in the early years.* Norwood, NJ: Ablex.

Corsaro, W. A. (1992). Interpretive reproduction in children's peer cultures. *Social Psychology Quarterly, 55,* 160–177.

Corsaro, W. A. (1994). Discussion, debate, and friendship processes: Peer discourse in U.S. and Italian nursery schools. *Sociology of Education, 67,* 1–26.

Corsaro, W. A. (2003). *We're friends, right?: Inside kids' culture.* Washington, DC: Joseph Henry Press.

Corsaro, W. A., & Molinari, L. (2000). Priming events and Italian children's transition from preschool to elementary school: Representations and action. *Social Psychology Quarterly, 63,* 16–33.

Corsaro, W. A., & Rizzo, T. A. (1990). Disputes in the peer culture of American and Italian nursery school children. In A. D. Grimshaw (Ed.), *Conflict talk: Sociolinguistic investigations of arguments in conversations* (pp. 21–66). New York: Cambridge University Press.

Costin, S. E., & Jones, D. C. (1992). Friendship as a facilitator of emotional responsiveness and prosocial interventions among young children. *Developmental Psychology, 28,* 941–947.

Cote, S. M., Vaillancourt, T., LeBlanc, J. C., Nagin, D. S., & Tremblay, R. E.

(2006). The development of physical aggression from toddlerhood to pre-adolescence: A nationwide longitudinal study of Canadian children. *Journal of Abnormal Child Psychology, 34*, 71–85.

Cotterell, J. (2007). *Social networks in youth and adolescence* (2nd ed.). New York: Routledge/Taylor & Francis.

Coyne, J. C. (1976). Depression and the response of others. *Journal of Abnormal Psychology, 85*, 186–193.

Crick, N. R., & Dodge, K. A. (1994). A review and reformulation of social information-processing mechanisms in children's social adjustment. *Psychological Bulletin, 115*, 74–101.

Crick, N. R., & Grotpeter, J. K. (1996). Children's treatment by peers: Victims of relational and overt aggression. *Development and Psychopathology, 8*, 367–380.

Crick, N. R., & Nelson, D. A. (2002). Relational and physical victimization within friendships: Nobody told me there'd be friends like these. *Journal of Abnormal Child Psychology, 30*, 599–607.

Criss, M. M., Pettit, G. S., Bates, J. E., Dodge, K. A., & Lapp, A. L. (2002). Family adversity, positive peer relationships, and children's externalizing behavior: A longitudinal perspective on risk and resilience. *Child Development, 73*, 1220–1237.

Crockett, L., Losoff, M., & Petersen, A. C. (1984). Perceptions of the peer group and friendships in early adolescence. *Journal of Early Adolescence, 4*, 155–181.

Crosnoe, R. (2000). Friendships in childhood and adolescence: The life course and new directions. *Social Psychology Quarterly, 63*, 377–391.

Cui, M., Conger, R. D., Bryant, C. M., & Elder, G. R. (2002). Parental behavior and the quality of adolescent friendships: A social contextual perspective. *Journal of Marriage and Family, 64*(3), 676–689.

Cutting, A. L., & Dunn, J. (1999). Theory of mind, emotion understanding, language, and family background: Individual differences. *Child Development, 70*, 853.

Cutting, A. L., & Dunn, J. (2006). Conversations with siblings and with friends: Links between relationship quality and social understanding. *British Journal of Developmental Psychology, 24*, 73–87.

Damon, W. (1977). *The social world of the child.* San Francisco: Jossey-Bass.

Damon, W., & Hart, D. (1982). The development of self-understanding from infancy through adolescence. *Child Development, 53*, 841–864.

Damon, W., & Hart, D. (1988). *Self-understanding in childhood and adolescence.* New York: Cambridge University Press.

Davies, P. T., Forman, E. M., Rasi, J. A., & Stevens, K. I. (2002). Assessing children's emotional security in the interparental relationship: The security in the interparental subsystem scales. *Child Development, 73*, 544–562.

De Goede, I. H. A., Branje, S. J. T., Delsing, M. J. M. H., & Meeus, W. H. J. (2009). Linkages over time between adolescents' relationships with parents and friends. *Journal of Youth and Adolescence, 38*, 1304–1315.

De Goede, I. H. A., Branje, S. J. T., & Meeus, W. H. J. (2009). Developmental changes and gender differences in adolescents' perceptions of friendships. *Journal of Adolescence, 32,* 1105–1123.

Demir, M., & Urberg, K. A. (2004). Friendship and adjustment among adolescents. *Journal of Experimental Child Psychology, 99,* 68–82.

Demorat, M. (1999, September). Emotion socialization in the classroom context: A functionalist analysis. *Dissertation Abstracts International Section A, 60.*

Denham, S., Mason, T., Caverly, S., Schmidt, M., Hackney, R., Caswell, C., et al. (2001). Preschoolers at play: Co-socialisers of emotional and social competence. *International Journal of Behavioral Development, 25,* 290–301.

Denham, S. A. (1998). *Emotional development in young children.* New York: Guilford Press.

Denham, S. A., Bassett, H. H., & Wyatt, T. (2007). The socialization of emotional competence. In J. E. Grusec & P. D. Hastings (Eds.), *Handbook of socialization: Theory and research* (pp. 614–637). New York: Guilford Press.

Denham, S. A., Blair, K. A., DeMulder, E., Levitas, J., Sawyer, K., Auerbach-Major, S., et al. (2003). Preschool emotional competence: Pathway to social competence. *Child Development, 74,* 238–256.

Denham, S. A., McKinley, M., Couchoud, E. A., & Holt, R. (1990). Emotional and behavioral predictors of preschool peer ratings. *Child Development, 61,* 1145–1152.

Denham, S. A., Renwick, S. M., & Holt, R. W. (1991). Working and playing together: Prediction of preschool social-emotional competence from mother–child interaction. *Child Development, 62,* 242–249.

Denham, S. A., von Salisch, M., Olthof, T., Kochanoff, A., & Caverly, S. (2002). Emotional and social development in childhood. In P. K. Smith & C. H. Hart (Eds.), *Blackwell handbook of childhood social development* (pp. 308–328). Malden, MA: Blackwell.

Denham, S. A., & Weissberg, R. P. (2004). Social-emotional learning in early childhood: What we know and where to go from here. In E. Chesebrough, P. King, T. P. Gullotta, & M. Bloom (Eds.), *A blueprint for the promotion of prosocial behavior in early childhood* (pp. 13–50). New York: Kluwer Academic/Plenum Press.

Denham, S. A., Zoller, D., & Couchoud, E. A. (1994). Socialization of preschoolers' emotion understanding. *Developmental Psychology, 30,* 928–936.

DeRosier, M., Kupersmidt, J., & Patterson, C. (1994). Children's academic and behavioral adjustment as a function of the chronicity and proximity of peer rejection. *Child Development, 65,* 1799–1813.

DeRosier, M. E. (2004). Building relationship and combating bullying: Effectiveness of a school-based social skills group intervention. *Journal of Clinical Child and Adolescent Psychology, 33,* 196–201.

DeRosier, M. E., & Kupersmidt, J. B. (1991). Costa Rican children's perceptions of their social networks. *Developmental Psychology, 27,* 656–662.

DeRosier, M. E., & Marcus, S. R. (2005). Building friendships and combating bullying: Effectiveness of S. S. Grin at one-year follow-up. *Journal of Clinical Child and Adolescent Psychology, 34,* 140–150.

Diamond, L. M., & Lucas, S. (2004). Sexual-minority and heterosexual youths' peer relationships: Experiences, expectations, and implications for well-being. *Journal of Research on Adolescence, 14,* 313–340.

Diamond, L. M., Savin-Williams, R. C., & Dubé, E. M. (1999). Sex, dating, passionate friendships, and romance: Intimate peer relations among lesbian, gay, and bisexual adolescents. In W. Furman, B. Brown, & C. Feiring (Eds.), *The development of romantic relationships in adolescence* (pp. 175–210). New York: Cambridge University Press.

DiIorio, C., Dudley, W. N., Kelly, M., Soet, J. E., Mbwara, J., & Potter, J. (2001). Social cognitive correlates of sexual experience and condom use among 13- through 15-year-old adolescents. *Journal of Adolescent Health, 29,* 208–216.

Dishion, T. J. (2000). Cross-setting consistency in early adolescent psychopathology: Deviant friendships and problem behavior sequelae. *Journal of Personality, 68,* 1109–1126.

Dishion, T. J., & Andrews, D. W. (1995). Preventing escalation in problem behaviors with high-risk young adolescents: Immediate and 1-year outcomes. *Journal of Consulting and Clinical Psychology, 63,* 538–548.

Dishion, T. J., Andrews, D. W., & Crosby, L. (1995). Antisocial boys and their friends in early adolescence: Relationship characteristics, quality, and interactional process. *Child Development, 66,* 139–151.

Dishion, T. J., Capaldi, D., Spracklen, K. M., & Li, F. (1995). Peer ecology of male adolescent drug use. *Development and Psychopathology, 7,* 803–824.

Dishion, T. J., Eddy, M., Haas, E., Li, F., & Spracklen, K. (1997). Friendships and violent behavior during adolescence. *Social Development, 6,* 207–223.

Dishion, T. J., McCord, J., & Poulin, F. (1999). When interventions harm: Peer groups and problem behavior. *American Psychologist, 54,* 755–764.

Dishion, T. J., Nelson, S. E., Winter, C. E., & Bullock, B. M. (2004). Adolescent friendship as a dynamic system: Entropy and deviance in the etiology and course of male antisocial behavior. *Journal of Abnormal Child Psychology, 32,* 651–663.

Dishion, T. J., & Owen, L. D. (2002). A longitudinal analysis of friendships and substance use: Bidirectional influence from adolescence to adulthood. *Developmental Psychology, 38,* 480–491.

Dishion, T. J., Patterson, G. R., & Griesler, P. C. (1994). Peer adaptations in the development of antisocial behavior: A confluence model. In L. R. Huesmann (Ed.), *Aggressive behavior: Current perspectives* (pp. 61–95). New York: Plenum Press.

Dishion, T. J., Spracklen, K. M., Andrews, D. W., & Patterson, G. R. (1996). Deviancy training in male adolescent friendships. *Behavior Therapy, 27,* 373–390.

Dobkin, P. L., Tremblay, R. E., Masse, L. C., & Vitaro, F. (1995). Individual and peer characteristics in predicting boys' early onset of substance abuse: A seven-year longitudinal study. *Child Development, 66,* 1198–1214.

Dodge, K. A. (1993). Social-cognitive mechanisms in the development of conduct disorder and depression. *Annual Review of Psychology, 44,* 559–584.

Dodge, K. A., Dishion, T. J., & Lansford, J. E. (Eds.). (2006). *Deviant peer influences in programs for youth: Problems and solutions.* New York: Guilford Press.

Dodge, K. A., Lansford, J. E., Burks, V. S., Bates, J. E., Pettit, G. S., Fontaine, R., et al. (2003). Peer rejection and social information-processing factors in the development of aggressive behavior problems in children. *Child Development, 74,* 374–393.

Dodge, K. A., Lansford, J. E., & Dishion, T. J. (2006). The problem of deviant peer influences in intervention programs. In K. A. Dodge, T. J. Dishion, & J. E. Lansford (Eds.), *Deviant peer influences in programs for youth: Problems and solutions* (pp. 3–13). New York: Guilford Press.

Dodge, K. A., Price, J. M., Coie, J. D., & Christopoulos, C. (1990). On the development of aggressive dyadic relationships in boys' peer groups. *Human Development, 33,* 260–270.

Doyle, A. B., Connolly, J., & Rivest, L-P. (1980). The effect of playmate familiarity on the social interactions of young children. *Child Development, 51,* 217–223.

Doyle, A. B., Lawford, H., & Markiewicz, D. (2009). Attachment style with mother, father, best friend, and romantic partner during adolescence. *Journal of Research on Adolescence, 19,* 690–714.

Doyle, A., & Markiewicz, D. (1996). Parents' interpersonal relationships and children's friendships. In W. M. Bukowski, A. F. Newcomb, & W. W. Hartup (Eds.), *The company they keep: Friendship in childhood and adolescence* (pp. 115–136). New York: Cambridge University Press.

Doyle, A. B., Markiewicz, D., & Hardy, C. (1994). Mothers' and children's friendships: Intergenerational associations. *Journal of Social and Personal Relationships, 11,* 363–377.

Duffy, A. L., & Nesdale, D. (2009). Peer groups, social identity, and children's bullying behavior. *Social Development, 18,* 121–139.

Dunn, J. (1988). *The beginnings of social understanding.* Cambridge, MA: Harvard University Press.

Dunn, J. (2004). *Children's friendships: The beginnings of intimacy.* Malden, MA: Blackwell.

Dunn, J., & Cutting, A. L. (1999). Understanding others, and individual differences in friendship interactions in young children. *Social Development, 8,* 201–219.

Dunphy, D. (1963). The social structure of urban adolescent peer groups. *Sociometry, 26,* 230–246.

Dunsmore, J. C., & Karn, M. A. (2004). The influence of peer relationships and maternal socialization on kindergartners' developing emotion knowledge. *Early Education and Development, 15,* 39–56.

Dykeman, B. F. (1995). The social cognitive treatment of anger and aggression in four adolescents with conduct disorder. *Journal of Instructional Psychology, 22,* 194–200.

East, P. L., & Rook, K. S. (1992). Compensatory patterns of support among children's peer relationships: A test using school friends, nonschool friends, and siblings. *Developmental Psychology, 28,* 163–172.

Eckerman, C. O. (1993). Toddlers' achievement of coordinated action with conspecifics: A dynamic systems perspective. In L. B. Smith & E. Thelen (Eds.), *A dynamic systems approach to development: Applications* (pp. 333–357). Cambridge, MA: MIT Press.

Eder, D. (1995). *School talk: Gender and adolescent culture.* New Brunswick, NJ: Rutgers University Press.

Edwards, C. P. (1992). Cross-cultural perspectives on family–peer relations. In R. D. Parke & G. W. Ladd (Eds.), *Family-peer relationships: Modes of linkage* (pp. 285–316). Hillsdale, NJ: Erlbaum.

Edwards, C. P., de Guzman, M. R. T., Brown, J., & Kumru, A. (2006). Children's social behaviors and peer interactions in diverse cultures. In X. Chen, D. C. French, & B. H. Schneider (Eds.), *Peer relationships in cultural context* (pp. 23–51). New York: Cambridge University Press.

Eisenberg, N., & Spinrad, T. L. (2004). Emotion-related regulation: Sharpening the definition. *Child Development, 75,* 334–339.

Elicker, J., Englund, M., & Sroufe, L. A. (1992). Predicting peer competence and peer relationships in childhood from early parent–child relationships. In R. D. Parke & G. W. Ladd (Eds.), *Family–peer relationships: Modes of linkage* (pp. 77–106). Hillsdale, NJ: Erlbaum.

Elkind, D. (1993). *Parenting your teenager.* New York: Ballantine Books.

Elliott, D. S., Huizinga, D., & Ageton, S. S. (1985). *Explaining delinquency and drug use.* Beverly Hills, CA: Sage.

Elliott, S. N., & Busse, R. T. (1991). Social skills assessment with children and adolescents. *School Psychology International, 12,* 63–83.

Ellis, W. E., & Zarbatany, L. (2007). Explaining friendship formation and friendship stability. *Merrill-Palmer Quarterly, 53,* 79–104.

Elman, N. M., & Kennedy-Moore, E. (2003). *The unwritten rules of friendship: Simple strategies to help your child make friends.* Boston: Little, Brown.

Emihovich, C. (1981). The intimacy of address: Friendship markers in children's social play. *Language in Society, 10,* 189–199.

Engels, S., & Sandstrom, M. (2010, July 22). There's only one way to stop a bully. *New York Times,* p. A23.

Epstein, J. L. (1983). Selection of friends in differently organized schools and classrooms. In J. L. Epstein & N. Karweit (Eds.), *Friends in school* (pp. 39–61). New York: Academic Press.

Erath, S. A., Flanagan, K. S., & Bierman, K. L. (2008). Early adolescent school adjustment: Associations with friendship and peer victimization. *Social Development, 17,* 853–870.

Erdley, C. A., Nangle, D. W., Newman, J. E., & Carpenter, E. M. (2001). Children's friendship experiences and psychological adjustment: Theory and research. In D. W. Nangle & C. A. Erdley (Eds.), *The role of friendship in psychological adjustment. New Directions for Child and Adolescent Development, 91,* 5–24.

Erikson, E. (1959). Identity and the life cycle: Selected papers. *Psychological Issues,* 11–171.

Erikson, E. (1968). *Identity: Youth and crisis.* New York: Norton.

Ervin-Tripp, S. M. (1986). Activity structure as scaffolding for children's second language learning. In J. Cook-Gumperz, W. A. Corsaro, & J. Streeck (Eds.), *Children's worlds and children's language* (pp. 327–358). New York: Mouton de Gruyter.

Espelage, D. L., Holt, M. K., & Henkel, R. R. (2003). Examination of peer-group contextual effects on aggression during early adolescence. *Child Development, 74,* 205–220.

Espelage, D. L., & Swearer, S. M. (2011). *Bullying in North American schools* (2nd ed). New York: Routledge.

Evans, S. W. (1999). Mental health services in schools: Utilization, effectiveness, and consent. *Clinical Psychology Review, 19,* 165–178.

Falvey, M. A., Forest, M. S., & Pearpoint, J. (2002). Building connections. In J. S. Thousand, R. A. Villa, & A. I. Nevin (Eds.), *Creativity and collaborative learning: The practical guide to empowering students, teachers, and families* (2nd ed., pp. 29–54). Baltimore: Brookes.

Fass, S., Briggs, J., & Cauthen, N. K. (2008). *Staying afloat in tough times: What states are and aren't doing to promote family economic security.* Report of the National Center for Children in Poverty. New York: Columbia University.

Federal Interagency Forum on Child and Family Statistics. (2008). *America's children in brief: Key National indicators of well-being, 2008.* Washington, DC: U.S. Government Printing Office.

Fehr, B. (1993). How do I love thee?: Let me consult my prototype. In S. Duck (Eds.), *Individuals in relationships* (pp. 87–120). Thousand Oaks, CA: Sage.

Fehr, B. (1996). *Friendship processes.* Thousand Oaks, CA: Sage.

Felsman, D. E., & Blustein, D. L. (1999). The role of peer relatedness in late adolescent career development. *Journal of Vocational Behavior, 54,* 279–295.

Fergusson, D. M., Vitaro, F., Wanner, B., & Brendgen, M. (2007). Protective and compensatory factors mitigating the influence of deviant friends on delinquent behaviours during early adolescence. *Journal of Adolescence, 30,* 33–50.

Field, T., Miller, J., & Field, T. (1994). How well preschool children know their friends. *Early Child Development and Care, 100,* 101–109.

Fine, G. A., & Sandstrom, K. L. (1988). *Knowing children: Participant observation with minors.* Newbury Park, CA: Sage.

Fonzi, A., Schneider, B. H., Tani, F., & Tomada, G. (1997). Predicting children's friendship status from their dyadic interaction in structured situations of potential conflict. *Child Development, 68,* 496–506.

Foot, H. C., Chapman, A. J., & Smith, J. R. (1977). Friendship and social responsiveness in boys and girls. *Journal of Personality and Social Psychology, 35,* 401–411.

Fordham, K., & Stevenson-Hinde, J. (1999). Shyness, friendship quality, and adjustment during middle childhood. *Journal of Child Psychology and Psychiatry, 40,* 757–768.

Fox, C. L., & Boulton, M. J. (2006). Friendship as a moderator of the relationship between social skills problems and peer victimisation. *Aggressive Behavior, 32,* 110–121.

Frankel, F. (2005). Parent-assisted children's friendship training. In E. D. Hibbs & P. S. Jensen (Eds.), *Psychosocial treatments for child and adolescent disorders: Empirically based approaches* (pp. 693–715). Washington, DC: American Psychological Association.

Frankel, F., Cantwell, D. P., & Myatt, R. (1996). Helping ostracized children: Social skills training and parent support for socially rejected children. In E. D. Hibbs & P. S. Jensen (Eds.), *Psychosocial treatments for child and adolescent disorders: Empirically based approaches* (pp. 595–617). Washington, DC: American Psychological Association.

Frankel, F., & Myatt, R. (2003). *Children's friendship training.* New York: Brunner-Routledge.

Frankel, F., Myatt, R., Cantwell, D. P., & Fineberg, D. T. (1997). Parent-assisted transfer of children's social skills training: Effects on children with and without attention-deficit hyperactivity disorder. *Journal of the American Academy of Child Psychiatry, 36,* 1056–1064.

Frankel, K. A. (1990). Girls' perceptions of peer relationship support and stress. *Journal of Early Adolescence, 10,* 69–88.

Frederickson, N., & Turner, N. (2003). Utilizing the classroom peer group to address children's social needs: An evaluation of the circle of friends intervention approach. *Journal of Special Education, 36,* 234–245.

Frederickson, N., Warren, L., & Turner, J. (2005). "Circle of friends"—An exploration of impact over time. *Educational Psychology in Practice, 21,* 197–217.

Freeman, H., & Brown, B. (2001). Primary attachment to parents and peers during adolescence: Differences by attachment style. *Journal of Youth and Adolescence, 30,* 653–674.

Freitag, M. K., Belsky, J., Grossmann, K., Grossmann, K. E., & Scheuerer-Englisch, H. (1996). Continuity in parent–child relationships from infancy to middle childhood and relations with friendship competence. *Child Development, 67,* 1437–1454.

French, D. C., Bae, A., Pidada, S., & Lee, O. (2006). Friendships of Indonesian, South Korean, and U.S. college students. *Personal Relationships, 13,* 69–81.

French, D. C., Jansen, E. A., Riansari, M., & Setiono, K. (2003). Friendships of Indonesian children: Adjustment of children who differ in friendship presence and similarity between mutual friends. *Social Development, 12,* 605–621.

French, D. C., Lee, O., & Pidada, S. U. (2006). Friendships of Indonesian, South Korean, and U.S. youth: Exclusivity, intimacy, enhancement of worth, and conflict. In X. Chen, D. C. French, & B. H. Schneider (Eds.), *Peer relationships in cultural context* (pp. 379–402). New York: Cambridge University Press.

French, D. C., Pidada, S., Denoma, J., McDonald, K., & Lawton, A. (2005). Reported peer conflicts of children in the United States and Indonesia. *Social Development, 14,* 458–472.

French, D. C., Pidada, S., & Victor, A. (2005). Friendships of Indonesian and United States youth. *International Journal of Behavioral Development, 29,* 304–313.

French, D. C., Rianasari, M., Pidada, S., Nelwan, P., & Buhrmester, D. (2001). Social support of Indonesian and U.S. children and adolescents by family members and friends. *Merrill-Palmer Quarterly, 47,* 377–394.

Freud, A. (1958). Adolescence. *The Psychoanalytic Study of the Child, 13,* 255–278.

Furman, W. (1982). Children's friendships. In T. M. Field, A. Huston, H. C. Quay, L. Troll, & G. E. Finley (Eds.), *Review of human development* (pp. 327–339). New York: Wiley.

Furman, W. (1984). Enhancing children's peer relations and friendships. In S. Duck (Ed.), *Personal relationships: Repairing personal relationships* (pp. 103–125). London: Academic Press.

Furman, W. (1996). The measurement of friendship perceptions: Conceptual and methodological issues. In W. M. Bukowski, A. F. Newcomb, & W. W. Hartup (Eds.), *The company they keep: Friendship in childhood and adolescence* (pp. 41–65). New York: Cambridge University Press.

Furman, W. (1999). Friends and lovers: The role of peer relationships in adolescent romantic relationships. In W. Collins & B. Laursen (Eds.), *Relationships as developmental contexts* (pp. 133–154). Mahwah, NJ: Erlbaum.

Furman, W. (2001). Working models of friendships. *Journal of Social and Personal Relationships, 18,* 583–602.

Furman, W., & Bierman, K. L. (1984). Children's conceptions of friendship: A multimethod study of developmental changes. *Developmental Psychology, 20,* 925–931.

Furman, W., & Buhrmester, D. (1985). Children's perceptions of the personal relationships in their social networks. *Developmental Psychology, 21,* 1016–1024.

Furman, W., & Buhrmester, D. (1992). Age and sex differences in perceptions of networks of personal relationships. *Child Development, 63,* 103–115.

Furman, W., & Buhrmester, D. (2009). Methods and measures: The Network of Relationships Inventory: Behavioral Systems Version. *International Journal of Behavioral Development, 33,* 470–478.

Furman, W., & Robbins, P. (1985). What's the point: Issues in the selection of treatment objectives. In B. Schneider, K. H. Rubin, & J. E. Ledingham (Eds.), *Children's peer relations: Issues in assessment and intervention* (pp. 41–54). New York: Springer-Verlag.

Furman, W., & Shaffer, L. (2003). The role of romantic relationships in adolescent development. In P. Florsheim (Eds.), *Adolescent romantic relations and sexual behavior: Theory, research, and practical implications* (pp. 3–22). Mahwah, NJ: Erlbaum.

Furman, W., Simon, V. A., Shaffer, L., & Bouchey, H. A. (2002). Adolescents' working models and styles for relationships with parents, friends, and romantic partners. *Child Development, 73,* 241–255.

Furman, W., & Wehner, E. A. (1994). Romantic views: Toward a theory of adolescent romantic relationships. In R. Montemayor, G. R. Adams, & T. P.

Gullotta (Eds.), *Advances in adolescent development: Vol. 6. Personal relationships in adolescence* (pp. 168–195). Thousand Oaks, CA: Sage.

Furman, W., & Wehner, E. A. (1997). Adolescent romantic relationships: A developmental perspective. In S. Shulman & W. A. Collins (Eds.). *Romantic relationships in adolescence: Developmental perspectives. New Directions for Child Development, 78,* 21–36.

Garmezy, N. (1983). Stressors of childhood. In N. Garmezy & M. Rutter (Eds.), *Stress, coping, and development in children* (pp. 43–85). New York: McGraw-Hill.

Garner, P. W., Dunsmore, J. C., & Southam-Gerrow, M. (2008). Mother–child conversations about emotions: Linkages to child aggression and prosocial behavior. *Social Development, 17*(2), 259–277.

Gaskins, S. (2006). The cultural organization of Yucatec Mayan children's social interactions. In X. Chen, D. C. French, & B. H. Schneider (Eds.), *Peer relationships in cultural context* (pp. 283–309). New York: Cambridge University Press.

Gauze, C., Bukowski, W. M., Aquan-Assee, J., & Sippola, L. K. (1996). Interactions between family environment and friendship and associations with self-perceived well-being during early adolescence. *Child Development, 67,* 2201–2216.

George, S. W., & Krantz, M. (1981). The effects of preferred play partnership on communication adequacy. *Journal of Psychology, 109,* 245–253.

George, T. P., & Hartmann, D. P. (1996). Friendship networks of unpopular, average, and popular children. *Child Development, 67,* 2301–2316.

Gershman, E. S., & Hayes, D. S. (1983). Differential stability of reciprocal friendships and unilateral relationships among preschool children. *Merrill-Palmer Quarterly, 29,* 169–177.

Gest, S. D. (2006). Teacher reports of children's friendships and social groups: Agreement with peer reports and implications for studying peer similarity. *Social Development, 15,* 248–259.

Gest, S. D., Farmer, T. W., Cairns, B. D., & Xie, H. (2003). Identifying children's peer social networks in school classrooms: Links between peer reports and observed interactions. *Social Development,12,* 513–529.

Gest, S. D., Graham-Bermann, S. A., & Hartup, W. W. (2001). Peer experience: Common and unique features of number of friendships, social network centrality, and sociometric status. *Social Development, 10,* 23–40.

Gini, G. (2008). Associations among overt and relational victimization and adolescents' satisfaction with friends: The moderating role of the need for affective relationships with friends. *Journal of Youth and Adolescence, 37,* 812–820.

Goldbaum, S., Craig, W. M., Pepler, D., & Connolly, J. (2003). Developmental trajectories of victimization: Identifying risk and protective factors. *Journal of Applied School Psychology, 19,* 139–156.

Goldstein, S., Field, T., & Healy, B. (1989). Concordance of play behavior and physiology in preschool friends. *Journal of Applied Developmental Psychology, 10,* 337–357.

Goncu, A. (1993). Development of intersubjectivity in the dyadic play of pre-schoolers. *Early Childhood Research Quarterly, 8,* 99–116.

González, Y. S., Moreno, D. S., & Schneider, B. H. (2004). Friendship expectations of early adolescents in Cuba and Canada. *Journal of Cross-Cultural Psychology, 35,* 436–445.

Gordon, S. L. (1989). The socialization of children's emotions: Emotional culture, competence, and exposure. In C. Saarni & P. L. Harris (Eds.), *Children's understanding of emotion* (pp. 319–349). New York: Cambridge University Press.

Gottfredson, M. R., & Hirschi, T. (1990). *A general theory of crime.* Stanford, CA: Stanford University Press.

Gottman, J. M. (1983). How children become friends. *Monographs of the Society for Research in Child Development, 48*(Serial No. 201).

Gottman, J. M., & Mettetal, G. (1986). Speculations about social and affective development of friendship and acquaintanceship through adolescence. In J. M. Gottman & J. Parker (Eds.), *Conversations of friends: Speculations on affective development* (pp. 192–237). New York: Cambridge University Press.

Graham, J. A., & Cohen, R. (1997). Race and sex as factors in children's sociometric ratings and friendship choices. *Social Development, 6,* 353–370.

Graham, J. A., Cohen, R., Zbikowski, S. M., & Secrist, M. E. (1998). A longitudinal investigation of race and sex as factors in children's classroom friendship choices. *Child Study Journal, 28,* 245–266.

Graham, S., Taylor, A. Z., & Ho, A. Y. (2009). Race and ethnicity in peer relations research. In K. H. Rubin, W. M. Bukowski, & B. Laursen (Eds.), *Handbook of peer interactions, relationships, and groups* (pp. 394–413). New York: Guilford Press.

Granic, I., & Dishion, T. J. (2003). Deviant talk in adolescent friendships: A step toward measuring a pathogenic attractor process. *Social Development, 12,* 314–334.

Graue, M. E., & Walsh, D. J. (1998). *Studying children in context: Theories, methods, and ethics.* Thousand Oaks, CA: Sage.

Greco, L. A., & Morris, T. L. (2005). Factors influencing the link between social anxiety and peer acceptance: Contributions of social skills and close friendships during middle childhood. *Behavior Therapy, 36,* 197–205.

Greenberger, E., Chen, C., Beam, M., Whang, S., & Dong, Q. (2000). The perceived social contexts of adolescents' misconduct: A comparative study of youths in three cultures. *Journal of Research on Adolescence, 10,* 365–388.

Greene, M. L., & Way, N. (2005). Self-esteem trajectories among ethnic minority adolescents: A growth curve analysis of the patterns and predictors of change. *Journal of Research on Adolescence, 15,* 151–178.

Greenway, C. (2000). Autism and Asperger syndrome: Strategies to promote prosocial behaviours. *Educational Psychology in Practice, 16,* 469–486.

Gresham, F. M., & Nagle, R. J. (1980). Social skills training with children: Responsiveness to modeling and coaching as a function of peer orientation. *Journal of Consulting and Clinical Psychology, 48,* 718–729.

Gross, E. F. (2004). Adolescent Internet use: What we expect, what teens report. *Developmental Psychology, 25,* 633–649.

Gross, J. J. (2008). Emotion and emotion regulation: Personality processes and individual differences. In O. P. John, R. W. Robins, & L. A. Pervin (Eds.), *Handbook of personality psychology: Theory and research* (3rd ed., pp. 701–724). New York: Guilford Press..

Gross, J. J., & Thompson, R. A. (2007). Emotion regulation: Conceptual foundations. In J. J. Gross (Ed.), *Handbook of emotion regulation* (pp. 3–24). New York: Guilford Press.

Grotevant, H. D. (1987). Toward a process model of identity formation. *Journal of Adolescent Research, 2,* 203–222.

Grotpeter, J. K., & Crick, N. R. (1996). Relational aggression, overt aggression, and friendship. *Child Development, 67,* 2328–2338.

Gummerum, M., & Keller, M. (2008). Affection, virtue, pleasure, and profit: Developing an understanding of friendship closeness and intimacy in western and Asian societies. *International Journal of Behavioral Development, 32,* 218–231.

Güroglu, B., van Lieshout, C. M., Haselager, G. T., & Scholte, R. J. (2007). Similarity and complementary of behavioral profiles of friendship types and types of friends: Friendships and psychosocial adjustment. *Journal of Research on Adolescence, 17,* 357–386.

Gus, L. (2000). Autism: Promoting peer understanding. *Educational Psychology in Practice, 16,* 461–468.

Haar, B. F., & Krahe, B. (1999). Strategies for resolving interpersonal conflicts in adolescence: A German–Indonesian comparison. *Journal of Cross-Cultural Psychology, 30,* 667–683.

Hafner, K. (2009, May 26). Texting may be taking a toll. *New York Times,* p. 1.

Haight, W., Black, J., Jacobsen, T., & Sheridan, K. (2006). Pretend play and emotion learning in traumatized mothers and children. In D. Singer, R. M. Golinkoff, & K. Hirsh-Pasek (Eds.), *Play = learning: How play motivates and enhances children's cognitive and social-emotional growth.* New York: Oxford University Press.

Halligan, S. L., & Philips, K. J. (2010). Are you thinking what I'm thinking?: Peer group similarities in adolescent hostile attribution tendencies. *Developmental Psychology, 46,* 1385–1388.

Hamm, J. V. (2000). Do birds of a feather flock together?: The variable bases for African American, Asian American, and European American adolescents' selection of similar friends. *Developmental Psychology, 36,* 209–219.

Hamm, J. V., Brown, B. B., & Heck, D. J. (2005). Bridging the ethnic divide: Student and school characteristics in American, Asian-descent, Latino, and White adolescents' cross-ethnic friend nominations. *Journal of Research on Adolescence, 15,* 21–46.

Hand, L., & Furman, W. (2009). Rewards and costs in adolescent other-sex friendships: Comparisons to same-sex friendships and romantic relationships. *Social Development, 18,* 270–287.

Hanish, L. D., Ryan, P., Martin, C. L., & Fabes, R. A. (2005). The social context of young children's peer victimization. *Social Development, 14,* 2–19.

Hardy, C. L., Bukowski, W. M., & Sippola, L. K. (2002). Stability and change in peer relationships during the transition to middle-level schools. *Journal of Early Adolescence, 22,* 117–142.

Harkness, S., & Super, C. M. (1983). The cultural construction of child development: A framework for the socialization of affect. *Ethos, 11,* 221–231.

Harkness, S., & Super, C. M. (1985). The cultural context of gender segregation in children's peer groups. *Child Development, 56,* 219–224.

Harris, J. R. (1995). Where is the child's environment?: A group socialization theory of development. *Psychological Review, 102,* 458–489.

Harrison, A. O., Stewart, R. B., Myambo, K., & Teveraishe, C. (1995). Perceptions of social networks among adolescents from Zimbabwe and the United States. *Journal of Black Psychology, 21,* 382–407.

Harrison, A. O., Stewart, R. B., Myambo, K., & Teveraishe, C. (1997). Social networks among early adolescent Zimbabweans in extended families. *Journal of Research on Adolescence, 7,* 153–172.

Harter, S. (1990). Self and identity development. In S. S. Feldman & G. R. Elliott (Eds.), *At the threshold: The developing adolescent* (pp. 352–387). Cambridge, MA: Harvard University Press.

Harter, S. (1998). The development of self-representations. In N. Eisenberg & W. Damon (Eds.), *Handbook of child psychology: Vol. 3. Social, emotional, and personality development* (5th ed., pp. 553–617). Hoboken, NJ: Wiley.

Harter, S. (2006). Developmental and individual difference perspectives on self-esteem. In D. K. Mroczek & T. D. Little (Eds.), *Handbook of personality development* (pp. 311–334). Mahwah, NJ: Erlbaum.

Harter, S., & Whitesell, N. (1989). Developmental changes in children's understanding of single, multiple, and blended emotion concepts. In C. Saarni & P. L. Harris (Eds.), *Children's understanding of emotion* (pp. 81–116). New York: Cambridge University Press.

Hartup, W. W. (1992a). Conflict and friendship relations. In C. U. Shantz & W. W. Hartup (Eds.), *Conflict in child and adolescent development* (pp. 186–215). New York: Cambridge University Press.

Hartup, W. W. (1992b). Friendships and their developmental significance. In H. McGurk (Ed.), *Childhood social development: Contemporary perspectives* (pp. 175–203). Hillsdale, NJ: Erlbaum.

Hartup, W. W. (1993). Adolescents and their friends. In B. Laursen (Ed.), *Close friendships in adolescence. New Directions for Child Development, 60,* 3–22.

Hartup, W. W. (1995). The three faces of friendship. *Journal of Social and Personal Relationships, 12,* 569–574.

Hartup, W. W. (1996a). The company they keep: Friendships and their developmental significance. *Child Development, 67,* 1–13.

Hartup, W. W. (1996b). Cooperation, close relationship, and cognitive development. In W. M. Bukowski, A. F. Newcomb, & W. W. Hartup (Eds.), *The company they keep: Friendship in childhood and adolescence* (pp. 213–237). New York: Cambridge University Press.

Hartup, W. W., French, D. C., Laursen, B., Johnston, M. K., & Ogawa, J. R.

(1993). Conflict and friendship relations in middle childhood: Behavior in a closed-field situation. *Child Development, 64,* 445–454.

Hartup, W. W., & Laursen, B. (1991). Relationships as developmental contexts. In R. Cohen & A. W. Siegel (Eds.), *Context and development* (pp. 253–279). Hillsdale, NJ: Erlbaum.

Hartup, W. W., & Laursen, B. (1999). Relationships as developmental contexts: Retrospective themes and contemporary issues. In W. A. Collins (Ed.), *Relationships as contexts: Vol. 30. The Minnesota symposia on child psychology* (pp. 13–35). Mahwah, NJ: Erlbaum.

Hartup, W. W., Laursen, B., Stewart, M. I., & Eastenson, A. (1988). Conflict and the friendship relations of young children. *Child Development, 59,* 1590–1600.

Hartup, W. W., & Stevens, N. (1997). Friendships and adaptation in the life course. *Psychological Bulletin, 121,* 355–370.

Hartup, W. W., & Stevens, N. (1999). Friendships and adaptation across the life span. *Current Directions in Psychological Science, 8,* 76–79.

Haselager, G. J. T., Hartup, W. W., van Lieshout, C. F. M., & Riksen-Walraven, J. M. A. (1998). Similarities between friends and nonfriends in middle childhood. *Child Development, 69,* 1198–1208.

Hawker, D. J., & Boulton, M. J. (2000). Twenty years' research on peer victimization and psychosocial maladjustment: A meta-analytic review of cross-sectional studies. *Journal of Child Psychology and Psychiatry, 41,* 441–455.

Hayes, D. S., Gershman, E. S., & Bolin, L. J. (1980). Friends and enemies: Cognitive bases for preschool children's unilateral and reciprocal relationships. *Child Development, 51,* 1276–1279.

Hazan, C., & Zeifman, D. (1994). Sex and the psychological tether. In K. Bartholomew & D. Perlman (Eds.), *Attachment processes in adulthood* (pp. 151–178). London: Kingsley.

Hendey, B., & Butter, E. J. (1981). Moral judgments by children of the intentional behavior of friends and strangers. *Journal of Genetic Psychology, 139,* 227–232.

Hendrick, S. S., & Hendrick, C. (1993). Lovers as friends. *Journal of Social and Personal Relationships, 10,* 459–466.

Herrera, C., & Dunn, J. (1997). Early experiences with family conflict: Implications for arguments with a close friend. *Developmental Psychology, 33,* 869–881.

Hinde, R. A. (1979). *Towards understanding relationships.* London: Academic Press.

Hinde, R. A. (1988). Continuities and discontinuities: Conceptual issues and methodological considerations. In M. Rutter (Ed.), *Studies of psychosocial risk: The power of longitudinal data* (pp. 367–383). New York: Cambridge University Press.

Hinde, R. A. (1997). *Relationships: A dialectical perspective.* East Sussex, UK: Psychology Press.

Hinde, R. A., Titmus, G., Easton, D., & Tamplin, A. (1985). Incidence of "friendship" and behavior toward strong associates versus nonassociates in preschoolers. *Child Development, 56,* 234–245.

Hirschfeld, L. A. (2002). Why don't anthropologists like children? *American Anthropologist, 14,* 611–627.

Hodges, E. V. E., Boivin, M., Vitaro, F., & Bukowski, W. M. (1999). The power of friendship: Protection against an escalating cycle of peer victimization. *Developmental Psychology, 75,* 94–101.

Hodges, E. V. E., Malone, M. J., & Perry, D. G. (1997). Individual risk and social risk as interacting determinants of victimization in the peer group. *Developmental Psychology, 33,* 1032–1039.

Hodges, E. V. E., & Perry, D. G. (1997, April). *Victimization by peers: The protective function of peer friendships.* Poster session presented at the meeting of the Society for Research in Child Development, Washington, DC.

Hodges, E. V. E., & Perry, D. G. (1999). Personal and interpersonal antecedents and consequences of victimization by peers. *Journal of Personality and Social Psychology, 76,* 677–685.

Hofstede, G. (1980). *Culture's consequences: International differences in work-related values.* Beverly Hills, CA: Sage.

Hofstede, G. (1994). Foreword. In U. Kim, H. C. Triandis, C. Kagitcibasi, S. Choi, & G. Yoon (Eds.), *Individualism and collectivism: Theory, method, and applications* (pp. ix–xiii). Thousand Oaks, CA: Sage.

Hofstede, G. (2001). *Culture's consequences: Comparing values, behaviors, institutions, and organizations across nations* (2nd ed.). Thousand Oaks, CA: Sage.

Hortacsu, N. (1997). Cross-cultural comparison of need importance and need satisfaction during adolescence: Turkey and the United States. *Journal of Genetic Psychology, 158,* 287–297.

Howe, N., Petrakos, H., Rinaldi, C. M., & LeFebvre, R. (2005). "This is a bad dog, you know ... ": Constructing shared meanings during sibling pretend play. *Child Development, 76,* 783–794.

Howes, C. (1983). Patterns of friendship. *Child Development, 54,* 1041–1053.

Howes, C. (1987). Social competence with peers in young children: Developmental sequences. *Developmental Review, 7,* 252–272.

Howes, C. (1988). Peer interaction of young children. *Monographs of the Society for Research in Child Development, 53*(Serial No. 217).

Howes, C. (1996). The earliest friendships. In W. M. Bukowski, A. F. Newcomb, & W. W. Hartup (Eds.), *The company they keep: Friendship in childhood and adolescence* (pp. 66–86). New York: Cambridge University Press.

Howes, C., Droege, K., & Matheson, C. C. (1994). Play and communicative processes within long- and short-term friendship dyads. *Journal of Social and Personal Relationships, 11,* 401–410.

Howes, C., Droege, K., & Phillipsen, L. (1992). Contribution of peers to socialization in early childhood. In M. Gettinger, S. N. Elliott, & T. R. Kratochwill (Eds.), *Preschool and early childhood treatment directions* (pp. 113–150). Hillsdale, NJ: Erlbaum.

Howes, C., & Farver, J. (1987). Toddlers' responses to the distress of their peers. *Journal of Applied Developmental Psychology, 8,* 441–452.

Howes, C., Hamilton, C. E., & Philipsen, L. C. (1998). Stability and continuity of child–caregiver and child–peer relationships. *Child Development, 69,* 418–426.

Howes, C., & Lee, L. (2006). Peer relations in young children. In L. Balter & C. S. Tamis-LeMonda (Eds.), *Child psychology: A handbook of contemporary issues* (2nd ed., pp. 135–151). New York: Psychology Press.

Howes, C., & Matheson, C. C. (1992). Sequences in the development of competent play with peers: Social and social pretend play. *Developmental Psychology, 28,* 961–974.

Howes, C., Matheson, C. C., & Wu, F. (1992). Friendships and social pretend play. In C. Howes, O. Unger, & C. C. Matheson (Eds.), *The collaborative construction of pretend.* Albany: State University of New York Press.

Hoza, B., Bukowski, W. M., & Beery, S. (2000). Assessing peer network and dyadic loneliness. *Journal of Clinical Child Psychology, 29,* 119–128.

Hoza, B., Gerdes, A. C., Hinshaw, S. P., Arnold, L. E., Pelham, Jr., W. E., Molina, B. S. G., et al. (2004). Self-perceptions of competence in children with ADHD and comparison children. *Journal of Consulting and Clinical Psychology, 72,* 382–391.

Hoza, B., Molina, B. S. G., Bukowski, W. M., & Sippola, L. (1995). Peer variables as predictors of later childhood adjustment. *Development and Psychopathology, 7,* 787–802.

Hoza, B., Mrug, S., Pelham, W. E., Greiner, A. R., & Gnagy, E. M. (2003). A friendship intervention for children with attention-deficit/hyperactivity disorder: Preliminary findings. *Journal of Attention Disorders, 6,* 87–98.

Hoza, B., Pelham, W. E., Dobbs, J., Owens, J. S., & Pillow, D. R. (2002). Do boys with attention-deficit/hyperactivity disorder have positive illusory self-concepts? *Journal of Abnormal Psychology, 111,* 268–278.

Hubbard, J. A. (2001). Emotion expression processes in children's peer interaction: The role of peer rejection, aggression, and gender. *Child Development, 72,* 1426.

Hughes, C. (2002). Executive functions and development: Emerging themes. *Infant and Child Development, 11,* 201–209.

Hughes, C., Cutting, A. L., & Dunn, J. (2001). Acting nasty in the face of failure?: Longitudinal observations of "hard-to-manage" children playing a rigged competitive game with a friend. *Journal of Abnormal Child Psychology, 29,* 403–416.

Hughes, C., & Dunn, J. (1997). "Pretend you didn't know": Preschoolers' talk about mental states in pretend play. *Cognitive Development, 12,* 381–403.

Hughes, C., & Dunn, J. (1998). Understanding mind and emotion: Longitudinal associations with mental-state talk between young friends. *Developmental Psychology, 34,* 1026–1037.

Hughes, C., & Ensor, R. (2007). Executive function and theory of mind: Predictive relations from ages 2 to 4. *Developmental Psychology, 43,* 1447–1459.

Hussong, A. M. (2000a). Distinguishing mean and structural sex differences in adolescent friendship quality. *Journal of Social and Personal Relationships, 17,* 223–243.

Hussong, A. M. (2000b). Perceived peer context and adolescent adjustment. *Journal of Research on Adolescence, 10,* 391–415.

Hymel, S., Rubin, K. H., Rowden, L., & LeMare, L. (1990). Children's peer relationships: Longitudinal predictions of internalizing and externalizing problems from middle to late childhood. *Child Development, 61,* 2004–2021.

Hymel, S., Woody, E., & Bowker, A. (1993). Social withdrawal in childhood: Considering the child's perspective. In K. H. Rubin & J. B. Asendorpf (Eds.), *Social withdrawal, inhibition, and shyness in childhood.* Hillsdale, NJ: Erlbaum.

Isakson, K., & Jarvis, P. (1999). The adjustment of adolescents during the transition into high school: A short term longitudinal study. *Journal of Youth and Adolescence, 28,* 1–26.

Jacobsen, T., & Hofmann, V. (1997). Children's attachment representations: Longitudinal relations to school behavior and academic competency in middle childhood and adolescence. *Developmental Psychology, 33,* 703–710.

James, A. (2007). Giving voice to children's voices: Practices and problems, pitfalls and potentials. *American Anthropologist, 109,* 261–272.

James, A., Jenks, C., & Prout, A. (1998). *Theorizing childhood.* New York: Teachers College Press.

James, A., & Leyden, G. (2010). Putting the circle back into circle of friends: A grounded theory study. *Educational and Child Psychology, 27,* 52–63.

Jenkins, J. M., & Astington, J. (2000). Theory of mind and social behavior: Causal models tested in a longitudinal study. *Merrill-Palmer Quarterly, 46,* 203–220.

Johnson, H. D. (2004). Gender, grade, and relationship differences in emotional closeness within adolescent friendships. *Adolescence, 39,* 243–255.

Jones, D. C. (1985). Persuasive appeals and responses to appeals among friends and acquaintances. *Child Development, 56,* 757–763.

Jones, D. C., Abbey, B., & Cumberland, A. (1998). The development of display rule knowledge: Linkages with family expressiveness and social competence. *Child Development, 69,* 1209–1222.

Jones, D. C., & Costin, S. E. (1995). Friendship quality during preadolescence and adolescence: The contributions of relationship orientations, instrumentality, and expressivity. *Merrill-Palmer Quarterly, 41,* 517–535.

Kalyva, E., & Avramidis, E. (2005). Improving communication between children with autism and their peers through the "circle of friends": A small-scale intervention study. *Journal of Applied Research in Intellectual Disabilities, 18,* 253–261.

Kandel, D. B. (1978). Homophily, selection, and socialization in adolescent friendships. *American Journal of Sociology, 84,* 427–436.

Kandel, D. B. (1986). Processes of peer influences in adolescence. In R. K. Silbereisen, K. Eyferth, & G. Rudinger (Eds.), *Development as action in context* (pp. 203–227). New York: Springer-Verlag.

Kandel, D. B. (1996). The parental and peer contexts of adolescent deviance: An algebra of interpersonal influences. *Journal of Drug Issues, 26,* 289–315.

Karcher, M. J. (1997). Perspective-taking to emotion-making in a middle school pair. In R. L. Selman, C. L. Watts, & L. H. Schultz (Eds.), *Fostering friendship: Pair therapy for treatment and prevention* (pp. 121–144). New York: Aldine.

Karweit, N., & Hansell, S. (1983). School organization and friendship selection. In J. L. Epstein & N. Karweit (Eds.), *Friends in school: Patterns of selection and influence in secondary schools* (pp. 29–38). San Diego, CA: Academic Press.

Kashy, D. A., & Kenny, D. A. (2000). The analysis of data from dyads and groups. In H. Reis & C. M. Judd (Eds.), *Handbook of research methods in social and personality psychology* (pp. 451–477). New York: Cambridge University Press.

Katz, L., & Woodin, E. M. (2002). Hostility, hostile detachment, and conflict engagement in marriages: Effects on child and family functioning. *Child Development, 73,* 636–651.

Kavanaugh, R. D. (2006). Pretend play and theory of mind. In L. Balter & C. S. Tamis-LeMonda (Eds.), *Child psychology: A handbook of contemporary issues* (2nd ed., pp. 153–166). New York: Psychology Press.

Kawabata, Y., & Crick, N. (2008). The role of cross-racial/ethnic friendships in social adjustment. *Developmental Psychology, 44,* 1177–1183.

Kawabata, Y., Crick, N. R., & Hamaguchi, Y. (2010). Forms of aggression, social-psychological adjustment, and peer victimization in a Japanese sample: The moderating role of positive and negative friendship quality. *Journal of Abnormal Child Psychology, 38,* 471–484.

Keats, J. A., Keats, D. M., Biddle, B. J., Bank, B. J., Hauge, R., Wan-Rafaei, A. R., et al. (1983). Parents, friends, siblings, and adults: Unfolding referent other importance data for adolescents. *International Journal of Psychology, 18,* 239–262.

Keefe, K., & Berndt, T. J. (1996). Relations of friendship quality to self-esteem in early adolescence. *Journal of Early Adolescence, 16,* 110–129.

Keenan, K., Loeber, R., Zhang, Q., Stouthamer-Loeber, M., & Van Kammen, W. B. (1995). The influence of deviant peers on the development of boys' disruptive and delinquent behavior: A temporal analysis. *Development and Psychopathology, 7,* 715–726.

Kelley, H. H., Berscheid, E., Christensen, A., Harvey, J. H., Huston, T. L., Levinger, G., et al. (1983). Analyzing close relationships. In H. H. Kelley, E. Berscheid, A. Christensen, J. H. Harvey, T. L. Huston, G. Levinger, et al. (Eds.), *Close relationships.* New York: Freeman.

Kelley, H. H., & Thibaut, J. W. (1978). *Interpersonal relations: A theory of interdependence.* New York: Wiley.

Kennedy, R. E. (1982). Cognitive-behavioral approaches to the modification of aggressive behavior in children. *School Psychology Review, 11,* 47–55.

Kenny, D. A. (1996). Models of non-independence in dyadic research. *Journal of Social and Personal Relationships, 13,* 279–294.

Kenny, D. A., Kashy, D. A., & Cook, W. L. (2006). *Dyadic data analysis.* New York: Guilford Press.

Kenny, D. A., Mohr, C. D., & Levesque, M. J. (2001). A social relations variance partitioning of dyadic behavior. *Psychological Bulletin, 127,* 128–141.

Kerns, K. A. (1996). Individual differences in friendship quality and their links to child–mother attachment. In W. M. Bukowski, A. F. Newcomb, & W. W.

Hartup (Eds.), *The company they keep: Friendship in childhood and adolescence* (pp. 137–157). Cambridge, UK: Cambridge University Press.

Kerns, K. A. (2000). Types of preschool friendships. *Personal Relationships, 7,* 311–324.

Kerns, K. A., Klepac, L., & Cole, A. K. (1996). Peer relationships and preadolescents' perceptions of security in the child–mother relationship. *Developmental Psychology, 32,* 457–466.

Kiesner, J., Kerr, M., & Stattin, H. (2004). "Very important persons" in adolescence: Going beyond in-school, single friendships in the study of peer homophily. *Journal of Adolescence, 27,* 545–560.

Kiesner, J., Poulin, F., & Dishion, T. J. (2010). Adolescent substance use with friends. *Merrill-Palmer Quarterly, 56,* 529–556.

Killen, M., & Sueyoshi, L. (1995). Conflict resolution in Japanese social interactions. *Early Education and Development, 6,* 317–334.

Kim, Y., & Leventhal, B. (2008). Bullying and suicide. A review. *International Journal of Adolescent Medicine and Health, 20,* 133–154.

Kindermann, T. A. (1993). Natural peer groups as contexts for individual development: The case of children's motivation in school. *Developmental Psychology, 29,* 970–977.

Kindermann, T. A. (1996). Strategies for the study of individual development within naturally-existing peer groups. *Social Development, 5,* 158–173.

Kindermann, T. A. (2007). Effects of naturally existing peer groups on changes in academic engagement in a cohort of sixth graders. *Child Development, 78,* 1186–1203.

Kingery, J. N., & Erdley, C. A. (2007). Peer experiences as predictors of adjustment across the middle school transition. *Education and Treatment of Children, 30,* 73–88.

Kirchler, E., Pombeni, M. L., & Palmonari, A. (1991). Sweet sixteen: Adolescents' problems and the peer group as source of support. *European Journal of Psychology of Education, 6,* 393–410.

Kistner, J., Balthazor, M., Risi, S., & Burton, C. (1999). Predicting dysphoria in adolescence from actual and perceived peer acceptance in childhood. *Journal of Clinical Child Psychology, 28,* 94–104.

Kitzmann, K. M., & Cohen, R. (2003). Parents' versus children's perceptions of interparental conflict as predictors of children' friendship quality. *Journal of Social and Personal Relationships, 20,* 689–700.

Kitzmann, K. M., Cohen, R., & Lockwood, R. L. (2002). Are only children missing out?: Comparison of the peer-related social competence of only children and siblings. *Journal of Social and Personal Relationships, 19,* 299–316.

Klass, P. (2009, June 9). At last, facing down bullies (and their enablers). *New York Times,* p. 5.

Klima, T., & Repetti, R. L. (2008). Children's peer relations and their psychological adjustment: Differences between close friendships and the larger peer group. *Merrill-Palmer Quarterly, 54,* 151–178.

Knecht, A., Snijders, T. A. B., Baerveldt, C., Steglich, C. E. G., & Raub, W. (2010). Friendship and delinquency: Selection and influence processes in early adolescence. *Social Development, 19,* 494–514.

Knight, G. P., & Chao, C. (1991). Cooperative, competitive, and individualistic social values among 8- to 12-year-old siblings, friends, and acquaintances. *Personality and Social Psychology Bulletin, 17,* 201–211.

Kobak, R., Rosenthal, N., Zajac, K., & Madsen, S. (2007). Adolescent attachment hierarchies and the search for an adult pair bond. In M. Scharf & O. Mayseless (Eds.), *Attachment in adolescence. New Directions for Child Development, 117,* 57–72.

Kochenderfer, B. J., & Ladd, G. W. (1997). Victimized children's responses to peers' aggression: Behaviors associated with reduced versus continued victimization. *Development and Psychopathology, 9,* 59–73.

Kochenderfer-Ladd, B., & Wardrop, J. L. (2001). Chronicity and instability of children's peer victimization experiences as predictors of loneliness and social satisfaction trajectories. *Child Development, 72,* 134.

Konner, M. J. (1981). Evolution of human behavior development. In R. H. Munroe, R. L. Munroe, & B. B. Whiting (Eds.), *Handbook of cross-cultural human development* (pp. 3–51). New York: Garland STPM Press.

Kovacs, D. M., Parker, J. G., & Hoffman, L. W. (1996). Behavioral, affective, and social correlates of involvement in cross-sex friendship in elementary school. *Child Development, 67,* 2269–2286.

Kramer, L., & Gottman, J. M. (1992). Becoming a sibling: With a little help from my friends. *Developmental Psychology, 28,* 685–699.

Krappmann, L. (1996). Amicitia, drujba, shin-yu, philia, freundschaft, friendship: On the cultural diversity of a human relationship. In W. M. Bukowski, A. F. Newcomb, & W. W. Hartup (Eds.), *The company they keep: Friendships in childhood and adolescence* (pp. 19–40). New York: Cambridge University Press.

Kruger, A. (1992). The effect of peer and adult–child transactive discussions on moral reasoning. *Merrill-Palmer Quarterly, 38,* 191–211.

Kubiszyn, T. (1999). Integrating health and mental health services in schools: Psychologists collaborating with primary care providers. *Clinical Psychology Review, 147,* 179–198.

Kumpulainen, K., & Kaartinen, S. (2003). The interpersonal dynamics of collaborative reasoning in peer interactive dyads. *Journal of Experimental Education, 71,* 333–370.

Kupersmidt, J. B., Burchinal, M., & Patterson, C. J. (1995). Developmental patterns of childhood peer relations as predictors of externalizing behavior problems. *Development and Psychopathology, 7,* 825–843.

Kupersmidt, J. B., DeRosier, M. E., & Patterson, C. P. (1995). Similarity as the basis for children's friendship: The roles of sociometric status, aggressive and withdrawn behavior, academic achievement and demographic characteristics. *Journal of Social and Personal Relationships, 12,* 439–452.

Kutnick, P., & Kington, A. (2005). Children's friendships and learning in school: Cognitive enhancement through social interaction? *British Journal of Educational Psychology, 75,* 521–538.

LaFromboise, T., Coleman, H. L. K., & Gerton, J. (1993). Psychological impact of biculturalism: Evidence and theory. *Psychological Bulletin, 114,* 395–412.

Ladd, G. W. (1981). Effectiveness of a social learning method for enhancing children's social interaction and peer acceptance. *Child Development, 52,* 171–178.

Ladd, G. W. (1983). Social networks of popular, average, and rejected children in school settings. *Merrill-Palmer Quarterly, 29,* 283–307.

Ladd, G. W. (1985). Documenting the effects of social skills training with children: Process and outcome assessment. In B. H. Schneider, K. H. Rubin, & J. E. Ledingham (Eds.), *Children's peer relations: Issues in assessment and intervention* (pp. 243–269). New York: Springer-Verlag.

Ladd, G. W. (1990). Having friends, keeping friends, making friends, and being liked by peers in the classroom: Predictors of children's early school adjustment? *Child Development, 61,* 1081–1100.

Ladd, G. W. (1999). Peer relationships and social competence during early and middle childhood. *Annual Review of Psychology, 50,* 333–359.

Ladd, G. W., Buhs, E. S., & Troop, W. (2002). Children's interpersonal skills and relationships in school settings: Adaptive significance and implications for school-based prevention and intervention programs. In P. K. Smith & C. H. Hart (Eds.), *Blackwell handbook of childhood social development* (pp. 394–415). Malden, MA: Blackwell.

Ladd, G. W., & Burgess, K. B. (1999). Charting the relationship trajectories of aggressive, withdrawn, and aggressive/withdrawn children during early grade school. *Child Development, 70,* 910–929.

Ladd, G. W., & Kochenderfer, B. J. (1996). Linkages between friendship and adjustment during early school transitions. In W. M. Bukowski, A. F. Newcomb, & W. W. Hartup (Eds.), *The company they keep: Friendships in childhood and adolescence* (pp. 322–345). New York: Cambridge University Press.

Ladd, G. W., Kochenderfer, B. J., & Coleman, C. C. (1996). Friendship quality as a predictor of young children's early school adjustment. *Child Development, 67,* 1103–1118.

Ladd, G. W., Kochenderfer, B. J., & Coleman, C. C. (1997). Classroom peer acceptance, friendship, and victimization: Distinct relational systems that contribute uniquely to children' school adjustment? *Child Development, 68,* 1181–1197.

Ladd, G. W., & Pettit, G. S. (2002). Parenting and the development of children's peer relationships. In M. H. Bornstein (Ed.), *Handbook of parenting: Vol. 5. Practical issues in parenting* (2nd ed., pp. 269–309). Mahwah, NJ: Erlbaum.

Ladd, G. W., & Troop-Gordon, W. (2003). The role of chronic peer difficulties in the development of children's psychological adjustment problems. *Child Development, 74,* 1344–1367.

LaFreniere, P. J., & Sroufe, L. (1985). Profiles of peer competence in the preschool: Interrelations between measures, influence of social ecology, and relation to attachment history. *Developmental Psychology, 21,* 56–69.

La Gaipa, J. J. (1979). A developmental study of the meaning of friendship in adolescence. *Journal of Adolescence, 2,* 201–213.

Lagattuta, K., & Wellman, H. M. (2001). Thinking about the past: Early knowledge about links between prior experience, thinking, and emotion. *Child Development, 72,* 82–102.

Lagattuta, K., & Wellman, H. M. (2002). Differences in early parent–child conversations about negative versus positive emotions: Implications for the development of psychological understanding. *Developmental Psychology, 38,* 564–580.

La Greca, A. M. (1993). Social skills training with children: Where do we go from here? *Journal of Clinical Child Psychology, 22,* 288–298.

La Greca, A. M., & Harrison, H. M. (2005). Adolescent peer relations, friendships, and romantic relationships: Do they predict social anxiety and depression? *Journal of Clinical Child and Adolescent Psychology, 34,* 49–61.

Laible, D. J., Carlo, G., & Raffaelli, M. (2000). The differential relations of parent and peer attachment to adolescent adjustment. *Journal of Youth and Adolescence, 29,* 45–59.

Laible, D. J., & Thompson, R. A. (2000). Mother–child discourse, attachment security, shared positive affect, and early conscience development. *Child Development, 71,* 1424–1440.

Laird, R. D., Jordan, K. Y., Dodge, K. A., Pettit, G. S., & Bates, J. E. (2001). Peer rejection in childhood, involvement with antisocial peers in early adolescence, and the development of externalizing behavior problems. *Development and Psychopathology, 13,* 337–354.

Lamarche, V., Brendgen, M., Boivin, M., Vitaro, F., Perusse, D., & Dionne, G. (2006). Do friendships and sibling relationships provide protection against peer victimization in a similar way? *Social Development, 15,* 373–393.

Laner, M., & Russell, J. (1998). Desired characteristics of spouses and best friends: Do they differ by sex and/or gender? *Sociological Inquiry, 68,* 186–202.

Lansford, J. E. (2004). Links between family relationships and best friendships in the United States and Japan. *International Journal of Aging and Human Development, 59,* 287–304.

Lansford, J. E., Capanna, C., Dodge, K. A., Caprara, G. V., Bates, J. E., Pettit, G. S., et al. (2007). Peer social preference and depressive symptoms of children in Italy and the United States. *International Journal of Behavioral Development, 31,* 274–283.

Lansford, J. E., Putallaz, M., Grimes, C. L., Schiro-Osman, K. A., Kupersmidt, J. B., & Coie, J. D. (2006). Perceptions of friendship quality and observed behaviors with friends: How do sociometrically rejected, average, and popular girls differ? *Merrill-Palmer Quarterly, 52,* 694–720.

Larose, S., & Bernier, A. (2001). Social support processes: Mediators of attachment state of mind and adjustment in late adolescence. *Attachment and Human Development, 3,* 96–120.

Larsen, H., Branje, S. J. T., van der Valk, I., & Meeus, W. H. J. (2007). Friendship quality as a moderator between perception of interparental conflicts and maladjustment in adolescence. *International Journal of Behavioral Development, 31,* 549–558.

Larson, R. W., Richards, M. H., Moneta, G., Holmbeck, G., & Duckett, E. (1996). Changes in adolescents' daily interactions with their families from ages 10 to 18: Disengagement and transformation. *Developmental Psychology, 32,* 744–754.

Laursen, B. (1993). Conflict management among close peers. In B. Laursen (Ed.), *Close friendships in adolescence* (pp. 39–54). San Francisco: Jossey-Bass.

Laursen, B. (2005). Dyadic and group perspectives on close relationships. *International Journal of Behavioral Development, 29,* 97–100.

Laursen, B., & Collins, W. A. (1994). Interpersonal conflict during adolescence. *Psychological Bulletin, 115,* 197–209.

Laursen, B., Finkelstein, B. D., & Betts, N. T. (2001). A developmental meta-analysis of peer conflict resolution. *Developmental Review, 21,* 423–449.

Laursen, B., Furman, W., & Mooney, K. S. (2006). Predicting Interpersonal competence and self-worth from adolescent relationships and relationship networks: Variable-centered and person-centered perspectives. *Merrill-Palmer Quarterly, 52,* 572–600.

Laursen, B., & Hafen, C. A. (2010). Future directions in the study of close relationships: Conflict is bad (except when it's not). *Social Development, 19,* 858–872.

Laursen, B., & Hartup, W. W. (1989). The dynamics of preschool children's conflicts. *Merrill-Palmer Quarterly, 35,* 281–297.

Laursen, B., Hartup, W. W., & Koplas, A. L. (1996). Towards understanding peer conflict. *Merrill-Palmer Quarterly, 42,* 76–102.

Laursen, B., & Mooney, K. S. (2005). Why do friends matter? *Human Development, 48,* 323–326.

Laursen, B., & Mooney, K. S. (2008). Relationship network quality: Adolescent adjustment and perceptions of relationships with parents and friends. *American Journal of Orthopsychiatry, 78,* 47–53.

Laursen, B., Wilder, D., Noack, P., & Williams, V. (2000). Adolescent perceptions of reciprocity, authority, and closeness in relationships with mothers, fathers, and friends. *International Journal of Behavioral Development, 24,* 464–471.

Laursen, B., & Williams, V. A. (1997). Perceptions of interdependence and closeness in family and peer relationships among adolescents with and without romantic partners. In S. Shulman & W. A. Collins (Eds.), *Romantic relationships in adolescence: Developmental perspectives* (pp. 3–20). San Francisco: Jossey-Bass.

Lavallee, K. L., Bierman, K. L., Nix, R. L., & Conduct Problems Prevention Research Group. (2005). The impact of first-grade "friendship group" experiences on child social outcomes in the fast track program. *Journal of Abnormal Child Psychology, 33,* 307–324.

Lavallee, K. L., & Parker, J. G. (2009). The role of inflexible friendship beliefs, rumination, and low self-worth in early adolescents' friendship jealousy and adjustment. *Journal of Abnormal Child Psychology, 37,* 873–885.

Lempers, J. D., & Clark-Lempers, D. S. (1993). A functional comparison of same-sex and opposite-sex friendships during adolescence. *Journal of Adolescent Research, 8,* 89–108.

Leung, K., & Wu, P. (1990). Dispute processing: A cross-cultural analysis. In R. W. Brislin (Ed.), *Applied cross-cultural psychology* (pp. 209–231). Thousand Oaks, CA: Sage.

LeVine, R. A. (2007). Ethnographic studies of childhood: A historical overview. *American Anthropologist, 109,* 247–260.

Levinger, G. (1983). Development and change. In H. H. Kelley, E. Berscheid, A. Christensen, J. H. Harvey, T. L. Huston, G. Levinger, et al. (Eds.), *Close relationships* (pp. 315–359). New York: Freeman.

Levy, G. D. (2000). Individual differences in race schematicity as predictors of African American and white children's race-relevant memories and peer preferences. *Journal of Genetic Psychology, 16,* 400–419.

Lewis, M., Young, C., Brooks, J., & Michalson, L. (1975). The beginning of friendship. In M. Lewis & L. A. Rosenblum (Eds.), *Friendship and peer relations: The origins of behavior* (Vol. 4). New York: Wiley.

Li, Z., Connolly, J., Jiang, D., Pepler, D., & Craig, W. (2010). Adolescent romantic relationships in China and Canada: A cross-national comparison. *International Journal of Behavioral Development, 34,* 113–120.

Lieberman, M., Doyle, A-B., & Markiewicz, D. (1999). Developmental patterns in security of attachment to mother and father in late childhood and early adolescence: Associations with peer relations. *Child Development, 70,* 202–213.

Lieberman, S. N., & Smith, L. B. (1991). Duo therapy: A bridge to the world of peers for the ego-impaired child. *Journal of Child and Adolescent Group Therapy, 1,* 243–252.

Lindsey, E. W. (2002). Preschool children's friendships and peer acceptance: Links to social competence. *Child Study Journal, 32,* 145–156.

Lindsey, E. W., Colwell, M. J., Frabutt, J. M., & MacKinnon-Lewis, C. (2006). Family conflict in divorced and non-divorced families: Potential consequences for boys' friendship status and friendship quality. *Journal of Social and Personal Relationships, 23,* 45–63.

Little, T. D., Brendgen, M., Wanner, B., & Krappmann, L. (1999). Children's reciprocal perceptions of friendship quality in the sociocultural contexts of East and West Berlin. *International Journal of Behavioral Development, 23,* 63–89.

Lochman, J. E. (1992). Cognitive-behavioral interventions with aggressive boys: Three year follow-up and preventative efforts. *Journal of Consulting and Clinical Psychology, 60,* 426–432.

Lochman, J. E., Burch, P. R., Curry, J. F., & Lampron, L. B. (1984). Treatment and generalization effects of cognitive-behavioral and goal-setting interventions with aggressive boys. *Journal of Consulting and Clinical Psychology, 52,* 915–916.

Lochman, J. E., Dunn, S. E., & Klimes-Dougan, B. (1993). An intervention and consultation model from a social cognitive perspective: A description of the anger coping program. *School Psychology Review, 22,* 458–471.

Lochman, J. E., Lampron, L. B., Gemmer, T. C., Harris, S. R., & Wyckoff, G. M. (1989). Teacher consultation and cognitive-behavioral interventions with aggressive boys. *Psychology in the Schools, 26,* 179–188.

Lochman, J. E., & Lenhart, L. A. (1993). Anger coping intervention for aggressive children: Conceptual models and outcome effects. *Clinical Psychology Review, 13,* 785–805.

Lochman, J. E., Nelson, W. M., III, & Sims, J. P. (1981). A cognitive-behavioral program for use with aggressive children. *Journal of Clinical Child Psychology, 13,* 527–538.

Lochman, J. E., & Wells, K. C. (1996). A social-cognitive intervention with aggressive children: Prevention effects and contextual implementation issues. In R. D. Peters & R. J. McMahon (Eds.), *Prevention and early intervention: Childhood disorders, substance use and delinquency* (pp. 111–143). Thousand Oaks, CA: Sage.

Lochman, J. E., & Wells, K. C. (2002a). Contextual social-cognitive mediators and child outcome: A test of the theoretical model in the coping power program. *Development and Psychopathology, 14,* 945–967.

Lochman, J. E., & Wells, K. C. (2002b). The coping power program at the middle-school transition: Universal and indicated prevention effects. *Psychology of Addictive Behaviors, 16,* S40–S54.

Lochman, J. E., & Wells, K. C. (2004). The coping power program for preadolescent aggressive boys and their parents: Outcome effects at the 1-year follow-up. *Journal of Consulting and Clinical Psychology, 72,* 571–578.

Lott, B. E., & Lott, A. J. (1960). The formation of positive attitudes toward group members. *Journal of Abnormal and Social Psychology, 61,* 297–300.

Lott, B. E., & Lott, A. J. (1974). The role of reward in the formation of positive interpersonal attitudes. In T. L. Huston (Ed.), *Foundations of interpersonal attraction* (pp. 171–192). New York: Academic Press.

Lucas-Thompson, R., & Clarke-Stewart, K. A. (2007). Forecasting friendship: How marital quality, maternal mood, and attachment security are linked to children's peer relationships. *Journal of Applied Developmental Psychology, 28,* 499–514.

Lyman, D. R., & Selman, R. L. (1985). Peer conflict in pair therapy: Clinical and developmental analyses. In M. W. Berkowitz (Ed.), *Peer conflict and psychological growth. New Directions for Child Development, 29,* 41–54.

Maccoby, E. E. (1998). *The two sexes: Growing up apart, coming together.* Cambridge, MA: Belknap Press of Harvard University Press.

Maguire, M. C., & Dunn, J. (1997). Friendships in early childhood, and social understanding. *International Journal of Behavioral Development, 21,* 669–686.

Main, M. (1991). Metacognitive knowledge, metacognitive monitoring, and singular (coherent) vs. multiple (incoherent) model of attachment: Findings and directions for future research. In C. Parkes, J. Stevenson-Hinde, & P. Marris (Eds.), *Attachment across the life cycle* (pp. 127–159). New York: Tavistock/Routledge.

Main, M., Kaplan, N., & Cassidy, J. (1985). Security in infancy, childhood, and adulthood: A move to the level of representation. *Monographs of the Society for Research in Child Development, 50,*(1–2), 66–104.

Malcolm, K. T., Jensen-Campbell, L. A., Rex-Lear, M., & Waldrip, A. M. (2006).

Divided we fall: Children's friendships and peer victimization. *Journal of Social and Personal Relationships, 23,* 721–740.

Malecki, C., & Demaray, M. (2003). What type of support do they need?: Investigating student adjustment as related to emotional, informational, appraisal, and instrumental support. *School Psychology Quarterly, 18,* 231–252.

Malik, N. M., & Furman, W. (1993). Practitioner review: Problems in children's peer relations: What can the clinician do? *Journal of Child Psychology and Psychiatry, 34,* 1303–1326.

Malone, M. J., & Perry, D. G. (1995, March). *Features of aggressive and victimized children's friendships and affiliative preferences.* Poster session presented at the meeting of the Society for Research in Child Development, Indianapolis, IN.

Mannarino, A. P. (1978). Friendship patterns and self-concept development in preadolescent males. *Journal of Genetic Psychology: Research and Theory on Human Development, 133,* 105–110.

Margie, N. G., Killen, M., Sinno, S., & McGlothlin, H. (2005). Minority children's intergroup attitudes about peer relationships. *British Journal of Developmental Psychology, 23,* 251–269.

Markiewicz, D., Doyle, A. B., & Brendgen, M. (2001). The quality of adolescents' friendships: Associations with mothers' interpersonal relationships, attachment to parents and friends, and prosocial behaviors. *Journal of Adolescence, 24,* 429–445.

Markiewicz, D., Lawford, H., Doyle, A., & Haggart, N. (2006). Developmental differences in adolescents' and young adults' use of mothers, fathers, best friends, and romantic partners to fulfill attachment needs. *Journal of Youth and Adolescence, 35,* 127–140.

Markus, H. R., & Kitayama, S. (1991). Culture and the self: Implications for cognition, emotion, and motivation. *Psychological Review, 98,* 224–253.

Markus, H. R., Kitayama, S., & Heiman, R. J. (1996). Culture and "basic" psychological principles. In E. T. Higgins & A. W. Kruglanski (Eds.), *Social psychology: Handbook of basic principles* (pp. 857–913). New York: Guilford Press.

Mascolo, M. F., & Fischer, K. W. (2002). Beyond the conduit: Prompting reflective learning about human development. *PsycCRITIQUES, 47,* 563–567.

Mashburn, A. J., Justice, L. M., Downer, J. T, & Pianta, R. C. (2009). Peer effects on children's language achievement during pre-kindergarten. *Child Development, 80,* 686–702.

Masten, A. S. (2005). Peer relationships and psychopathology in developmental perspective: Reflections on progress and promise. *Journal of Clinical Child and Adolescent Psychology, 34,* 87–92.

Mathur, R., & Berndt, T. J. (2006). Relations of friends' activities to friendship quality. *Journal of Early Adolescence, 26,* 365–388.

Mayer, J. D., & Beltz, C. M. (1998). Socialization, society's "emotional contract," and emotional intelligence. *Psychological Inquiry, 9,* 300–303.

McCandless, B. R., & Marshall, H. R. (1957). A picture sociometric technique for preschool children and its relation to teacher judgments of friendship. *Child Development, 28,* 139–147.

McDowell, D. J., & Parke, R. D. (2009). Parental correlates of children's peer relations: An empirical test of a tripartite model. *Developmental Psychology, 45,* 224–235.

McElhaney, K. B., Immele, A., Smith, F. D., & Allen, J. P. (2006). Attachment organization as a moderator of the link between friendship quality and adolescent delinquency. *Attachment and Human Development, 8,* 33–46.

McElwain, N. L., Cox, M. J., Burchinal, M. R., & Macfie, J. (2003). Differentiating among insecure mother–infant attachment classifications: A focus on child–friend interaction and exploration during solitary play at 36 months. *Attachment and Human Development, 5,* 136–164.

McGlothin, H., Killen, M., & Edmonds, C. (2005). European-American children's intergroup attitudes about peer relationships. *British Journal of Developmental Psychology, 23,* 227–249.

McNelles, L. R., & Connolly, J. A. (1999). Intimacy between adolescent friends: Age and gender differences in shared affect and behavioral form. *Journal of Research on Adolescence, 9,* 143–159.

Mead, G. H. (1934). *Mind, self, and society.* Chicago: University of Chicago Press.

Meeus, W., Oosterwegel, A., & Vollebergh, W. (2002). Parental and peer attachment and identity development in adolescence. *Journal of Adolescence, 25,* 93–106.

Mendelson, M. J., & Aboud, F. E. (1999). Measuring friendship quality in late adolescents and young adults: McGill friendship questionnaires. *Canadian Journal of Behavioural Science, 31,* 130–132.

Mendelson, M. J., Aboud, F. E., & Lanthier, R. P. (1994). Kindergartners' relationships with siblings, peers, and friends. *Merrill-Palmer Quarterly, 40,* 416–435.

Menesini, E. (1997). Behavioural correlates of friendship status among Italian schoolchildren. *Journal of Social and Personal Relationships, 14,* 109–121.

Miell, D., & MacDonald, R. (2000). Children's creative collaborations: The importance of friendship when working together on a musical composition. *Social Development, 9,* 348–369.

Mikami, A. Y., Lerner, M. D., Griggs, M. S., McGrath, A., & Calhoun, C. D. (2010). Parental influence on children with attention-deficit/hyperactivity disorder: II. Results of a pilot intervention training parents as friendship coaches for children. *Journal of Abnormal Child Psychology, 38,* 737–749.

Mikami, A. Y., Szwedo, D. E., Allen, J. P., Evans, M. A., & Hare, A. L. (2010). Adolescent peer relationships and behavior problems predict young adults' communication on social networking websites. *Developmental Psychology, 46,* 46–56.

Minuchin, P. (1988). Relationships within the family: A systems perspective on development. In R. A. Hinde & J. Stevenson-Hinde (Eds.), *Relationships within families: Mutual influences* (pp. 7–26). Oxford, UK: Clarendon Press.

Minuchin, S. (1974). *Families and family therapy.* Cambridge, MA: Harvard University Press.

Mishna, F., Wiener, J., & Pepler, D. (2008). Some of my best friends—Experiences of bullying within friendships. *School Psychology International, 29,* 549–573.

Mize, J., & Ladd, G. W. (1990). A cognitive-social learning approach to social skill training with low-status preschool children. *Developmental Psychology, 26,* 388–397.

Moffitt, T. E. (1993). Adolescence-limited and life-course-persistent antisocial behavior: A developmental taxonomy. *Psychological Review, 100,* 674–701.

Monahan, K. C., Steinberg, L., & Cauffman, E. (2009). Affiliation with antisocial peers, susceptibility to peer influence, and antisocial behavior during the transition to adulthood. *Developmental Psychology, 2009,* 1520–1530.

Mounts, N. S. (2004). Adolescents' perceptions of parental management of peer relationships in an ethnically diverse sample. *Journal of Adolescent Research, 19,* 446–467.

Mouttapa, M., Valente, T., Gallaher, P., Rohrback, L. A., & Unger, J. B. (2004). Social network predictors of bullying and victimization. *Adolescence, 39,* 315–335.

Mrug, S., Hoza, B., & Bukowski, W. M. (2004). Choosing or being chosen by aggressive-disruptive peers: Do they contribute to children's externalizing and internalizing problems? *Journal of Abnormal Child Psychology, 32,* 53–65.

Mrug, S., Hoza, B., & Gerdes, A. C. (2001). Children with attention-deficit/hyperactivity disorder: Peer relationships and peer-oriented interventions. In D. Nangle & C. Erdley (Eds.), *The role of friendship in psychological adjustment. New Directions for Child and Adolescent Development, 91,* 51–77.

Muris, P., Meesters, C., Vincken, M., & Eijkelenboom, A. (2005). Reducing children's aggressive and opposition behaviors in the schools: Preliminary results on the effectiveness of a social-cognitive group intervention program. *Child and Family Behavior Therapy, 27,* 17–32.

Nagy, E., Loveland, K. A., Kopp, M., Orvos, H., Pal, A., & Molnar, P. (2001). Different emergence of fear expressions in infant boys and girls. *Infant Behavior and Development, 24,* 189–194.

Nangle, D. W., Erdley, C. A., & Gold, J. A. (1996). A reflection on the popularity construct: The importance of who likes or dislikes a child. *Behavior Therapy, 27,* 337–352.

Nangle, D. W., Erdley, C. A., Newman, J. E., Mason, C. A., & Carpenter, E. M. (2003). Popularity, friendship quantity, and friendship quality: Interactive influences on children's loneliness and depression. *Journal of Clinical Child and Adolescent Psychology, 32,* 546–555.

New, R. S. (1994). Child's play—una cosa naturale: An Italian perspective. In J. L. Roopnarine, J. E. Johnson, & F. H. Hooper (Eds.), *Children's play in diverse cultures* (pp. 123–147). Albany: State University of New York Press.

Newcomb, A. F., & Bagwell, C. L. (1995). Children's friendship relations: A meta-analytic review. *Psychological Bulletin, 117,* 306–347.

Newcomb, A. F., & Bagwell, C. L. (1996). The developmental significance of children's friendship relations. In W. M. Bukowski, A. F. Newcomb, & W.

W. Hartup (Eds.), *The company they keep: Friendship in childhood and adolescence* (pp. 289–321). New York: Cambridge University Press.

Newcomb, A. F., & Brady, J. E. (1982). Mutuality in boys' friendship relations. *Child Development, 53,* 392–395.

Newcomb, A. F., & Bukowski, W. M. (1983). Social impact and social preference as determinants of children's peer group status. *Developmental Psychology, 19,* 856–867.

Newcomb, A. F., Bukowski, W. M., & Bagwell, C. L. (1999). Knowing the sounds: Friendship as a developmental context. In W. A. Collins & B. Laursen (Eds.), *Relationships as developmental contexts* (pp. 63–84). Mahwah, NJ: Erlbaum.

Newcomb, A. F., Bukowski, W. M., & Pattee, L. (1993). Children's peer relations: A meta-analytic review of popular, rejected, neglected, controversial, and average sociometric status. *Psychological Bulletin, 113,* 99–128.

Newton, C., Taylor, G., & Wilson, D. (1996). Circle of friends: An inclusive approach to meeting emotional and behavioral needs. *Educational Psychology, 11,* 41–48.

Nomaguchi, K. M. (2008). Gender, family structure, and adolescents' primary confidants. *Journal of Marriage and Family, 70,* 1213–1227.

Oden, S., & Asher, S. R. (1977). Coaching children in social skills for friendship making. *Child Development, 48,* 495–506.

Oden, S., Hertzberger, S. D., Mangaine, P. L., & Wheeler, V. A. (1984). Children's peer relationship: An examination of social processes. In J. C. Masters & K. Yarkin-Levin (Eds.), *Boundary areas in social and developmental psychology* (pp. 182–213). New York: Academic Press.

Ojanen, T., Sijtsema, J. J., Hawley, P. H., & Little, T. D. (2010). Intrinsic and extrinsic motivation in early adolescents' friendship development: Friendship selection, influence, and prospective friendship quality. *Journal of Adolescence, 33,* 837–851.

Oldenberg, C. M., & Kerns, K. A. (1997). Associations between peer relationships and depressive symptoms: Testing moderator effects of gender and age. *Journal of Early Adolescence, 17,* 319–337.

Oliveri, M. E., & Reiss, D. (1987). Social networks of family members: Distinctive roles of mothers and fathers. *Sex Roles, 17,* 719–738.

Ollendick, T. H., Weist, M. D., Borden, M. G., & Greene, R. W. (1992). Sociometric status and academic, behavioral, and psychological adjustment: A 5-year longitudinal study. *Journal of Consulting and Clinical Psychology, 60,* 80–87.

Olweus, D. (1993). Bully/victim problems among schoolchildren: Long-term consequences and an effective intervention program. In S. Hodgins (Ed.), *Mental disorder and crime* (pp. 317–349). Thousand Oaks, CA: Sage.

Olweus, D. (2004). The Olweus bullying prevention programme: Design and implementation issues and a new national initiative in Norway. In P. K. Smith, D. Pepler, & K. Rigby (Eds.), *Bullying in schools: How successful can interventions be?* (pp. 13–36). New York: Cambridge University Press.

Olweus, D., & Limber, S. P. (2010). The Olweus bullying prevention program. In S. R. Jimerson, S. M. Swearer, & D. L. Espelage (Eds.), *Handbook of bullying in schools: An international perspective* (pp. 377–401). New York: Routledge.

Oppenheim, D., Nir, A., Warren, S., & Emde, R. N. (1997). Emotion regulation in mother–child narrative co-construction: Associations with children's narratives and adaptation. *Developmental Psychology, 33,* 284–294.

Oyserman, D., Coon, H. M., & Kemmelmeier, M. (2002). Rethinking individualism and collectivism: Evaluation of theoretical assumptions and meta-analyses. *Psychological Bulletin, 128,* 3–72.

Pagel, M. D., Erdly, W. W., & Becker, J. (1987). Social networks: We get by with (and in spite of) a little help from our friends. *Journal of Personality and Social Psychology, 53,* 793–804.

Paley, V. (2004). *A child's work: The importance of fantasy play.* Chicago: University of Chicago Press.

Panak, W. F., & Garber, J. (1992). Role of aggression, rejection, and attributions in the prediction of depression in children. *Development and Psychopathology, 4,* 145–165.

Panella, D., & Henggeler, S. W. (1986). Peer interactions of conduct-disordered, anxious-withdrawn, and well-adjusted black adolescents. *Journal of Abnormal Child Psychology, 14,* 1–11.

Park, K. A., Lay, K. L., & Ramsay, L. (1993). Individual differences and developmental changes in preschoolers' friendships. *Developmental Psychology, 29,* 264–270.

Park, K. A., & Waters, E. (1989). Security of attachment and preschool friendships. *Child Development, 60,* 1076.

Parke, R. D., & Buriel, R. (1998). Socialization in the family: Ethnic and ecological perspectives. In W. Damon (Series Ed.) & N. Eisenberg (Vol. Ed.), *Handbook of child psychology: Vol. 3. Social, emotional, and personality development* (5th ed., pp. 463–552). New York: Wiley.

Parke, R. D., Burks, V. M., Carson, J. L., Neville, B., & Boyum, L. A. (1994). Family–peer relationships: A tripartite model. In R. D. Parke & S. G. Kellam (Eds.), *Exploring family relationships with other social contexts* (pp. 115–145). Hillsdale, NJ: Erlbaum.

Parke, R. D., & Ladd, G. W. (Eds.). (1992). *Family–peer relationships: Modes of linkage.* Hillsdale, NJ: Erlbaum.

Parke, R. D., Simpkins, S. D., McDowell, D. J., Kim, M., Killian, C., Dennis, J., et al. (2002). Relative contributions of families and peers to children's social development. In P. K. Smith & C. H. Hart (Eds.), *Blackwell handbook of childhood social development* (pp. 156–177). Malden, MA: Blackwell.

Parker, J. G., & Asher, S. R. (1987). Peer relations and later personal adjustment: Are low-accepted children at risk? *Psychological Bulletin, 102,* 357–389.

Parker, J. G., & Asher, S. R. (1993). Friendship and friendship quality in middle childhood: Links with peer group acceptance and feelings of loneliness and social dissatisfaction. *Developmental Psychology, 29,* 611–621.

Parker, J. G., & Gottman, J. M. (1989). Social and emotional development in a relational context: Friendship interaction from early childhood to adolescence. In T. J. Berndt & G. W. Ladd (Eds.), *Peer relationships in child development* (pp. 95–131). Oxford, UK: Wiley.

Parker, J. G., Kruse, S. A., & Aikins, J. W. (2010). When friends have other friends: Friendship jealousy in childhood and early adolescence. In S. L. Hart & M. Legerstee (Eds.), *Handbook of jealousy: Theory, research, and multidisciplinary approaches* (pp. 516–546). New York: Wiley-Blackwell.

Parker, J. G., Rubin, K., Price, J., & DeRosier, M. (1995). Peer relationships, child development, and adjustment. In D. Cicchetti & D. Cohen (Eds.), *Developmental psychopathology: Vol. 2. Risk, disorder, and adaptation* (pp. 96–161). New York: Wiley.

Parker, J. G., & Seal, J. (1996). Forming, losing, renewing, and replacing friendships: Applying temporal parameters to the assessment of children's friendship experiences. *Child Development, 67,* 2248–2268.

Parkhurst, J. T., & Asher, S. R. (1992). Peer rejection in middle school: Subgroup differences in behavior, loneliness, and interpersonal concerns. *Developmental Psychology, 28,* 231–241.

Patterson, G. R. (1995). Coercion as a basis for early age of onset for arrest. In J. McCord (Ed.), *Coercion and punishment in long-term perspectives* (pp. 81–105). New York: Cambridge University Press.

Patterson, G. R. (2002). The early development of coercive family process. In J. B. Reid, G. R. Patterson, & J. Snyder (Eds.), *Antisocial behavior in children and adolescents: A developmental analysis and model for intervention* (pp. 25–44). Washington, DC: American Psychological Association.

Patterson, G. R., Capaldi, D. M., & Bank, L. (1991). An early starter model for predicting delinquency. In D. J. Pepler & K. H. Rubin (Eds.), *The development and treatment of childhood aggression* (pp. 139–168). Hillsdale, NJ: Erlbaum.

Patterson, G. R., Dishion, T. J., & Yoerger, K. (2000). Adolescent growth in new forms of problem behavior: Macro- and micro-peer dynamics. *Prevention Science, 1,* 3–13.

Patterson, G. R., Littman, R. A., & Bricker, W. (1967). Assertive behavior in children: A step toward a theory of aggression. *Monographs of the Society for Research in Child Development, 32,* No. 5(Serial No. 113).

Patterson, G. R., & Yoerger, K. (2002). A developmental model for early- and late-onset delinquency. In J. B. Reid, G. R. Patterson, & J. Snyder (Eds.), *Antisocial behavior in children and adolescents: A developmental analysis and model for intervention* (pp. 147–172). Washington, DC: American Psychological Association.

Paul, E. L., & White, K. M. (1990). The development of intimate relationships in late adolescence. *Adolescence, 25,* 375–400.

Pearpoint, J., Forest, M., & O'Brien, J. (1996). MAPs, circles of friends, and PATH: Powerful tools to help build caring communities. In S. B. Stainback & W. C. Stainback (Eds.), *Inclusion: A guide for educators* (pp. 67–86). Baltimore: Brookes.

Pelham, W. E., Jr., & Hoza, B. (1996). Intensive treatment: A summer treatment program for children with ADHD. In E. D. Hibbs & P. S. Jensen (Eds.), *Psychosocial treatments for child and adolescent disorders: Empirically based strategies for clinical practice* (pp. 311–340). Washington, DC: American Psychological Association.

Pellegrini, A. D., Bartini, M., & Brooks, F. (1999). School bullies, victims, and aggressive victims: Factors relating to group affiliation and victimization in early adolescence. *Journal of Educational Psychology, 91,* 216–224.

Pellegrini, A. D., & Galda, L. (2001). "I'm so glad I'm glad": The role of emotions and close relationships in children's play and narrative language. In A. Goncu & E. L. Klein (Eds.), *Children in play, story, and school* (pp. 204–219). New York: Guilford Press.

Pellegrini, A. D., Galda, L., Bartini, M., & Charak, D. (1998). Oral language and literacy language in context: The role of social relationships. *Merrill-Palmer Quarterly, 44,* 38–54.

Pellegrini, A. D., & Long, J. D. (2002). A longitudinal study of bullying, dominance, and victimization during the transition from primary school through secondary school. *British Journal of Developmental Psychology, 20,* 259–280.

Pellegrini, D. S., & Urbain, E. S. (1985). An evaluation of interpersonal problem solving training with children. *Journal of Child Psychology and Psychiatry, 26,* 17–41.

Perlman, D., & Fehr, B. (1986). Theories of friendship: The analysis of interpersonal attraction. In V. J. Derlega & B. A. Winstead (Eds.), *Friendship and social interaction* (pp. 9–40). New York: Springer-Verlag.

Peterson, L., Mullins, L. L., & Ridley-Johnson, R. (1985). Childhood depression: Peer reactions to depression and life stress. *Journal of Abnormal Child Psychology, 13,* 597–609.

Pettit, G. (1997). The untold story of childhood friendships. *PsycCRITIQUES, 42,* 807–808.

Phillipsen, L. C. (1999). Associations between age, gender, and group acceptance and three components of friendship quality. *Journal of Early Adolescence, 19,* 438–464.

Piaget, J. (1926). *The language and thought of a child.* Oxford, UK: Harcourt, Brace.

Piaget, J. (1932). *The moral judgment of the child.* New York: Free Press.

Piehler, T. F., & Dishion, T. J. (2007). Interpersonal dynamics within adolescent friendships: Dyadic mutuality, deviant talk, and patterns of antisocial behavior. *Child Development, 78,* 1611–1624.

Pike, A., & Atzaba-Poria, N. (2003). Do sibling and friend relationships share the same temperamental origins? A twin study. *Journal of Child Psychology and Psychiatry, 44,* 598–611.

Pike, A., & Eley, T. C. (2009). Links between parenting and extra-familial relationships: Nature or nurture? *Journal of Adolescence, 32,* 519–533.

Pilgrim, C., & Rueda-Riedle, A. (2002). The importance of social context in cross-cultural comparisons: First graders in Colombia and the United States. *Journal of Genetic Psychology, 163,* 283–295.

Pinto, G., Bombi, A. S., & Cordioli, A. (1997). Similarity of friends in three countries: A study of children's drawings. *International Journal of Behavioral Development, 20,* 453–469.

Poe, J., Dishion, T. J., Griesler, P., & Andrews, D. W. (1990). *Topic code.* Unpublished coding manual, Oregon Social Learning Center, Eugene, OR.

Popp, D., Laursen, B., Kerr, M., Stattin, H., & Burk, W. K. (2008). Modeling homophily over time with an actor-partner interdependence model. *Developmental Psychology, 44*, 1028–1039.

Poulin, F., & Boivin, M. (1999). Proactive and reactive aggression and boys' friendship quality in mainstream classrooms. *Journal of Emotional and Behavioral Disorders, 7*, 168–177.

Poulin, F., Dishion, T. J., & Haas, E. (1999). The peer influence paradox: Friendship quality and deviancy training within male adolescent friendships. *Merrill-Palmer Quarterly, 45*, 42–61.

Preissler, M. (2006). Play and autism: Facilitating symbolic understanding. In D. G. Singer, R. Golinkoff, & K. Hirsh-Pasek (Eds.), *Play = learning: How play motivates and enhances children's cognitive and social-emotional growth* (pp. 231–250). New York: Oxford University Press.

Prinstein, M. J., Boergers, J., Spirito, A., Little, T. D., & Grapentine. W. L. (2000). Peer functioning, family dysfunction, and psychological symptoms in a risk factor model for adolescent inpatients' suicidal ideation severity. *Journal of Clinical Child Psychology, 29*, 392–405.

Prinstein, M. J., & Dodge, K. A. (Eds.). (2008). *Understanding peer influence in children and adolescents.* New York: Guilford Press.

Prinstein, M. J., Heilbron, N., Guerry, J. D., Franklin, J. C., Rancourt, D., Simon, V., et al. (2010). Peer influence and nonsuicidal self injury: Longitudinal results in community and clinically-referred adolescent samples. *Journal of Abnormal Child Psychology, 38*, 669–682.

Prinstein, M. J., Meade, C. S., & Cohen, G. L. (2003). Adolescent oral sex, peer popularity, and perceptions of best friends's sexual behavior. *Journal of Pediatric Psychology, 28*(4), 243–249.

Putallaz, M. (1987). Maternal behavior and children's sociometric status. *Child Development, 58*, 324.

Quinn, M., Kavale, K., Mathur, S., Rutherford, R., & Forness, S. (1999). A meta-analysis of social skill interventions for students with emotional or behavioral disorders. *Journal of Emotional and Behavioral Disorders, 7*, 1478–1487.

Rabiner, D., & Coie, J. D. (1989). Effect of expectancy inductions on rejected children's acceptance by unfamiliar peers. *Developmental Psychology, 25*, 450–457.

Radmacher, K., & Azmitia, M. (2006). Are there gendered pathways to intimacy in early adolescents' and emerging adults' friendships? *Journal of Adolescent Research, 21*, 415–448.

Rao, N., & Stewart, S. M. (1999). Cultural influences on sharer and recipient behavior: Sharing in Chinese and Indian preschool children. *Journal of Cross-Cultural Psychology, 30*, 219–241.

Rathunde, K., & Csikszentmihalyi, M. (2005). The social context of middle school: Teachers, friends, and activities in Montessori and traditional school environments. *Elementary School Journal, 106*, 59–79.

Rawlins, W. K. (1992). *Friendship matters: Communication, dialectics, and the life course.* New York: Aldine.

Reavis, R. D., Keane, S. P., & Calkins, S. D. (2010). Trajectories of peer victimization: The role of multiple relationships. *Merrill-Palmer Quarterly, 56,* 303–332.

Reed-Danahay, D. (1999). Friendship, kinship and the life course in rural Auvergne. In S. Bell & S. Coleman (Eds.), *The anthropology of friendship* (pp. 137–154). New York: Berg.

Reid, M., Landesman, S., Treder, R., & Jaccard, J. (1989). "My family and friends": Six- to twelve-year-old children's perceptions of social support. *Child Development, 60,* 896–910.

Reis, H. T., Collins, W. A., & Berscheid, E. (2000). The relationship context of human behavior and development. *Psychological Bulletin, 126,* 844–872.

Renshaw, P. D. (1981). The roots of current peer interaction research: A historical analysis of the 1930s. In S. R. Asher & J. M. Gottman (Eds.), *The development of children's friendships* (pp. 1–28). New York: Cambridge University Press.

Renshaw, P. D., & Brown, P. J. (1993). Loneliness in middle childhood: Concurrent and longitudinal predictors. *Child Development, 64,* 1271–1284.

Repinski, D. J., & Zook, J. M. (2005). Three measures of closeness in adolescents' relationships with parents and friends: Variations and developmental significance. *Personal Relationships, 12,* 79–102.

Rezende, C. B. (1999). Building affinity through friendship. In S. Bell & S. Coleman (Eds.), *The anthropology of friendship* (pp. 79–97). New York: Berg.

Richards, M. H., Crowe, P. A., Larson, R., & Swarr, A. (1998). Developmental patterns and gender differences in the experience of peer companionship during adolescence. *Child Development, 69,* 154–163.

Riegle-Crumb, C., & Callahan, R. (2009). Exploring the academic benefits of friendship ties for latino boys and girls. *Social Science Quarterly, 90,* 611–631.

Rizzo, T. A. (1989). *Friendship development among children in school.* Norwood, NJ: Ablex.

Rodkin, P. C., & Ahn, H. (2009). Social networks derived from affiliations and friendships, multi-informant and self-reports: Stability, concordance, placement of aggressive and unpopular children, and centrality. *Social Development, 18,* 556–576.

Rodkin, P. C., & Hanish, L. D. (Eds.). (2007). *Social network analysis and children's peer relationships.* San Francisco: Jossey-Bass.

Rogoff, B. (1990). *Apprenticeship in thinking: Cognitive development in social context.* New York: Oxford University Press.

Rogoff, B. (1998). Cognition as a collaborative process. In W. Damon (Ed.), *Handbook of child psychology: Vol. 2: Cognition, perception, and language* (pp. 679–744). Hoboken, NJ: Wiley

Rook, K. S. (1984). The negative side of social interaction: Impact on psychological well-being. *Journal of Personality and Social Psychology, 46,* 1097–1108.

Rose, A. J. (2002). Co-rumination in the friendships of girls and boys. *Child Development, 73,* 1830–1843.

Rose, A. J., & Asher, S. R. (1999). Children's goals and strategies in response to conflicts within a friendship. *Developmental Psychology, 35,* 69–79.

Rose, A. J., & Asher, S. R. (2004). Children's strategies and goals in response to help-giving and help-seeking tasks within a friendship. *Child Development, 75,* 749–763.

Rose, A. J., Carlson, W., & Waller, E. M. (2007). Prospective associations of co-rumination with friendship and emotional adjustment: Considering the socioemotional trade-offs of co-rumination. *Developmental Psychology, 43,* 1019–1031.

Rose, A. J., & Rudolph, K. D. (2006). A review of sex differences in peer relationship processes: Potential trade-offs for the emotional and behavioral development of girls and boys. *Psychological Bulletin, 132,* 98–131.

Ross, H. S., & Lollis, S. P. (1989). A social relations analysis of toddler peer relationships. *Child Development, 60,* 1082–1091.

Rotenberg, K. J., & Sliz, D. (1988). Children's restrictive disclosure to friends. *Merrill-Palmer Quarterly, 34,* 203–215.

Rubin, K. H. (2004). Three things to know about friendship. *International Society for the Study of Behavioral Development Newsletter, 46,* 5–7.

Rubin, K. H., Bukowski, W. M., & Laursen, B. (Eds.). (2009). *Handbook of peer interactions, relationships, and groups.* New York: Guilford Press.

Rubin, K. H., Bukowski, W. M., & Parker, J. G. (2006). Peer interactions, relationships, and groups. In N. Eisenberg, W. Damon, & R. M. Lerner (Eds.), *Handbook of child psychology: Vol. 3. Social, emotional, and personality development* (6th ed.), (pp. 571–645). Hoboken, NJ: Wiley.

Rubin, K. H., Dwyer, K. M., Booth-LaForce, C., Kim, A. H., Burgess, K. B., & Rose-Krasnor, L. (2004). Attachment, friendship, and psychosocial functioning in early adolescence. *Journal of Early Adolescence, 24,* 326–356.

Rubin, K. H., & Thompson, A. (2002). *The friendship factor: Helping our children navigate their social world and why it matters for their success and happiness.* New York: Penguin Books.

Rueger, S., Malecki, C., & Demaray, M. (2008). Gender differences in the relationship between perceived social support and student adjustment during early adolescence. *School Psychology Quarterly, 23,* 496–514.

Rusbult, C. (1980). Commitment and satisfaction in romantic associations: A test of the investment model. *Journal of Experimental Social Psychology, 16,* 172–186.

Russell, S. T., Kosciw, J., Horn, S., & Saewyc, E. (2010). Safe schools policy for LGBTQ students. *Society for Research in Child Development Social Policy Report, 24,* 1–20.

Rys, G. S., & Bear, G. G. (1997). Relational aggression and peer relations: Gender and developmental issues. *Merrill-Palmer Quarterly, 43,* 87–106.

Saarni, C. (1990). Emotional competence: How emotions and relationships become integrated. In R. A. Thompson (Ed.), *Nebraska Symposium on Motivation, 1988: Socioemotional development* (pp. 115–182). Lincoln: University of Nebraska Press.

Saarni, C. (1999). *The development of emotional competence.* New York: Guilford Press.

Saarni, C. (2007). The development of emotional competence: Pathways for helping children to become emotionally intelligent. In R. Bar-On, J. G. Maree, &

M. Elias (Eds.), *Educating people to be emotionally intelligent* (pp. 15–35). Westport, CT: Praeger.

Saarni, C. (2008). The interface of emotional development with social context. In M. Lewis, J. M. Haviland-Jones, & L. F. Barrett (Eds.), *Handbook of emotions* (3rd ed., pp. 332–347). New York: Guilford Press.

Saarni, C., Mumme, D. L., & Campos, J. J. (1998). Emotional development: Action, communication, and understanding. In N. Eisenberg & W. Damon (Eds.), *Handbook of child psychology: Vol. 3. Social, emotional, and personality development* (5th ed., pp. 237–309). Hoboken, NJ: Wiley.

Salmivalli, C., Huttunen, A., & Lagerspetz, K. M. J. (1997). Peer networks and bullying in schools. *Scandinavian Journal of Psychology, 38*, 305–312.

Salmivalli, C., & Isaacs, J. (2005). Prospective relations among victimization, rejection, friendlessness, and children's self- and peer-perceptions. *Child Development, 76*, 1161–1171.

Salmivalli, C., Lagerspetz, K., Bjorkqvist, K., Kaukiainen, A., & Osterman, K. (1996). Bullying as a group process: Participant roles and their relations to social status within the group. *Aggressive Behavior, 22*, 1–15.

Sanderson, C. A., Rahm, K. B., & Beigbeder, S. A. (2005). The link between the pursuit of intimacy goals and satisfaction in close same-sex friendships: An examination of the underlying processes. *Journal of Social and Personal Relationships, 22*, 75–98.

Sanderson, J. A., & Siegal, M. (1995). Loneliness and stable friendship in rejected and nonrejected preschoolers. *Journal of Applied Developmental Psychology, 16*, 555–567.

Sandler, I. N., Miller, P., Short, J., & Wolchik, S. A. (1989). Social support as a protective factor for children in stress. In D. Belle (Ed.), *Children's social networks and social supports* (pp. 277–307). New York: Wiley.

Sandstrom, M. J., & Cillessen, A. H. N. (2003). Sociometric status and children's peer experiences: Use of the daily diary method. *Merrill-Palmer Quarterly, 49*, 427–452.

Sandstrom, M. J., & Zakriski, A. L. (2004). Understanding the experience of peer rejection. In J. B. Kupersmidt & K. A. Dodge (Eds.), *Children's peer relations: From development to intervention* (pp. 101–118). Washington, DC: American Psychological Association.

Sarason, I. G., & Sarason, B. R. (1985). Life change, social support, coping, and health. In R. M. Kaplan & M. H. Criqui (Eds.), *Behavioral epidemiology and disease prevention* (pp. 219–236). New York: Plenum Press.

Savin-Williams, R. C., & Berndt, T. J. (1990). Friendships and peer relations during adolescence. In S. S. Feldman & G. Eliott (Eds.), *At the threshold: The developing adolescent* (pp. 277–307). Cambridge, MA: Harvard University Press.

Scharf, M., & Hertz-Lazarowitz, R. (2003). Social networks in the school context: Effects of culture and gender. *Journal of Social and Personal Relationships, 20*, 843–858.

Schmidt, M. E., & Bagwell, C. L. (2007). The protective role of friendship in overtly and relationally victimized boys and girls. *Merrill-Palmer Quarterly, 53*, 439–460.

Schneider, B. H. (1992). Didactic methods for enhancing children's peer relations: A quantitative review. *Clinical Psychology Review, 12,* 363–382.

Schneider, B. H. (1998). Cross-cultural comparison as doorkeeper in research on the social and emotional adjustment of children and adolescents. *Developmental Psychology, 34,* 793–797.

Schneider, B. H., Atkinson, L., & Tardif, C. (2001). Child–parent attachment and children's peer relations: A quantitative review. *Developmental Psychology, 37,* 86–100.

Schneider, B. H., Fonzi, A., Tani, F., & Tomada, G. (1997). A cross-cultural exploration of the stability of children's friendships and the predictors of their continuation. *Social Development, 6,* 322–339.

Schneider, B. H., Fonzi, A., Tomada, G., & Tani, F. (2000). A cross-national comparison of children's behavior with their friends in situations of potential conflict. *Journal of Cross-Cultural Psychology, 31,* 259–266.

Schneider, B. H., Smith, A., Poisson, S. E., & Kwan, A. B. (1997). Cultural dimensions of children's peer relations. In S. Duck (Ed.), *Handbook of personal relationships: Theory, research, and interventions* (2nd ed., pp. 121–146). Hoboken, NJ: Wiley.

Schneider, B. H., Wiener, J., & Murphy, K. (1994). Children's friendships: The giant step beyond peer acceptance. *Journal of Social and Personal Relationships, 11,* 323–340.

Schneider, B. H., Woodburn, S., Soteras del Toro, M., & Udvari, S. J. (2005). Cultural and gender differences in the implications of competition for early adolescent friendship. *Merrill-Palmer Quarterly, 51,* 163–192.

Schofield, J. W., & Eurich-Fulcer, R. (2004). When and how school desegregation improves intergroup relations. In M. B. Brewer & M. Hewstone (Eds.), *Applied social psychology* (pp. 186–205). Malden, MA: Blackwell.

Scholte, R. J., Overbeek, G., ten Brink, G., Rommes, E., de Kemp, R. A. T., Goossens, L., et al. (2009). The significance of reciprocal and unilateral friendships for peer victimization in adolescence. *Journal of Youth and Adolescence, 38,* 89–100.

Scholte, R. J., van Lieshout, C. M., & van Aken, M. G. (2001). Perceived relational support in adolescence: Dimensions, configurations, and adolescent adjustment. *Journal of Research on Adolescence, 11,* 71–94.

Schug, J., Yuki, M., Horikawa, H., & Takemura, K. (2009). Similarity attraction and actually selecting similar others: How cross-societal differences in relational mobility affect interpersonal similarity in Japan and the USA. *Asian Journal of Social Psychology, 12,* 95–103.

Schultz, L. H. (1997). A developmental and thematic analysis of pair counseling with preadolescent school-girls. In R. L. Selman, C. L. Watts, & L. H. Schultz (Eds.), *Fostering friendship: Pair therapy for treatment and prevention* (pp. 251–271). New York: Aldine.

Schwartz, D., Dodge, K. A., Pettit, G. S., Bates, J. E., & Conduct Problems Prevention Research Group. (2000). Friendship as a moderating factor in the pathway between early harsh home environment and later victimization in the peer group. *Developmental Psychology, 36,* 646–662.

Schwartz, D., Gorman, A., Dodge, K. A., Pettit, G. S., & Bates, J. E. (2008). Friendships with peers who are low or high in aggression as moderators of the link between peer victimization and declines in academic functioning. *Journal of Abnormal Child Psychology, 36,* 719–730.

Schwartz, D., McFadyen-Ketchum, S., Dodge, K. A., Pettit, G. S., & Bates, J. E. (1999). Early behaviour problems as a predictor of later peer group victimization: Moderators and mediators in the pathways of social risk. *Journal of Abnormal Child Psychology, 27,* 191–201.

Sebanc, A. M. (2003). The friendship features of preschool children: Links with prosocial behavior and aggression. *Social Development, 12,* 249–268.

Selfhout, M. H. W., Branje, S. J. T., Delsing, M., ter Bogt, T. F. M., & Meeus, W. H. J. (2009). Different types of internet use, depression, and social anxiety: The role of perceived friendship quality. *Journal of Adolescence, 32,* 819–833.

Selfhout, M. H. W., Branje, S. J. T., & Meeus, W. H. J. (2009). Developmental trajectories of perceived friendship intimacy, constructive problem solving, and depression from early to late adolescence. *Journal of Abnormal Child Psychology, 37,* 251–264.

Selman, R. L. (1980). *The growth of interpersonal understanding: Developmental and clinical analyses.* New York: Academic Press.

Selman, R. L. (1981). The development of interpersonal competence: The role of understanding in conduct. *Developmental Review, 1,* 401–422.

Selman, R. L. (1989). Fostering intimacy and autonomy. In W. Damon (Ed.), *Child development today and tomorrow* (pp. 409–435). San Francisco: Jossey-Bass.

Selman, R. L. (1997). The evolution of pair therapy. In R. L. Selman, C. L. Watts, & L. H. Schultz (Eds.), *Fostering friendship: Pair therapy for treatment and prevention* (pp. 3–18). New York: Aldine.

Selman, R. L., & Demorest, A. P. (1984). Observing troubled children's interpersonal negotiation strategies: Implications of and for a developmental model. *Child Development, 55,* 288–304.

Selman, R. L., & Schultz, L. H. (1990). *Making a friend in youth: Developmental theory and pair therapy.* Chicago: University of Chicago Press.

Selman, R. L., Schultz, L. H., Caplan, B., & Schantz, K. (1989). The development of close relationships: Implications from therapy with two early adolescent boys. In M. J. Packer & R. B. Addison (Eds.), *Entering the circle: Hermeneutic investigation in psychology* (pp. 59–93). New York: State University of New York Press.

Selman, R. L., Schultz, L. H., Nakkula, M., Barr, D., Watts, C., & Richmond, J. B. (1992). Friendship and fighting: A developmental approach to the study of risk and prevention of violence. *Development and Psychopathology, 4,* 529–558.

Shantz, C. U. (1983). Social cognition. In P. H. Mussen (Ed.), *Carmichael's manual of child psychology* (pp. 495–555). New York: Wiley.

Shantz, C. U. (1987). Conflicts between children. *Child Development, 58,* 283–305.

Shantz, C. U. (1993). Children's conflicts: Representations and lessons learned.

In R. R. Cocking & K. Renninger (Eds.), *The development and meaning of psychological distance* (pp. 185–202). Hillsdale, NJ: Erlbaum.

Shantz, C. U., & Hobart, C. J. (1989). Social conflict and development: Peers and siblings. In T. J. Berndt & G. W. Ladd (Eds.), *Peer relationships in child development* (pp. 71–94). Oxford, UK: Wiley.

Sharabany, R. (2006). The cultural context of children and adolescents: Peer relationships and intimate friendships among Arab and Jewish children in Israel. In X. Chen, D. C. French, & B. H. Schneider (Eds.), *Peer relationships in cultural context* (pp. 452–478). New York: Cambridge University Press.

Sharabany, R., Eshel, Y., & Hakim, C. (2008). Boyfriend, girlfriend in a traditional society: Parenting styles and development of intimate friendships among Arabs in school. *International Journal of Behavioral Development, 32,* 66–75.

Sharabany, R., Gershoni, R., & Hofman, J. E. (1981). Girlfriend, boyfriend: Age and sex differences in intimate friendship. *Developmental Psychology, 17,* 800–808.

Sharabany, R., & Wiseman, H. (1993). Close relationships in adolescence: The case of the kibbutz. *Journal of Youth and Adolescence, 22,* 671–695.

Shechtman, Z., Freidman, Y., Kashti, Y., & Sharabany, R. (2002). Group counseling to enhance adolescents' close friendships. *International Journal of Group Psychotherapy, 52,* 537–553.

Shin, Y. (2007). Peer relationships, social behaviours, academic performance and loneliness in Korean primary school children. *School Psychology International, 28,* 220–236.

Shipman, K. L., Zeman, J., Nesin, A. E., & Fitzgerald, M. (2003). Children's strategies for displaying anger and sadness: What works with whom? *Merrill-Palmer Quarterly, 49,* 100–122.

Shomaker, L. B., & Furman, W. (2009). Parent–adolescent relationship qualities, internal working models, and attachment styles as predictors of adolescents' interactions with friends. *Journal of Social and Personal Relationships, 2,* 579–603.

Shortt, J. W., Capaldi, D. M., Dishion, T. J., Bank, L., & Owen, L. D. (2003). The role of adolescent friends, romantic partners, and siblings in the emergence of the adult antisocial lifestyle. *Journal of Family Psychology, 17,* 521–533.

Shotton, G. (1998). A circle of friends approach with socially neglected children. *Educational Psychology in Practice, 14,* 22–25.

Shulman, S. (1993). Close friendships in early and middle adolescence: Typology and friendship reasoning. In B. Laursen (Ed.), *Close friendships in adolescence. New Directions for Child Development, 60,* 56–71.

Shulman, S., Laursen, B., Kalman, Z., & Karpovsky, S. (1997). Adolescent intimacy revisited. *Journal of Youth and Adolescence, 26,* 597–617.

Shute, R., De Blasio, T., & Williamson, P. (2002). Social support satisfaction of Australian children. *International Journal of Behavioral Development, 26,* 318–326.

Sijtsema, J. J., Lindenberg, S. M., & Veenstra, R. (2010). Do they get what they want or are they stuck with what they get?: Testing homophily against default selection for friendships of highly aggressive boys. The TRAILS study. *Journal of Abnormal Child Psychology, 38*, 803–813.

Sijtsema, J. J., Ojanen, T., Veenstra, R., Lindenberg, S., Hawley, P. H., & Little, T. D. (2010). Forms and functions of aggression in adolescent friendship selection and influence: A longitudinal social network analysis. *Social Development, 19*, 515–534.

Simmons, R. G., & Blyth, D. A. (1987). *Moving into adolescence: The impact of pubertal change and school context.* Hawthorne NY: Aldine.

Simmons, R. G., Carlton-Ford, S. L., & Blyth, D. A. (1987). Predicting how a child will cope with the transition to junior high school. In R. M. Lerner & T. T. Foch (Eds.), *Biological and psychosocial interactions in early adolescence* (pp. 325–375). Hillsdale, NJ: Erlbaum.

Simons, R. L., Wu, C., Conger, R. D., & Lorenz, F. O. (1994). Two routes to delinquency: Differences between early and late starters in the impact of parenting and deviant peers. *Criminology, 32*, 247–276.

Simpkins, S. D., & Parke, R. D. (2001). The relations between parental friendships and children's friendships: Self-report and observational analysis. *Child Development, 72*, 569–582.

Simpkins, S. D., & Parke, R. D. (2002a). Do friends and nonfriends behave differently?: A social relations analysis of children's behavior. *Merrill-Palmer Quarterly, 48*, 263–283.

Simpkins, S. D., & Parke, R. D. (2002b). Maternal monitoring and rules as correlates of children's social adjustment. *Merrill-Palmer Quarterly, 48*, 360–377.

Slomkowski, C., & Dunn, J. (1996). Young children's understanding of other people's beliefs and feelings and their connected communication with friends. *Developmental Psychology, 32*, 442–447.

Slomkowski, C. L., & Killen, M. (1992). Young children's conceptions of transgressions with friends and nonfriends. *International Journal of Behavioral Development, 15*, 247–258.

Smart, A. (1999). Expressions of interest: Friendship and *guanxi* in Chinese societies. In S. Bell & S. Coleman (Eds.), *The anthropology of friendship* (pp. 119–136). New York: Berg.

Smith, C., & Cooke, T. (2000). Collaboratively managing the behavior of a reception class pupil. *Educational Psychology in Practice, 16*, 235–242.

Smokowski, P. R., Bacallao, M., & Buchanan, R. L. (2009). Interpersonal mediators linking acculturalization stressors to subsequent internalizing symptoms and self-esteem in Latino adolescents. *Journal of Community Psychology, 37*, 1024–1045.

Snyder, J., Schrepferman, L., Oeser, J., Patterson, G., Stoolmiller, M., Johnson, K., et al. (2005). Deviancy training and association with deviant peers in young children: Occurrence and contribution to early-onset conduct problems. *Development and Psychopathology, 17*, 397–413.

Snyder, J., Stoolmiller, M., Wilson, M., & Yamamoto, M. (2003). Child anger regulation, parental responses to children's anger displays, and early child antisocial behavior. *Social Development, 12*, 335–360.

Spencer, M., Noll, E., Stoltzfus, J., & Harpalani, V. (2001). Identity and school adjustment: Revisiting the "acting white" assumption. *Educational Psychologist, 36,* 21–30.

Spinrad, T. L., Stifter, C. A., Donelan-McCall, N., & Turner, L. (2004). Mothers' regulation strategies in response to toddlers' affect: Links to later emotion self-regulation. *Social Development, 13,* 40–55.

Sroufe, L. A., & Fleeson, J. (1986). Attachment and the construction of relationships. In W. W. Hartup & Z. Rubin (Eds.), *Relationship and development* (pp. 239–252). Hillsdale, NJ: Erlbaum.

Steinberg, L. (1990). Autonomy, conflict, and harmony in the family relationship. In S. Feldman & G. R. Elliott (Eds.), *At the threshold: The developing adolescent* (pp. 255–276). Cambridge, MA: Harvard University Press.

Stocker, C., & Dunn, J. (1990). Sibling relationships in childhood: Links with friendships and peer relationships. *British Journal of Developmental Psychology, 8,* 227–244.

Stocker, C. M. (1994). Children's perceptions of relationships with siblings, friends, and mothers: Compensatory processes and links with adjustment. *Journal of Child Psychology and Psychiatry, 35,* 1447–1459.

Stout, H. (2010, June 17). A best friend? You must be kidding. *New York Times,* p. 1.

Strayer, F. F. (1989). Co-adaptation within the early peer group: A psychobiological study of social competence. In B. H. Schneider, G. Attili, J. Nadd, & R. P. Weissberg (Eds.), *Social competence in developmental perspective* (pp. 145–174). Norwell, MA: Kluwer.

Strough, J., Swenson, L. M., & Cheng, S. (2001). Friendship, gender, and preadolescents' representations of peer collaboration. *Merrill-Palmer Quarterly, 47,* 475–499.

Suarez-Orozco, C., & Suarez-Orozco, M. M. (2001). *Children of immigration.* Cambridge, MA: Harvard University Press.

Sullivan, H. S. (1953). *The interpersonal theory of psychiatry.* New York: Norton.

Sutherland, E. (1947). *Principles of criminology* (3rd ed.), Philadelphia: Lippincott.

Swenson, L. P., & Rose, A. J. (2009). Friends' knowledge of youth internalizing and externalizing adjustment: Accuracy, bias, and the influence of gender, grade, positive friendship quality, and self-disclosure. *Journal of Abnormal Child Psychology, 37,* 887–901.

Taylor, S. E., & Brown, J. D. (1988). Illusion and well-being: A social psychological perspective on mental health. *Psychological Bulletin, 103,* 193–210.

Thibaut, J. W., & Kelley, H. (1959). *The social psychology of groups.* New York: Wiley.

Thompson, M., Grace, C., & Cohen, L. (2001). *Best friends, worst enemies: Understanding the social lives of children.* New York: Ballantine Books.

Thompson, R. A. (1994). Emotion regulation: A theme in search of definition. In N. A. Fox (Ed.), The development of emotion regulation: Biological and behavioral considerations. *Monographs of the Society for Research in Child Development, 59*(2–3, Serial No. 240), 25–52.

Thompson, R. A., & Goodvin, R. (2007). Taming the tempest in the teapot:

Emotion regulation in toddlers. In C. A. Brownell & C. B. Kopp (Eds.), *Socioemotional development in the toddler years: Transitions and transformations* (pp. 320–341). New York: Guilford Press.

Thompson, R. A., & Meyer, S. (2007). Socialization of emotion regulation in the family. In J. J. Gross (Ed.), *Handbook of emotion regulation* (pp. 249–268). New York: Guilford Press.

Thornberry, T. P., & Krohn, M. D. (1997). Peers, drug use, and delinquency. In D. Stoff, J. Breiling, & J. D. Maser (Eds.), *Handbook of antisocial behavior* (pp. 218–233). New York: Wiley.

Thorne, B. (1993). *Gender play: Girls and boys in school.* New Brunswick, NJ: Rutgers University Press.

Thornton, T. N., Craft, C. A., Dahlberg, L. L., Lynch, B. S., & Baer, K. (2000). *Best practices of youth violence prevention: A sourcebook for community action.* Atlanta, GA: Centers for Disease Control and Prevention.

Tierney, T., & Dowd, R. (2000). The use of social skills groups to support girls with emotional difficulties in secondary schools. *Support for Learning, 15,* 82–85.

Tietjen, A. (1989). The ecology of children's social support networks. In D. Belle (Ed.), *Children's social networks and social supports* (pp. 37–69). New York: Wiley.

Tiffen, K., & Spence, S. H. (1986). Responsiveness of isolated versus rejected children to social skills training. *Journal of Child Psychology and Psychiatry, 27,* 343–355.

Tomada, G., Schneider, B. H., de Domini, P., Greenman, P. S., & Fonzi, A. (2005). Friendship as a predictor of adjustment following a transition to formal academic instruction and evaluation. *International Journal of Behavioral Development, 29,* 314–322.

Tomada, G., Schneider, B. H., & Fonzi, A. (2002). Verbal and nonverbal interactions of four-and five-year-old friends in potential conflict situations. *Journal of Genetic Psychology, 163,* 327–339.

Tooby, J., & Cosmides, L. (1996). Friendship and the banker's paradox: Other pathways to the evolution of adaptations for altruism. In W. G. Runciman, J. Smith, & R. M. Dunbar (Eds.), *Evolution of social behaviour patterns in primates and man* (pp. 119–143). New York: Oxford University Press.

Tremblay, R. E., Masse, L. C., Vitaro, F., & Dobkin, P. L. (1995). The impact of friends' deviant behavior on early onset of delinquency: Longitudinal data from 6 to 13 years of age. *Development and Psychopathology, 7,* 649–667.

Triandis, H. C. (1990). Theoretical concepts that are applicable to the analysis of ethnocentrism. In R. W. Brislin (Ed.), *Applied cross-cultural psychology* (pp. 34–55). Newbury Park, CA: Sage.

Triandis, H. C. (1995). *Individualism and collectivism.* Boulder, CO: Westview Press.

Triandis, H. C., Bontempo, R., Villareal, M. J., Asai, M., & Lucca, N. (1988). Individualism and collectivism: Cross-cultural perspectives on self-ingroup relationships. *Journal of Personality and Social Psychology, 54,* 323–338.

Tsethlikai, M. (2010). The influence of a friend's perspective on American Indian children's recall of previously misconstrued events. *Developmental Psychology, 46,* 1481–1496.

Tudge, J., & Rogoff, B. (1989). Peer influences on cognitive development: Piagetian and Vygotskian perspectives. In M. H. Bornstein & J. S. Bruner (Eds.), *Interaction in human development* (pp. 17–40). Hillsdale, NJ: Erlbaum.

Underwood, M. K. (2003). *Social aggression among girls.* New York: Guilford Press.

Urberg, K. A. (1999). Introduction: Some thoughts about studying the influence of peers on children and adolescents. *Merrill-Palmer Quarterly, 45,* 1–12.

Urberg, K. A., Değirmencioğlu, S. M., & Tolson, J. M. (1998). Adolescent friendship selection and termination: The role of similarity. *Journal of Social and Personal Relationships, 15,* 703–710.

Urberg, K. A., Değirmencioğlu, S. M., Tolson, J. M., & Halliday-Scher, K. (1995). The structure of adolescent peer networks. *Developmental Psychology, 31,* 540–547.

Urberg, K. A., Değirmencioğlu, S. M., Tolson, J. M., & Halliday-Scher, K. (2000). Adolescent social crowds: Measurement and relationship to friendships. *Journal of Adolescent Research, 15,* 427–445.

Valdivia, I. A., Schneider, B. H., Chavez, K. L., & Chen, X. (2005). Social withdrawal and maladjustment in a very group-oriented society. *International Journal of Behavioral Development, 29,* 219–228.

Valkenburg, P. M., & Peter, J. (2007). Preadolescents' and adolescents' online communication and their closeness to friends. *Developmental Psychology, 43,* 267–277.

van Aken, M. A. G., & Asendorpf, J. B. (1997). Support by parents, classmates, friends and siblings in preadolescence: Covariation and compensation across relationships. *Journal of Social and Personal Relationships, 14,* 79–93.

Van Horn, K. R., & Marques, J. C. (2000). Interpersonal relationships in Brazilian adolescents. *International Journal of Behavioral Development, 24,* 199–203.

van Lier, P., Boivin, M., Dionne, G., Vitaro, F., Brendgen, M., Koot, H., et al. (2007). Kindergarten children's genetic vulnerabilities interact with friends' aggression to promote children's own aggression. *Journal of the American Academy of Child and Adolescent Psychiatry, 46,* 1080–1087.

van Lier, P. A. C., Vitaro, F., Wanner, B., Vuijk, P., & Crijnen, A. A. M. (2005). Gender differences in developmental links among antisocial behavior, friends' antisocial behavior, and peer rejection in childhood: Results from two cultures. *Child Development, 76,* 841–855.

van Lier, P. A. C., Vuijk, P., & Crijnen, A. A. M. (2005). Understanding mechanisms of change in the development of antisocial behavior: The impact of a universal intervention. *Journal of Abnormal Child Psychology, 33,* 521–535.

van Manen, T. G., Prins, P. J. M., & Emmelkamp, P. M. G. (2004). Reducing aggressive behavior in boys with a social cognitive group treatment: Results of a randomized, controlled trial. *Journal of the American Academy of Child and Adolescent Psychiatry, 43,* 1478–1487.

Van Zalk, M. H. W., Kerr, M., Branje, S. J. T., Stattin, H., & Meeus, W. H. J. (2010). It takes three: Selection, influence, and de-selection processes of depression in adolescent friendship networks. *Developmental Psychology, 46,* 927–938.

Vandell, D. L., & Mueller, E. C. (1980). Peer play and friendships during the first two years. In H. C. Foot, A. J. Chapman, & J. R. Smith (Eds.), *Friendship and social relations in children* (pp. 191–208). London: Wiley.

Vaughan, C. A., Foshee, V. A., & Ennett, S. T. (2010). Protective effects of maternal and peer support on depressive symptoms during adolescence. *Journal of Abnormal Child Psychology, 38,* 261–272.

Verkuyten, M., & Masson, K. (1996). Culture and gender differences in the perception of friendship by adolescents. *International Journal of Psychology, 31,* 207–217.

Vernberg, E. M. (1990). Psychological adjustment and experiences with peers during early adolescence: Reciprocal, incidental, or unidirectional relationships? *Journal of Abnormal Child Psychology, 18,* 187–198.

Vernberg, E. M., Abwender, D. A., Ewell, K. K., & Beery, S. H. (1992). Social anxiety and peer relationships in early adolescence: A prospective analysis. *Journal of Clinical Child Psychology, 21,* 189–196.

Véronneau, M., Vitaro, F., Brendgen, M., Dishion, T. J., & Tremblay, R. E. (2010). Transactional analysis of the reciprocal links between peer experiences and academic achievement from middle childhood to early adolescence. *Developmental Psychology, 46,* 773–790.

Verschueren, K., & Marcoen, A. (2005). Perceived security of attachment to mother and father in 8- to 11-year-olds: Developmental differences and relations to self-worth and peer relationships at school. In K. A. Kerns & R. A. Richardson (Eds.), *Attachment in middle childhood* (pp. 212–230). New York: Guilford Press.

Vespo, J. E. (1991). Features of preschoolers' relationships. *Early Child Development and Care, 68,* 19–26.

Vitaro, F., Brendgen, M., & Tremblay, R. E. (2000). Influence of deviant friends on delinquency: Searching for moderator variables. *Journal of Abnormal Child Psychology, 28,* 313–325.

Vitaro, F., Brendgen, M., & Wanner, B. (2005). Patterns of affiliation with delinquent friends during late childhood and early adolescence: Correlates and consequences. *Social Development, 14,* 82–108.

Vitaro, F., Pedersen, S., & Brendgen, M. (2007). Children's disruptiveness, peer rejection, friends' deviancy, and delinquent behaviors: A process-oriented approach. *Development and Psychopathology, 19,* 433–453.

Vitaro, F., Tremblay, R. E., & Bukowski, W. M. (2001). Friends, friendships, and conduct disorders. In J. Hill & B. Maughan (Eds.), *Conduct disorders in childhood and adolescence* (pp. 346–378). New York: Cambridge University Press.

Vitaro, F., Tremblay, R. E., Kerr, M., Pagani, L., & Bukowski, W. M. (1997). Disruptiveness, friends' characteristics, and delinquency in early adolescence: A test of two competing models of development. *Child Development, 68,* 676–689.

Voss, K., Markiewicz, D., & Doyle, A. (1999). Friendship, marriage and self-esteem. *Journal of Social and Personal Relationships, 16,* 103–122.

Vygotsky, L. S. (1978). *Mind and society: The development of higher psychological processes.* Cambridge, MA: Harvard University Press.

Vygotsky, L. S. (1986). *Thought and language* (A. Kozulin, Trans.). Cambridge, MA: MIT Press.

Wang, A., Peterson, G. W., & Morphey, L. (2007). Who is more important for early adolescents' developmental choices? Peers or parents? *Marriage and Family Review, 42,* 95–122.

Waters, E., Kondo-Ikemura, K., Posada, G., & Richters, J. E. (1991). Learning to love: Mechanisms and milestones. In M. R. Gunnar & L. Sroufe (Eds.), *Self processes and development* (pp. 217–255). Hillsdale, NJ: Erlbaum.

Way, N. (2006). The cultural practice of close friendships among urban adolescents in the United States. In X. Chen, D. C. French, & B. H. Schneider (Eds.), *Peer relationships in cultural context* (pp. 403–425). New York: Cambridge University Press.

Way, N., & Chen, L. (2000). Close and general friendships among African American, Latino, and Asian American adolescents from low-income families. *Journal of Adolescent Research, 15,* 274–301.

Way, N., & Greene, M. L. (2006). Trajectories of perceived friendship quality during adolescence: The patterns and contextual predictors. *Journal of Research on Adolescence, 16,* 293–320.

Weisfeld, G. E., Weisfeld, C. C., & Callaghan, J. W. (1984). Peer and self perceptions in Hopi and Afro-American third- and sixth-graders. *Ethos, 12,* 64–84.

Weiss, L., & Lowenthal, M. F. (1975). Life-course perspectives on friendship. In M. F. Lowenthal, M. Thurnher, & D. Chiriboga (Eds.), *Four stages of life: A comparative study of women and men facing transitions* (pp. 48–61). San Francisco: Jossey-Bass.

Weiss, R. S. (1973). *Loneliness: The experience of emotional and social isolation.* Cambridge, MA: MIT Press.

Weiss, R. S. (1974). The provisions of social relationships. In Z. Rubin (Ed.), *Doing unto others* (pp. 17–26). Englewood Cliffs, NJ: Prentice-Hall.

Werner, N. E., & Crick, N. R. (2004). Maladaptive peer relationships and the development of relational and physical aggression during middle childhood. *Social Development, 13,* 495–514.

Whaley, K. L, & Rubenstein, T. S. (1994). How toddlers "do" friendship: A descriptive analysis of naturally occurring friendships in a group child care setting. *Journal of Social and Personal Relationships, 11,* 383–400.

Wheeler, L., Reis, H. T., & Bond, M. H. (1989). Collectivism–individualism in everyday life: The middle kingdom and the melting pot. *Journal of Personality and Social Psychology, 57,* 79–86.

Whiting, B., Edwards, C., Ember, C. R., Erchak, G. M., Harkness, S., Munroe, R. L., et al. (1988). *Children of different worlds: The formation of social behavior.* Cambridge, MA: Harvard University Press.

Wight, V. R., Chau, M., & Aratani, Y. (2011). *Who are America's poor children?:*

The official story. Report of the National Center for Children in Poverty. New York: Columbia University.

Wilcox, S., & Udry, J. R. (1986). Autism and accuracy in adolescent perceptions of friends' sexual attitudes and behavior. *Journal of Applied Social Psychology, 16,* 361–374.

Wilkinson, R. B. (2010). Best friend attachment versus peer attachment in the prediction of adolescent psychological adjustment. *Journal of Adolescence, 33,* 709–717.

Witvliet, M., van Lier, P. A. C., Cuijpers, P., & Koot, H. M. (2009). Testing links between childhood positive peer relations and externalizing outcomes through a randomized controlled intervention study. *Journal of Consulting and Clinical Psychology, 77,* 905–915.

Wolak, J., Mitchell, K. J., & Finkelhor, D. (2003). Escaping or connecting?: Characteristics of youth who form close online relationships. *Journal of Adolescence, 26,* 105–119.

Wolchik, S. A., Beals, J., & Sandler, I. N. (1989). Mapping children's support networks: Conceptual and methodological issues. In D. Belle (Ed.), *Children's social networks and social supports* (pp. 277–307). Oxford, UK: Wiley.

Wood, J. J., Emmerson, N. A., & Cowan, P. A. (2004). Is early attachment security carried forward into relationships with preschool peers? *British Journal of Developmental Psychology, 22,* 245–253.

Woodward, L. J., & Fergusson, D. M. (1999). Childhood peer relationship problems and psychosocial adjustment in late adolescence. *Journal of Abnormal Child Psychology, 27,* 87–104.

Yeates, K. O., Schultz, L. H., & Selman, R. L. (1991). The development of interpersonal negotiation strategies in thought and action: A social-cognitive link to behavioral adjustment and social status. *Merrill-Palmer Quarterly, 37,* 369–405.

Youniss, J. (1980). *Parents and peers in social development: A Sullivan–Piaget perspective.* Chicago: University of Chicago Press.

Youniss, J., & Smollar, J. (1985). *Adolescent relations with mothers, fathers, and friends.* Chicago: University of Chicago Press.

Yu, P., Harris, G. E., Solovitz, B. L., & Franklin, J. L. (1986). A social problem-solving intervention for children at high risk for later psychopathology. *Journal of Clinical Child Psychology, 15,* 30–40.

Zakriski, A. L., & Coie, J. D. (1996). A comparison of aggressive-rejected and nonaggressive-rejected children's interpretations of self-directed and other-directed rejection. *Child Development, 67,* 1048–1070.

Zeman, J., & Garber, J. (1996). Display rules for anger, sadness, and pain: It depends on who is watching. *Child Development, 67,* 957–973.

Zeman, J., & Shipman, K. (1996). Children's expression of negative affect: Reasons and methods. *Developmental Psychology, 32,* 842–849.

Zerwas, S. C., & Brownell, C. A. (2003, April). *Partners in pretend play.* Paper presented at the Society for Research in Child Development, Tampa, FL.

Zimmer-Gembeck, M. J., & Collins, W. (2003). Autonomy development during adolescence. In G. R. Adams & M. D. Berzonsky (Eds.), *Blackwell handbook of adolescence* (pp. 175–204). Malden MA: Blackwell.

Index

381